BSAVA Manual of Canine and Feline Head, Neck and Thoracic Surgery
second edition

Editors:

Daniel J. Brockman
BVSc Cert VR CertSAO DipACVS DipECVS FHEA MRCVS
The Royal Veterinary College, Hawkshead Lane,
North Mymms, Hatfield, Hertfordshire AL9 7TA, UK

David E. Holt
BVSc DipACVS
University of Pennsylvania, School of Veterinary Medicine,
3900 Delancey Street, Philadelphia, PA 19104-6010, USA

Gert ter Haar
DVM PhD DipECVS
Specialist Veterinary Clinic Utrecht,
Middenwetering 19, 3543 AR, Utrecht, the Netherlands

Published by:

British Small Animal Veterinary Association
Woodrow House, 1 Telford Way,
Waterwells Business Park, Quedgeley,
Gloucester GL2 2AB

A Company Limited by Guarantee in England
Registered Company No. 2837793
Registered as a Charity

4447PUBS18

Titles in the BSAVA Manuals series

For further information on these and all BSAVA publications, please visit our website: **www.bsava.com**

Contents

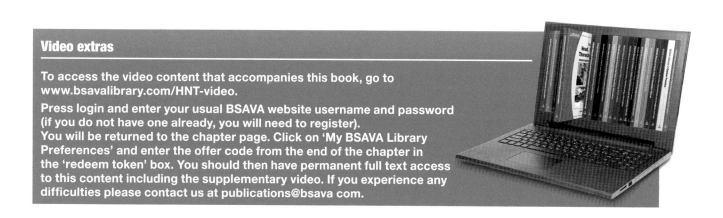

Video extras

To access the video content that accompanies this book, go to
www.bsavalibrary.com/HNT-video.

Press login and enter your usual BSAVA website username and password
(if you do not have one already, you will need to register).
You will be returned to the chapter page. Click on 'My BSAVA Library
Preferences' and enter the offer code from the end of the chapter in
the 'redeem token' box. You should then have permanent full text access
to this content including the supplementary video. If you experience any
difficulties please contact us at publications@bsava com.

Contributors

Davina Anderson
MA VetMB PhD DipSAS(ST) DipECVS MRCVS
Anderson Moores Veterinary Specialists,
The Granary, Bunstead Barns, Poles Lane, Hursley,
Winchester, Hampshire SO21 2LL, UK

Stephen Baines
MA VetMB PhD CertVR CertSAS DipECVS DipClinOnc MRCVS
Willows Veterinary Centre and Referral Service,
Highlands Road, Shirley, Solihull,
West Midlands B90 4NH, UK

Daniel J. Brockman
BVSc Cert VR CertSAO DipACVS DipECVS FHEA MRCVS
The Royal Veterinary College,
Hawkshead Lane, North Mymms,
Hatfield, Hertfordshire AL9 7TA, UK

Carolyn Burton
BVetMed PhD CertVA CertSAS DipECVS MRCVS
Davies Veterinary Specialists Limited,
Manor Farm Business Park,
Higham Gobion, Hitchen,
Hertfordshire SG5 3HR, UK

Christine Cain
DVM BS DipACVD
University of Pennsylvania,
School of Veterinary Medicine,
3900 Delancey Street, Philadelphia,
PA 19104-6010, USA

Kenneth Drobatz
DVM MS BS BA DipACVIM DipACVECC
University of Pennsylvania,
School of Veterinary Medicine,
3900 Delancey Street, Philadelphia,
PA 19104-6010, USA

Gert ter Haar
DVM PhD DipECVS
Specialist Veterinary Clinic Utrecht,
Middenwetering 19, 3543 AR,
Utrecht, the Netherlands

Zoë J. Halfacree
MA VetMB CertVDI CertSAS FHEA DipECVS MRCVS
The Royal Veterinary College,
Hawkshead Lane, North Mymms,
Hatfield, Hertfordshire AL9 7TA, UK

Cheryl S. Hedlund
DVM MS DipACVS
Iowa State University,
Department of Veterinary Clinical Sciences,
1809 South Riverside Drive, Ames,
Iowa 50011-3619, USA

Daniel Holden
BVetMed DVA DipECVAA CertSAM MRCVS
County Veterinary Clinic,
137 Kingston Road, Taunton,
Somerset TA2 7SR, UK

David E. Holt
BVSc DipACVS
University of Pennsylvania,
School of Veterinary Medicine,
3900 Delancey Street, Philadelphia,
PA 19104-6010, USA

Arthur K. House
BSc BVMS CertSAS PhD DipDECVS
Veterinary Referral Hospital Melbourne,
18/151–159 Princes Hwy Hallam,
3803 Victoria, Australia

Jennifer Huck
DVM DipACVS
University of Pennsylvania,
School of Veterinary Medicine,
3900 Delancey Street, Philadelphia,
PA 19104-6010, USA

Andrew E. Kyles
BVMS PhD DipACVS
BluePearl Veterinary Partners,
410 West 55th Street,
New York, NY 10019, USA

Victoria Lipscomb
MA VetMB CertSAS DipECVS MRCVS
The Royal Veterinary College,
Hawkshead Lane, North Mymms,
Hatfield, Hertfordshire AL9 7TA, UK

Julius M. Liptak
BVSc MVetClinStud FACVSc DipACVS DipECVS
VCA Canada – Alta Vista Animal Hospital,
2616 Bank Street, Ottawa,
Ontario K1T1M9, Canada

Philipp D. Mayhew
BVM&S DipACVS
Surgical and Radiological Sciences,
UC Davis School of Veterinary Medicine,
1418 Tupper Hall, Davis, CA 95616-8745, USA

Michael B. Mison
DVM BS DipACVS
University of Pennsylvania,
School of Veterinary Medicine,
3900 Delancey Street, Philadelphia,
PA 19104-6010, USA

Eric Monnet
DVM PhD DipACVS DipECVS
Veterinary Teaching Hospital/Animal Care Center,
300 West Drake Road, Fort Collins,
CO 80525, USA

Gerhard U. Oechtering
Prof.DrMedVet DipECVAA
University of Leipzig,
Small Animal Department, An den Tierkliniken 23,
D-04103 Leipzig, Germany

David A. Puerto
DVM DipACVS
Center for Animal Referral and Emergency Services,
2010 Cabot Blvd. West, Suite D,
Langhorne, PA 19047, USA

Alexander M. Reiter
DipTzt DrMedVet DipAVDC DipEVDC
University of Pennsylvania,
School of Veterinary Medicine,
3900 Delancey Street, Philadelphia,
PA 19104-6010, USA

Mark M. Smith
VMD DipACVS DipAVDC
Center for Veterinary Dentistry and Oral Surgery,
9041 Gaither Road, Gaithersburg, MD 20877, USA

Karen M. Tobias
DVM MS DipACVS
Department of Small Animal Clinical Sciences,
C247 Veterinary Teaching Hospital,
University of Tennessee, Knoxville,
TN 37996-4544, USA

Nicholas J. Trout
MA VetMB DipACVS DipECVS
Angell Animal Medical Center,
350 South Huntington Avenue,
Boston, MA 02130, USA

Lori S. Waddell
DVM DipACVECC
University of Pennsylvania,
School of Veterinary Medicine,
3900 Delancey Street, Philadelphia,
PA 19104-6010, USA

Chick Weisse
BA VMD DipACVS
Animal Medical Center,
510 East 62nd Street, New York,
NY 10065, USA

Foreword

Very early on, my surgical career narrowed to the head, neck and chest of dogs and cats. Dr Anjop Venker van Haagen and I established the International Veterinary Ear Nose and Throat Association (IVENTA) in the early 1980s. However, further focusing of my academic career on dentistry and oro-maxillofacial surgery did not allow me time to continue with ear, nose and throat work, which was handed on to my Penn Vet colleague Dr David Holt, one of the editors of the *BSAVA Manual of Canine and Feline Head, Neck and Thoracic Surgery*.

The invitation to write this Foreword has provided the opportunity for me to consider the substantial progress that has been made in this field, of which there are several major presentation themes warranting consideration, which have been addressed in this latest edition. The challenges of treating airway abnormalities linked to brachycephalism, the constraints of complex bony anatomy and rich vascularity of the head when performing radical surgery for neoplasia in these areas, and the treatment of trauma headlined, of course, by 'high-rise syndrome' in cats and road traffic accidents, have all been covered.

The challenge when performing surgery for any of these conditions is ensuring airway function from the moment the endotracheal tube is removed. The establishment of the first Veterinary Intensive Care Unit, at the University of Pennsylvania, allowed my early work in airway surgery to be much more successful. Airway procedures should not be undertaken unless the requisite level of anesthetic management and postoperative monitoring and care is available. This requirement is, of course, a critical factor in the work that Dr Dan Brockman and colleagues have been pursuing in clinical open heart surgery in dogs; a well-trained team is needed.

The authors of this second edition of the *BSAVA Manual of Canine and Feline Head, Neck and Thoracic Surgery* have been selected to ensure that the most recent techniques, and associated diagnostic information and clinical care, are available in an authoritative, well-organized and illustrated format. I have no doubt this edition will serve practicing veterinarians well.

Colin Harvey BVSc DipACVS DipAVDC DipEVDC FRCVS
Emeritus Professor of Surgery and Dentistry,
University of Pennsylvania

Preface

Diseases of the head, neck, and thorax are often multifaceted cases that require technically precise surgery in areas with complex anatomy. For the second edition of this Manual we have assembled a wide range of experts for the various chapters; we would like to thank these authors for sharing their knowledge and experience with us. We would also like to acknowledge the many clinicians who have pioneered these fields, including Dr Venker-van Haagen, Dr Spreull, Dr Lane, Dr Little, Dr White, Dr Buchanan and many others, and thank them for their years of work and contributions to our understanding. We would especially like to acknowledge and thank Dr Colin Harvey for his willingness to write the Foreword to this edition. All of these clinicians have served as teachers and mentors to many veterinarians and have made huge contributions to these fields.

All three of the editors had the good fortune of residency training and mentors to guide us through difficult cases. We realize that specialist training is not possible for many veterinarians and hope this manual provides the information and guidance needed for managing these cases that are sometimes challenging but often very rewarding.

Dan Brockman
David Holt
Gert ter Haar
August 2018

Chapter 1

Surgical principles and instrumentation

Stephen Baines, Victoria Lipscomb and Alexander M. Reiter

Introduction

Surgery of the head, neck and thorax forms a large part of soft tissue surgery. It is indicated for a variety of disease processes affecting a number of different organ systems, with many surgical procedures described for their management. As ever, the standard principles of good surgical practice are relevant to surgical procedures in these areas. There are, however, a few distinguishing features that set the practice of surgery of the head, neck and thorax apart from other regions (e.g. general surgery of the abdomen). These include:

- Proximity of vital structures, primarily nerves and vessels, to the surgical site
- The organs involved in the disease process are vitally important (e.g. heart, lungs, airways)
- The patient may show few clinical signs, and yet be severely compromised
- The patient may present in severe distress (e.g. acute upper respiratory tract obstruction)
- Intensive preoperative stabilization and postoperative care are often required
- There is limited surgical access to some organs and structures (e.g. soft palate)
- Many of these patients represent an increased anaesthetic risk
- The anaesthetic management of these cases may be more complex
- There is the need for the surgeon and anaesthetist to work closely together.

The surgical techniques described in this manual fall into six broad categories, based on location:

- The ear
- The oral cavity
- The airways
- The head and neck, excluding the airways
- The thoracic wall
- The thoracic cavity and viscera.

As a general rule, patients with diseases affecting the ear or the head and neck, excluding the airways, are relatively free of severe systemic signs or physical compromise. This is not true for all patients; those animals, for example, with vestibular signs, hyperthyroidism or chronic regurgitation from oesophageal disease will have their own systemic problems that need to be addressed. On the other hand, patients with diseases affecting the airway or thorax tend to have the potential for serious cardiorespiratory compromise.

Patient assessment

It is essential that an accurate assessment of the patient is made to allow a preoperative diagnosis, wherever possible. This includes an assessment of the nature and stage of the disease and an assessment of how the patient is affected by the disease. The contribution of the various diagnostic aids available will differ according to the region affected. Nevertheless, an attempt should be made to achieve a preoperative diagnosis so that the surgical procedure and anaesthetic management can be carefully planned. Anaesthetizing a patient for surgery of the airways and thorax requires particular knowledge of the physiology of the cardiorespiratory system, and preoperative evaluation should focus on this system. For the patient that represents an anaesthetic risk, it is advisable that surgical correction of the lesion, where appropriate, should follow on directly from anaesthesia for diagnosis. The likely outcome, potential complications and long-term prognosis should be identified and communicated to the client before the surgery is performed. A correct evaluation of the problem and careful assessment of the patient is the key to a successful anaesthetic and surgical procedure.

Signalment

The signalment of the patient may aid the diagnosis. The incidence of disease differs between species (e.g. dogs develop laryngeal paralysis more frequently than cats, whereas a cranial mediastinal mass is more common in cats). Many disorders have strong breed predilections (e.g. brachycephalic airway disease), many are congenital and will be noted in the young animal (e.g. cleft palate) and many are neoplastic and occur in the older animal (e.g. squamous cell carcinoma of the nasal planum). Entire animals are more likely to stray and are at increased risk of trauma.

History

Consideration of the clinical signs shown by the animal may point towards a diagnosis and, more importantly, may allow the severity of the disease process to be identified. For instance, regurgitation is the most common clinical sign in patients with a vascular ring anomaly. However, the presence of emaciation indicates that the animal is nutritionally compromised and is a poor candidate for anaesthesia and surgery. Clinical signs indicating cardiorespiratory system involvement should be given priority.

The client's description of the clinical signs shown should be noted. The time of onset, duration and progression of the signs should be established. The possible association with other events at the time of onset should be determined. Trauma is a relatively common cause of disorders of the head, neck and thorax, and the possibility of a traumatic aetiology should always be considered even if no event has been observed. Factors that exacerbate the clinical signs (e.g. exercise, excitement or increased environmental temperature) should be noted. The current health status of the animal should be ascertained.

The previous medical history of the patient should be reviewed. For instance, an animal that suffered a traumatic episode some time ago may have developed a diaphragmatic rupture, which is now causing clinical signs due to incarceration of a liver lobe and pleural effusion. Diseases may be acute in onset (e.g. thoracic wall trauma following a road traffic accident) or chronic (e.g. otitis externa). However, the potential for an acute exacerbation of a chronic disease should always be considered (e.g. tracheal collapse or laryngeal paralysis).

Physical examination

Although a complete general physical examination should be performed, it will necessarily focus on those anatomical regions suspected of being involved. Once again, because of its critical importance to the animal and the likelihood of it being involved in the disease process, the cardiorespiratory system should receive particular attention. The physical examination findings associated with diseases of the ear, oral cavity and structures of the head and neck, excluding the airways, are dealt with in individual chapters. A review of the important clinical findings in animals with cardiorespiratory disease is presented here.

The following points are of critical importance for those patients with disorders of the cardiorespiratory system:

- Abnormal posture
- Abnormal respiratory sounds
- Abnormal response to handling
- Abnormal breathing pattern
- Abnormal mucous membrane colour
- Abnormal peripheral pulses
- Thoracic auscultation
- Thoracic inspection and palpation
- Thoracic percussion.

Patients with cardiorespiratory disease may show compromise of the organs involved, and care should be taken to avoid exacerbating these signs. The patient should be initially observed from a distance with minimal restraint. If there are any clinical signs indicating respiratory or cardiovascular compromise, admitting and stabilizing the animal immediately, before proceeding any further, may be appropriate. Minimal restraint should be used for severely dyspnoeic patients and they should be allowed to adopt the position they find most comfortable. The emergency management of the patient in respiratory distress is described in Chapter 2.

Abnormal posture

Open-mouth breathing, abducted forelimbs and restlessness indicate moderate to severe respiratory distress that may require emergency intervention. Severely dyspnoeic patients may be reluctant to adopt a recumbent position.

Abnormal respiratory sounds

The following information may be gained from listening to the patient:

- Inspiratory stridor (a whistling-type noise) is common in upper airway obstruction (e.g. laryngeal paralysis, brachycephalic airway disease)
- Stertor (a snoring-type noise) suggests a (naso)pharyngeal disorder (e.g. overlong soft palate, nasopharyngeal stenosis)
- Gagging and regurgitation are common with (naso)pharyngeal, laryngeal and some tracheal diseases
- Dysphonia (a change in the voice) may be present in patients with laryngeal disease.

Abnormal response to handling

The patient in severe respiratory distress may be oblivious to the presence of the clinician, but will tend to resent any kind of manipulation or attempts to change its posture.

Abnormal breathing pattern

The following information may be gained from watching the patient breathe.

- Inspiratory dyspnoea is seen as difficulty in expanding the lungs, with a relatively easy expiratory effort. The lips are drawn back, the neck is extended, costal margins protrude, the abdomen is drawn in (paradoxical abdominal movement) and inspiration is prolonged. It is observed in upper respiratory tract obstruction, where it is often accompanied by stertor and/or stridor.
- Expiratory dyspnoea is seen as difficulty expelling air from the lungs, with a prolonged expiratory time. The abdomen is actively lifted and plays a more active role in expiration. The anus may protrude. It is seen most frequently in intrathoracic tracheal collapse and obstructive lung disease; the obstruction may be inside the bronchial lumen (bronchiectasis, aspiration of fluid), in the bronchial wall (bronchial asthma, oedema) or in the region surrounding the bronchi (emphysema).
- Inspiratory and expiratory dyspnoea may be observed together in various diseases affecting the pulmonary parenchyma and in disorders resulting in a fixed upper airway obstruction (e.g. laryngeal mass) rather than a dynamic airway obstruction (e.g. laryngeal paralysis). Pulmonary oedema is often characterized by both inspiratory and expiratory dyspnoea.
- Rapid, shallow, choppy breathing is seen in animals with disease affecting the pleural space (e.g. pneumothorax and pleural effusion) or the pulmonary parenchyma (e.g. pulmonary fibrosis), and in animals with painful lesions of the chest wall (e.g. rib fractures).
- Tachypnoea, dyspnoea and exercise intolerance may be found in more markedly affected individuals.
- Severely affected patients may exhibit marked dyspnoea, cyanosis and syncope.
- Coughing indicates a disease affecting the larynx and/or tracheobronchial tree (tracheal collapse) or the pulmonary parenchyma (e.g. pneumonia, pulmonary oedema, trauma, tumour or foreign body).

- Progressive post-traumatic dyspnoea may be present with pneumothorax, pulmonary contusions or progression of a diaphragmatic rupture (e.g. incarceration of a liver lobe with resulting pleural effusion or gastric tympany).
- A hyperinflated, expanded chest with little or no movement may be seen in tension pneumothorax.
- Paradoxical movement of a segment of chest wall is seen in flail chest.
- Decreased expansion of the hemithorax may be seen with mainstem bronchus obstruction or a unilateral ruptured diaphragm.
- Central nervous system (CNS) respiratory centre disturbance may result in slow, feeble, irregular breathing, or periods of normal respiration or hyperventilation followed by apnoea (Cheyne–Stokes breathing).
- Deep sighing movements (Kussmaul's hyperventilation) may indicate metabolic acidosis, diabetic acidosis or renal disease.

Abnormal mucous membrane colour

The colour of the mucous membranes may be altered in certain diseases:

- Pale: seen with anaemia, hypothermia, hypovolaemia and sympathetic response
- Cyanotic: seen with upper respiratory tract obstruction and tetralogy of Fallot
- Differential cyanosis: seen with reverse-shunting patent ductus arteriosus
- Brick red: seen with sepsis.

Abnormal peripheral pulses

The peripheral pulse should be assessed for:

- Rate
- Quality
- Rhythm
- Deficits between peripheral pulse rate and heart rate (from auscultation).

Thoracic auscultation

Auscultation of the lungs may reveal:

- Change in the quality of normal lung sounds (e.g. harsher in chronic bronchitis)
- Areas where no sound is heard (e.g. pneumothorax, pleural effusion, diaphragmatic rupture, mass lesion)
- Abnormal distribution (e.g. bronchial sounds peripherally indicate lung consolidation)
- Adventitious sounds.

Adventitious sounds may be:

- Crackles (e.g. pulmonary fibrosis, oedema)
- Wheezes (e.g. narrowing of the airway)
- Pleural friction rub (e.g. inflammatory disease of the pleural space).

Auscultation of the heart may reveal:

- Murmurs
- Additional heart sounds creating a gallop rhythm
- Arrhythmias
- Muffling of heart sounds and displacement of the apex beat.

Thoracic inspection and palpation

Thoracic palpation may reveal:

- Fractured ribs
- Chest wall mass
- Subcutaneous emphysema
- Pectus excavatum
- Sternal anomalies associated with peritoneal– pericardial diaphragmatic hernia
- Apex shift of the heart (e.g. ruptured diaphragm or lateralized cranial mediastinal mass)
- Precordial thrill (e.g. patent ductus arteriosus)
- Non-compressible cranial thorax (e.g. cranial mediastinal mass).

Thoracic percussion

Findings on thoracic percussion may be hyporesonance, hyperresonance or normal.

Hyporesonance may indicate:

- Pleural effusion
- Pulmonary consolidation
- Ruptured diaphragm
- Peritoneal–pericardial diaphragmatic hernia
- Thoracic cavity/thoracic wall neoplasia
- Marked cardiomegaly.

Hyperresonance may indicate:

- Pneumothorax
- Gas-filled viscus in the thoracic cavity (e.g. ruptured diaphragm and gastric tympany).

Other findings

Other signs of cardiovascular disease that may be found on physical examination include:

- Hepatosplenomegaly
- Ascites
- Jugular distension or pulsation.

Clinical pathology

Laboratory data are not commonly required for the diagnosis of disorders of the ear or upper respiratory tract. However, even in these patients, routine blood screens are of use to detect underlying diseases or diseases secondary to the primary disorder, and to assess the general fitness for anaesthesia and postoperative therapy. In patients with systemic disease, an assessment of routine haematological and biochemical parameters along with urinalysis is essential to identify haematological and metabolic derangements that may require management prior to anaesthesia and surgery.

Poor jugular venepuncture technique may result in iatrogenic damage to vital structures in the neck. In addition, the resulting haematoma may interfere with the surgical approach. In patients scheduled for unilateral procedures involving the neck (e.g. arytenoid lateralization, thyroidectomy, parathyroidectomy) it may be prudent to collect blood from the contralateral jugular vein or another peripheral vessel. Arterial blood gas analysis forms an important part of the assessment of the respiratory system and the adequacy of ventilation and oxygenation.

Diagnostic imaging

Radiography

Radiography is of limited use in the evaluation of aural disease. Radiographs may reveal ear canal stenosis and calcification of the ear canal cartilage, when it is present. The tympanic bulla may have a soft tissue opacity, indicating the presence of fluid or soft tissue. Bony proliferation or erosion of the bulla may be present with otitis media or if a tumour is present. However, the changes seen in the external canal may all be appreciated clinically and, apart from documenting bony lysis or proliferation, radiography is insensitive in identifying the presence of otitis media, and it does not play a large part in decision-making. However, substantial bone lysis, for instance of the bulla, when dealing with aural neoplasia suggests that a total ear canal ablation/lateral bulla osteotomy is unlikely to obtain a surgical margin. Therefore, if ear canal neoplasia is suspected, imaging of the skull, and the thorax, is indicated.

The pharynx and cervical trachea are suitable for radiographic examination because of the presence of air within the lumina of these structures, giving a high contrast. However, superimposition of other structures, particularly the vertebral column, limits the examination to a lateral view. Lesions affecting the bony parts of the skull and neck (e.g. oral tumours) are good candidates for radiographic evaluation. The remainder of the structures are generally soft tissue and in close proximity to each other with no contrasting substance (e.g. fat or air) between them, so the value of radiographic examination is limited to the identification of radiodense foreign material.

Radiography is an excellent tool for the evaluation of thoracic disease. Right and left lateral thoracic radiographs should also be obtained if neoplasia is suspected. A standard lateral and dorsoventral (DV) or ventrodorsal (VD) view are recommended for most conditions.

Contrast radiography: This imaging modality is not commonly used. The upper airways have inherent natural contrast because of the air they contain, and contrast studies of the lower airways yield relatively little information for the potential hazard they represent. Ultrasonography of the heart has largely replaced angiocardiography, and direct visualization of the airways is more useful than a contrast examination. The role of contrast radiography in the evaluation of ear disease is minimal.

Three techniques may be of use, however:

* Sialography – may be used to identify the location of leakage of saliva in a patient with a salivary mucocele
* Fistulography/sinusography – may be of use in identifying the nature and extent of a cutaneous draining tract and the connection with other structures
* Oesophagography – this is a valuable technique for the evaluation of oesophageal disease. Its usefulness is increased if real-time images are obtained with fluoroscopy.

Ultrasonography

Ultrasonographic imaging complements radiographic imaging as it allows an assessment of patients in which the region of interest consists of areas of similar radiopacity in close proximity (e.g. pleural effusion, neck mass); radiography is unable to differentiate between structures of similar radiopacity. Use of ultrasonography in the evaluation of diseases of the ear, oral cavity and pharynx is limited.

The other soft tissues of the neck (e.g. oesophagus, salivary glands, thyroid and parathyroid glands) may be imaged with ultrasonography. However, apart from examination of the thyroid and parathyroid glands, the clinical utility is limited.

In animals with disorders of the upper respiratory tract (e.g. laryngeal paralysis, tracheal collapse), ultrasonography allows some information to be gained in the conscious animal. This enables the clinician to be ready for the likely diagnosis prior to anaesthesia.

Ultrasonography is most useful for:

* Evaluation of cardiac disease
* Examination of the pleural space in animals with a pleural effusion
* Evaluation of a lung mass or mediastinal mass if a suitable acoustic window exists (e.g. the mass is in contact with the chest wall, heart or diaphragm, or there is a pleural effusion).

Advanced imaging

Computed tomography (CT) and magnetic resonance imaging (MRI) are becoming more widely available and are particularly useful for areas of complex anatomy because they eliminate superimposition. Although they generate images differently, they both produce a cross-sectional tomographic image. These modalities are both suitable for examination of the head and neck. CT is more suited to the assessment of bony lesions, particularly where destruction is present (e.g. middle ear), and for evaluation of the thorax (Figure 1.1). MRI offers superior soft tissue differentiation (e.g. soft tissue sarcoma) and is more appropriate for the evaluation of the central nervous system (e.g. in animals with central vestibular syndrome). Both of these techniques may be used for the evaluation of the nasal passages and the sinuses, pharynx and larynx.

Scintigraphy

Scintigraphy has relatively few indications in small animal practice. It may be used for investigation of ectopic thyroid tissue in hyperthyroid cats and for a skeletal survey for occult metastases from a malignant lesion (e.g. osteosarcoma of the rib).

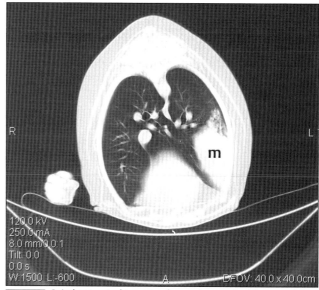

1.1 Spiral computed tomography creates excellent images of the pulmonary parenchyma. A hyperdense mass (m) is present in the periphery of the left lung.

Endoscopy

Direct inspection of the oral cavity and respiratory tract under general anaesthesia via rhinoscopy, laryngoscopy or bronchoscopy, using a flexible or rigid endoscope, is the most common means of achieving a definitive diagnosis of disorders affecting these regions.

The most useful endoscopes include:

- A small-diameter rigid endoscope for rhinoscopy and otoscopy
- A small-diameter flexible endoscope for nasopharyngoscopy
- A laryngoscope for laryngoscopy
- A larger-diameter rigid or flexible endoscope for tracheoscopy and bronchoscopy
- A larger-diameter flexible or rigid endoscope for oesophagoscopy.

The perioperative use of anti-inflammatory doses of corticosteroids (e.g. dexamethasone sodium phosphate 0.1–1 mg/kg i.v. or methylprednisolone sodium succinate 0.5–2 mg/kg i.v.) may help to reduce the oedema associated with such diagnostic interventions, particularly intralaryngeal procedures. In animals that represent an anaesthetic risk, diagnostic endoscopy should be followed with a definitive surgical procedure under the same anaesthetic, whenever possible.

Thoracoscopy: Advances in equipment and expertise have allowed the development of thoracoscopy as a suitable diagnostic and therapeutic technique for diseases of the thoracic cavity. The entire thoracic cavity may be visualized from appropriately placed portals and this allows evaluation of the pleura, pleural space, mediastinum, lungs, heart and pericardium, trachea and thoracic duct.

Fine-needle aspiration and biopsy

A cytological or histological diagnosis for all lesions of unknown aetiology should ideally be obtained prior to planning treatment. Exceptions to this include where it will not change the treatment plan (e.g. lung lobectomy for a solitary lung mass) or where it will not change the client's willingness to treat the patient.

Fine-needle aspiration cytology is a simple and quick procedure. It is suitable for the diagnosis of external lesions (e.g. cutaneous tumours) at first presentation and for deeper lesions under ultrasound guidance (e.g. cranial mediastinal mass). Fine-needle aspiration cytology may differentiate tumours from inflammatory and other lesions (e.g. salivary mucocele). It may also differentiate tumour types (e.g. epithelial tumour, mesenchymal tumour or round cell tumour) and determine chronicity (e.g. acute *versus* chronic inflammation).

Biopsy preserves tissue architecture and should yield a definitive diagnosis. It should be performed preoperatively if fine-needle aspiration cytology cannot be performed or is non-diagnostic. Tissue samples may be obtained via grab biopsy with forceps (e.g. nasal passages), skin biopsy punch (e.g. cutaneous masses), Tru-cut biopsy needles (e.g. subcutaneous mass lesions) and wedge incision (e.g. oral masses). Biopsy should be performed postoperatively on all excised tissue where a definitive diagnosis has not been achieved preoperatively, and on all tumours, even those with a preoperative diagnosis, to assess tumour type, grade, degree of vessel and lymphatic invasion, and margins of excision.

Diagnosis, staging, prognosis and intended procedure

At this point a definitive diagnosis should have been achieved, along with an assessment of the severity of the disease or staging, and the presence of concurrent disease.

A plan should be developed to outline the following:

- Pre-anaesthetic stabilization
- Anaesthesia
- Diagnostic procedures to be performed
- Surgical procedure to be performed
- Perioperative and postoperative analgesia
- Postoperative care and monitoring
- Postoperative nutritional support
- Expected long-term prognosis.

The diagnosis, potential complications and expected long-term prognosis should be communicated to the client. It should be ensured that the client understands the nature of the disease and its current severity and has reasonable expectations for the long-term outcome.

Anaesthesia and analgesia

All dogs and cats undergoing head, neck and thoracic surgery require cardiovascular support in the form of intravenous fluid therapy and must be provided with an appropriate level of anaesthesia and analgesia. These techniques are discussed in detail in the *BSAVA Manual of Canine and Feline Anaesthesia and Analgesia* and the *BSAVA Manual of Canine and Feline Surgical Principles*.

Patient positioning

For each surgical procedure there is an optimal position for the patient to allow the best access to, and visibility of, the surgical site, to create tension on the tissues to be incised, thus allowing safer dissection, and to allow safe anaesthesia and monitoring. Positioning the patient for some procedures, particularly those that require access via the mouth (Figure 1.2), may be awkward, but it is critical that the best access is gained and that the patient stays in this position. A little extra time spent ensuring proper patient positioning will pay dividends.

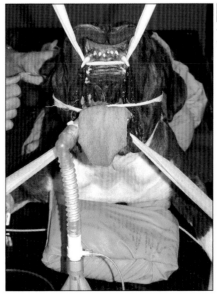

1.2 Positioning of a Bulldog for an oral approach to the airway.

Equipment and surgical instrumentation

Biopsy

The following instruments are used for biopsy sample collection:

- **Fine needles:** These are used to obtain tissue samples for cytological examination by means of inserting the needle with or without aspiration ('woodpecker method')
- **Needle core instruments:** These recover substantially more cells than fine needles
- **Biopsy punch:** This is commonly used for the collection of biopsy specimens from the intraoral and extraoral tissues of the head
- **Straight round or oval cup forceps:** These are used to collect biopsy samples from the nasal cavity and oropharynx.

Tooth extraction

The following instruments are used for tooth extraction:

- **Dental luxators:** These have sharp, flat-tipped blades and are used to penetrate into and cut the periodontal ligament between the tooth and alveolar bone
- **Dental elevators:** These are less sharp, more curved blades that fit the circumference of the tooth and are designed to exert a rotational force for weakening the periodontal ligament
- **Extraction forceps:** These are used to grasp and remove an already mobile tooth.

Surgical instruments

Types of general surgical instruments, their manufacture, maintenance, repair and correct use are covered in the *BSAVA Manual of Canine and Feline Surgical Principles*. Further information on dental instruments is available in the *BSAVA Manual of Canine and Feline Dentistry and Oral Surgery*.

Scalpel blades and handles

A scalpel is the best instrument for incising tissue with minimal trauma. The Bard–Parker No. 3 handle is standard and can be obtained with ruler markings along the handle. It will accept the commonly used No. 10, 11 and 15 blades, as well as No. 12D and 15C blades designed for certain procedures in the oral cavity. The Bard–Parker No. 5 and 7 handles accept the same blades, but they are long narrow handles that may be easier to use inside a deep cavity or for delicate incisions.

Scissors

Scissors (Figure 1.3) are used for cutting or blunt dissection. All Mayo and Metzenbaum scissors should be sharp enough to easily cut four layers of gauze swab (smaller scissors should be able to cut through at least two layers).

- **Mayo scissors:** These are available either curved or straight and in a variety of sizes. Mayo scissors are robust instruments useful for cutting thick tissue, connective tissue, fascia and cartilage. A designated pair of Mayo scissors in each surgical pack should be reserved for cutting sutures.

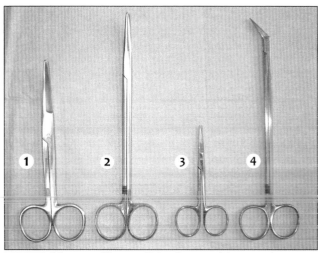

1.3 Scissors. 1 = Mayo; 2 = Metzenbaum; 3 = Iris; 4 = 45-degree Potts.

- **Metzenbaum scissors:** These are fine scissors used for dissecting soft tissues. The curved scissors improve visibility and control and are available in a variety of sizes. A good pair of Metzenbaum scissors is essential for head, neck and thoracic surgery. Gold-handled Metzenbaum scissors have a tungsten carbide cutting edge, resulting in very durable sharp blades. Smaller curved blunt-ended versions with serrated blades are most useful in oral surgery.

> **WARNING**
>
> Never use Metzenbaum scissors to cut suture material, as they will quickly become blunt, and the blades will loosen

- **Iris scissors:** These are small sharp straight scissors that allow precise small cuts to be made.
- **Potts scissors:** These scissors have a short sharp angled straight blade that may be very useful in cardiovascular, laryngeal and otological surgery. They are commonly used with a 45-degree angled blade, but are available with various angled blades ranging from 0 to 90 degrees.

Thumb forceps

Thumb forceps (Figure 1.4) are used to stabilize and expose tissue during dissection and suturing. They should be able to grasp tissue securely with minimal trauma to delicate tissue. Thumb forceps should not be used to grasp needles as this may damage the tips. The tips should meet and any intermeshing striations or teeth should align perfectly.

- **DeBakey forceps:** These have long, narrow jaws with longitudinally ribbed tips that intermesh to hold tissue very delicately but securely. They are available in various sizes, with 1 or 2 mm tip widths. A fine pair of DeBakey forceps is an essential instrument for delicate soft tissue handling in the neck and chest.
- **Adson forceps:** These have fine rat-toothed tips, which cause minimal trauma to tissue. Adson forceps are particularly useful for manipulating oral mucosa flaps.
- **Adson–Brown forceps:** These have fine intermeshing teeth at the tips, which provide a slightly broader but delicate grip on tissue.

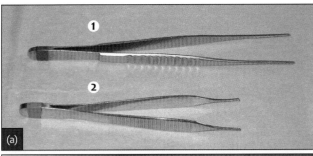

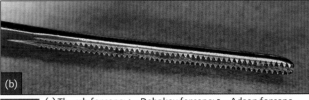

1.4 (a) Thumb forceps: 1 = Debakey forceps; 2 = Adson forceps. (b) Debakey detail.

Tissue forceps

- **Allis forceps:** These have traumatic gripping teeth (Figure 1.5) and should never be used on delicate tissue. They may be used on tissue that is definitely to be excised and to secure suction, diathermy and power lines to drapes.
- **Babcock forceps:** These have a smoother grasping surface (Figure 1.5) with curved longitudinal striations, and may be used to stabilize soft tissues (e.g. pericardium or mediastinum in the chest), although the use of stay sutures is even less traumatic.
- **Backhaus towel clamps:** These are available in small (9 cm) and large (13 cm) sizes and are generally used to secure drapes to the skin. They are penetrating towel clamps, so once they have been placed they are non-sterile. The tips of these clamps end in a fine point, so they do not have a wide crushing area. They may also be used to grasp small bones or flaps for manipulation during elevation and apposition prior to suturing (Reiter, 2013).

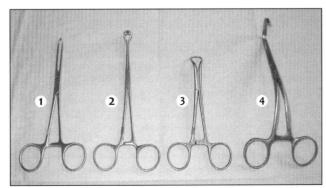

1.5 Tissue forceps and clamps. 1 = Allis; 2 = Babcock; 3 = Backhaus; 4 = Lane's.

Haemostatic forceps

Haemostatic forceps are crushing instruments. Many different types are available in varying sizes, curved or straight, with longitudinal or transverse serrations. Grasping too much tissue or inappropriate material with delicate artery forceps will lead to damage of the tips and overload of the ratchet mechanism. Haemostatic forceps should not spring open when clamped on to the first tooth of the ratchet and the jaws should align properly.

- **Halsted mosquito forceps:** These are small (9–12.5 cm) fine-tipped artery forceps useful for grasping a bleeding vessel. They can also be used to gently separate and explore delicate areas of tissue or tissue containing important structures. They have transverse serrations and are available with regular or extra fine tips.
- **Kelly or Crile forceps:** These are sturdier, larger (14 cm) artery forceps that can be used on thicker portions of tissue, as well as for the placement of stay sutures. Both have transverse serrations, but Kelly forceps have serrations over only the distal half of the jaw.
- **Rochester–Pean forceps:** These are strong artery forceps, available in a variety of sizes (14–30 cm). They have similar uses to Kelly and Crile forceps but may also be used to clamp larger pedicles of tissue.
- **Rochester–Carmalt and Schnidt forceps:** These curved forceps can be used for oesophagostomy tube placement. The forceps should be advanced from the oral cavity into the mid-cervical oesophagus and the curved tips pushed laterally until they can be seen and felt on the skin to be incised (Reiter, 2013).

Angled forceps

Angled forceps (Figure 1.6) that can be used to dissect around large vessels and pass ligatures are important instruments in cardiothoracic surgery. The tips should be inspected before each use to ensure that they are smooth and free of burrs.

- **Mixter forceps:** These are dissecting forceps with transverse serrations and a ratchet. They are available in a selection of sizes (14–23 cm) with standard or delicate tips. Right-angled Mixter forceps are commonly used in cardiothoracic surgery, but forceps with varying curvatures <90 degrees may be useful. Right-angled Mixter forceps can also be used to dissect free and encompass the inferior alveolar neurovascular bundle in preparation for ligation just before it enters the mandibular canal at the mandibular foramen on the caudomedial aspect of the mandible. In addition, curved Mixter forceps can be used to aid oesophagostomy tube placement (see above).
- **Lahey bile duct forceps:** These dissecting right-angled forceps have longitudinal serrations and a blunt tip.
- **Waterston forceps:** These ligature forceps have smooth rounded blunt tips, which reduce the risk of puncturing a vessel. They are available with 45-degree and 90-degree angles. Ligature forceps have no ratchet and only the tips of the instrument meet, which prevents accidental clamping or tearing of the vessel wall when passing a ligature around it.

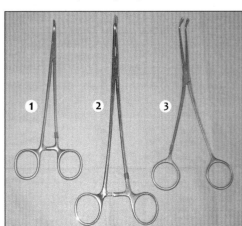

1.6 Angled forceps. 1 = Mixter; 2 = Lahey bile duct; 3 = Waterston.

Retractors

Appropriate retraction decreases surgical time and reduces the risk of surgical complications.

Hand-held retractors:

- **Senn retractors:** These retractors have three sharp prongs at one end and a right-angled fingerplate at the other end (Figure 1.7). They are delicate instruments, useful for retracting skin and superficial soft tissues (e.g. in the neck).
- **Seldin retractors:** These are large and sturdy periosteal elevator-like instruments; also useful to break any remaining bony attachments after osteotomy during mandibulectomy or maxillectomy procedures.
- **Army–Navy, Parker–Kerr and Langenbeck retractors:** These are larger instruments with variously angled ends, enabling retraction of more tissue in deeper cavities. They are available in a selection of sizes. Army–Navy and Parker–Kerr retractors are double-ended, whereas Langenbeck retractors have a single end (Figure 1.7).
- **Skin hooks:** These hooks are used for the retraction of delicate tissues.
- **Malleable retractors:** These retractors are versatile because they can be moulded to the shape desired. They are useful for retracting organs within the chest (organs are protected with a saline-soaked swab). Malleable retractors are available in a variety of blade widths (2–5 cm).

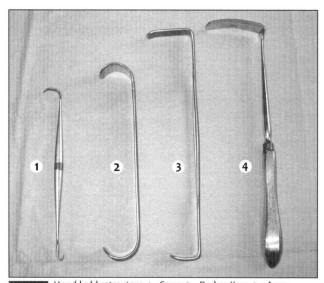

1.7 Hand-held retractors. 1 = Senn; 2 = Parker-Kerr; 3 = Army–Navy; 4 = Langenbeck.

Self-retaining retractors: These instruments are able to maintain themselves in a spread position and are very useful during head and neck surgery (Figure 1.8).

- **Gelpi retractors:** These retractors have single-pronged outwardly turning tips. Gelpi retractors maintain tension using a grip-lock mechanism and are available in small (14 cm) or large (17 cm) sizes, with pointed or blunt tips. The blunt tips are preferable if they are to be placed next to important nerves or vessels.
- **West, Weitlaner and Travers retractors:** These retractors have multiple tips, offering a wider surface area for retraction. The tips can be pointed or blunt. Travers retractors are larger (20 cm) than West or Weitlaner retractors (14–16 cm).

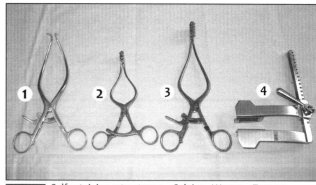

1.8 Self-retaining retractors. 1 = Gelpi; 2 = West; 3 = Travers; 4 = Finochietto.

- **Finochietto retractors:** These rib retractors have a ratchet and can be used for both intercostal and sternotomy approaches. These retractors need to be extremely robust with deep, wide blades to spread open the ribs and maintain rib retraction. Small, medium and large sizes are available, so they may be used in cats as well as large dogs.

Lip, cheek and tongue retractors:

- **Lip retractors:** The tips of these retractors are plastic-coated to minimize trauma to the labial mucosa and lip skin and can be adjusted by lightly bending. Lips can be retracted for clear access to the upper and lower jaw.
- **Cawood–Minnesota retractors:** One end is straight and flat, the other end is curved as a broad hook, allowing retraction of the lip, cheek, tongue and tissue flaps.
- A dental mirror or moistened tongue depressor can also be used for retraction of the tongue and cheek.

Periosteal elevators

These are small narrow-tipped (2–6 mm) instruments (Figure 1.9) used to deflect tissues that have adhered to bone. They are very helpful in mobilizing and reflecting the mucoperiosteum during periodontal flap procedures, mandibulectomies, maxillectomies and palate surgeries. The blade portion is used with the convex side against the soft tissue, reducing the chance of tearing or puncturing the flap. Larger instruments may be used to deflect tissue from the field of operation and improve visibility. Periosteal elevators come in various sizes and blade shapes (e.g. Molt, West, Williger, Glickman, Seldin).

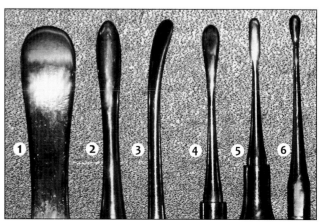

1.9 Periosteal elevators. 1 = Senn; 2 = Molt; 3 = Freer; 4 = Goldman-Fox; 5 and 6 = feline.

Rongeurs

Lateral or ventral bulla osteotomy may require the use of rongeurs (Figure 1.10) to aid precise removal of bone. Double-action rongeurs are more powerful and have a smoother action than single-action rongeurs. The ideal rongeurs for middle ear surgery would have a powerful mechanism and relatively delicate jaws. Rongeurs may also be useful for the collection of specimens when performing a biopsy of soft and hard tissues in the oral cavity.

- **Lempert rongeurs:** These are standard single-action small rongeurs with 2–3 mm wide jaws, available straight or curved.
- **Ruskin rongeurs:** These are double-action rongeurs with 3, 5 or 7 mm wide jaws.
- **Kerrison rongeurs:** These are double-action rongeurs with a long delicate blade that operates with a unique action. The upper blade is cutting and slides along the lower blade, which ends in a protective footplate.

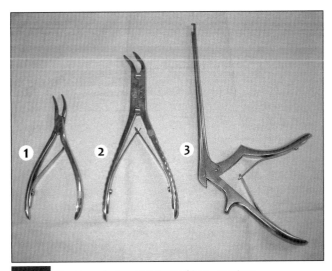

1.10 Rongeurs. 1 = Lempert; 2 = Ruskin; 3 = Kerrison.

Needle holders

Needle holders are used to grasp and manipulate curved needles. It is important to choose the correct size for the needle being used. Large needle holders can distort or break small needles. Using too large a needle in delicate needle holders will damage the instrument. Gold-handled needle holders have a tungsten carbide insert in the jaws, which provides increased durability and an excellent grip. Needle holders that can be locked on to the needle, usually by a ratchet mechanism, are recommended to prevent slippage of the needle. The needle should not be able to move in the jaws of the instrument when the ratchet is locked to the second tooth. A needle holder without a ratchet mechanism may be used for very delicate or microvascular surgery to prevent any motion at the instrument tip.

- **Mayo–Hegar needle holders:** These are standard sturdy needle holders, which are available in a variety of sizes.
- **Olsen–Hegar needle holders:** These needle holders have an integral scissor blade, which enables them to cut sutures.
- **Halsey needle holders:** These are sturdier needle holders with serrated jaws, often used in head and neck surgery.

- **DeBakey needle holders:** These are more delicate needle holders with serrated jaws for finer surgery.
- **Ryder (micro) needle holders:** These are extremely delicate needle holders for use with very small needles.
- **Castroviejo needle holders:** These are round-handled needle holders with extremely fine tips and no ratchet mechanism, suitable for microvascular surgery.

Vascular clamps

Vascular clamps (Figure 1.11) are non-crushing clamps that may be used for temporary occlusion of large vessels. These clamps are available in small and large sizes and may be straight, curved, right-angled or tangential. The DeBakey pattern is commonly used to provide an atraumatic tip for vascular clamps. Other atraumatic tip configurations are available, including the Cooley pattern.

Tangential clamps (e.g. Satinsky clamps) provide partial occlusion of a vessel wall whilst allowing blood to flow through the remaining portion. They may also be useful for placing across a right atrial appendage that requires resection. DeBakey tangential vascular clamps can be placed on an elongated soft palate for resection of excess tissue or along the palatine tonsil attachment for tonsillectomy. Doyen intestinal forceps are useful to clamp the body of the tongue to provide temporary haemostasis whilst the distal tissue portion is resected and the cut edge repaired.

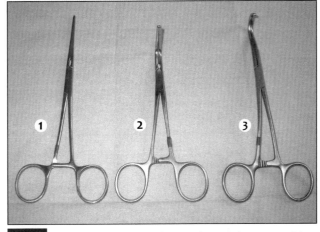

1.11 Vascular clamps. 1 = straight; 2 = right-angled; 3 = tangential.

Surgical curettes

Curettes may be used for the removal of debris and granulation tissue from a soft tissue wound, a bone surface or defect, an alveolar socket after tooth extraction, during ear surgery to remove tissue remaining inside the tympanic bulla and for turbinectomy during rhinotomy procedures.

- **Spratt curette:** These curettes have round cups and are available in various sizes.
- **Volkmann curette:** These curettes are double-ended with round or oval cups and are available in various sizes.

Dental explorer and periodontal probe

A dental explorer is used to assess the structural integrity of a tooth and explore the presence of pulp exposure. A periodontal probe is used to measure the depth of periodontal pockets and the height of excess gingiva (Reiter, 2013).

Mallet and osteotome

A mallet and osteotome are needed to separate the two mandibles at the symphysis or to make precise bone cuts (e.g. during mandibulectomy, maxillectomy, dorsal rhinotomy or ventral bulla osteotomy).

Rib shears

It is occasionally necessary to remove a rib to improve the access obtained via an intercostal thoracotomy. Standard bone cutters, used with care, are capable of performing this task. However, rib shears are available that have a single blade that apposes a curved protective edge, which reduces the risk of iatrogenic thoracic damage.

Saws

Power saws remove the physical effort of cutting through bone and are essential because of the control and accuracy of cut they afford. The blades are available in various sizes and move back and forth (reciprocating) in an arc of 5 or 6 degrees parallel to (sagittal) or at a right angle to (oscillating) the drive shaft (Figure 1.12). The cutting teeth move only a small distance on the bone and adjacent soft tissues are usually unaffected. The saw, blades and power cable can be dismantled and sterilized. The heat produced by friction may cause heat necrosis of the bone and this is minimized by cooling the blade with sterile saline during use. Sagittal and oscillating saws are used for dorsal rhinotomies, mandibulectomies, maxillectomies and zygoma surgeries. It is mandatory to use a sagittal or oscillating saw for a median sternotomy to divide the sternebrae accurately in the midline. Dedicated sternotomy saws are available, which have a protective underplate to reduce the risk of the blade inadvertently lacerating adjacent structures upon entry into the chest. Piezoelectric surgery utilizes tips that vibrate (distances range from 60 to 200 μm) when precisely cutting through hard tissue, whilst leaving soft tissue untouched by the process (Reiter, 2013).

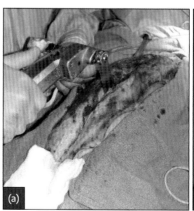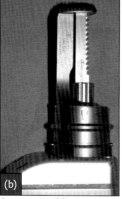

1.12 The sternebrae of a large dog may be cut using (a) an oscillating saw or (b) a sagittal saw.

Surgical biomaterials

Suture materials

Many of the synthetic absorbable suture materials are appropriate for use in soft tissue surgery. Poliglecaprone 25, polyglactin 910 and polyglycolic acid lose a significant portion of their tensile strength relatively rapidly (1–2 weeks) and are suitable for subcutaneous tissues and muscle. The oesophagus, similar to the rest of the gastrointestinal tract, heals rapidly, and use of a monofilament absorbable suture material (e.g. poliglecaprone 25 or polydioxanone) is recommended because it produces low tissue drag and does not have interstices that can potentially harbour bacteria. Polydioxanone provides extended support for 1–2 months and may be chosen in a compromised patient when it is suspected that oesophageal healing may be prolonged.

Repair of a diaphragmatic rupture and intercostal thoracotomy closure necessitate the use of suture material that provides prolonged wound support, such as polydioxanone or non-absorbable monofilament nylon. Median sternotomy closure must be very secure and is achieved using large-gauge polydioxanone or stainless steel wire sutures, which have the highest tensile strength of all the suture materials. Non-absorbable suture material, traditionally polypropylene, is used for securing the laryngeal cartilages during arytenoid lateralization surgery. Polypropylene is the least thrombogenic suture material and is the material of choice for vascular surgery. Monofilament nylon with a swaged-on reverse-cutting needle is preferred for skin sutures, including those apposing cartilage during closure of aural surgical procedures. Tying secure knots is an essential surgical skill, which may be particularly challenging within a deep thoracic cavity with the added distraction of the heart and lung movements.

An absorbable suture material is preferred for wound closure in the oral cavity and oropharynx so that sedation or anaesthesia for suture removal can be avoided. Chromic catgut persists in the oral cavity for approximately 4–7 days, which is considered to be ideal in humans. However, a longer-lasting synthetic material is preferred in dogs and cats to avoid early wound breakdown. Polyglactin 910 and polyglycolic acid are good for procedures in which healing is relatively rapid, but they may elicit an inflammatory reaction in oral tissue, due to their multifilament nature. Synthetic monofilament sutures induce the least foreign body reaction in oral tissues. Poliglecaprone 25 (1 metric (5/0 USP), 1.5 metric (4/0 USP) or 2 metric (3/0 USP), depending on the size of the animal and the type of procedure being performed) has become a very popular suture material and may persist in the oral cavity for approximately 3–5 weeks. Polydioxanone is used where prolonged suture strength is required (e.g. palate surgery) and may persist in the oral cavity for 6–8 weeks (LaBagnara, 1995). Square or surgeon's knots should be followed by at least three more throws to ensure knot security in the oral cavity (Reiter, 2013).

Surgical needles

Swaged needles glide smoothly and efficiently through tissue and are considered mandatory for atraumatic soft tissue surgery. Needles with varying curvatures (e.g. ⅜ to ½ circle) are most versatile and commonly used. Taper-point needles are non-cutting round needles, which are used for viscera, muscle, fat and cardiovascular tissues. They are also preferred for wound closure in the oral cavity and oropharynx, thus reducing trauma to already inflamed or friable tissues. Certain cardiovascular procedures require the use of suture material with a needle swaged on to both ends. Small, swaged-on ⅜ circle, reverse-cutting needles may cause minimal tissue drag, but have the potential to tear through delicate or inflamed tissue.

Surgical staplers

Mechanical staplers are an efficient alternative to manual suturing for a variety of intrathoracic procedures. When applied correctly, surgical staplers provide consistent and secure haemostasis and are particularly useful in areas that may be difficult to access. Linear (also known as thoracoabdominal) staplers are the most applicable to thoracic surgery. They are available in a variety of lengths between 30 and 90 mm. Cartridges corresponding to the width of the stapler produce a double staggered row of titanium staples in two standard sizes:

- 'Medium' cartridges have 3.5 mm staples, which compress tissue to a width of 1.5 mm
- 'Large' cartridges have 4.8 mm staples, which compress tissue to a width of 2 mm.

A 30 mm width linear stapler is also available, which accepts 'small/vascular' cartridges that have the added security of three staggered rows of 3 mm staples and compress tissue to a width of 1 mm. This vascular stapler is particularly useful for placing across the hilus of a lung for complete lung lobectomy or resection of an atrial appendage mass. Partial lung lobectomy may be performed with linear or linear cutter staplers. Linear cutter staplers fire four rows of staggered staples and cut between the second and third rows, eliminating the need to resect the redundant tissue with a blade. Further in-depth information on the types and use of surgical staplers is available in the *BSAVA Manual of Canine and Feline Surgical Principles*.

Generally, complications associated with the use of surgical staplers are few providing the instruments are used correctly. The tissue to be stapled should be viable and all layers of the tissue must be penetrated. It is very important not to try to force an excessive amount of tissue into the stapler. The stapled line must be inspected carefully to detect any potential failure of the staples to engage the tissue properly.

Orthopaedic equipment

Instruments and materials include orthopaedic wire (for interdental, circumferential or intraosseous wiring), hypodermic needles (to guide the wire), resin material (for building splints), Kirschner wire and Steinman pins (for external skeletal fixation), and a plating system with supporting tools (Reiter, 2013).

Additional surgical equipment

Drapes

In most surgical procedures four 'quarter' drapes are placed at the periphery of the sterile field. A single large drape with a central fenestration may also be placed over the entire surgical field. Some surgeons additionally sew or clip drapes to the skin incision edges to provide extra protection against wound contamination from bacteria, which migrate to the skin surface from within the hair follicles during surgery. Once the drapes are placed they must not be repositioned. Disposable synthetic or reusable cloth drapes may be used. There are advantages and disadvantages to both and the choice is based on economics, laundering facilities and convenience. However, if a cloth drape becomes wet it is no longer sterile owing to inevitable 'strikethrough'. Compared with surgical procedures that advance through the skin into deeper structures, the surface linings of the oral cavity and oropharynx are non-sterile environments that cannot be prepared adequately with antiseptics to provide a sterile field. Nevertheless, flushing the mucosal surfaces with dilute chlorhexidine prior to surgery and draping the surrounding areas are useful in preventing excessive contamination of cut surfaces, particularly when they involve the lips and adjacent oral tissues.

Surgical marker pen and plastic ruler

A marker pen and ruler are used for planning and outlining skin or mucosal incisions for the creation of flaps, repair of defects and removal of tissue (Reiter, 2013).

Wedge props and mouth gags

Props and gags aid in keeping the mouth open to allow access to surgical sites in the oral cavity and oropharynx (Figure 1.13). Custom-made devices (such as needle caps and syringe cases) are also useful. Note that keeping the mouth stretched open for prolonged periods of time may cause strain to the masticatory muscles or injury to the temporomandibular joints, and could detrimentally affect maxillary arterial blood flow (particularly in cats) (Reiter, 2014).

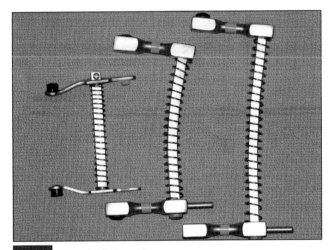

1.13 Spring-loaded mouth gags.

Swabs

Laparotomy swabs: Laparotomy swabs can be very useful for temporary packing of the oropharynx in dogs during surgical procedures of the oral cavity and surrounding structures, as they provide additional protection against aspiration of foreign material. A cord attaches the swabs to the endotracheal tube, ensuring that they are not left in place once the procedure is complete and the patient is recovered from anaesthesia. Moistened laparotomy swabs are useful in thoracic surgery for packing off areas of lung and protecting the edges of thoracotomy incisions from retractors.

Gauze swabs: The standard swabs used in general surgery are 10 x 10 cm (4 x 4 inches). Gauze swabs of 7.5 x 7.5 cm (3 x 3 inches) are most commonly used for surgical procedures in the oral cavity and oropharynx. Gauze swabs and small sponges can also be used for temporary packing of the oropharynx in smaller dogs and cats.

> **WARNING**
>
> Swabs must be counted at the beginning and end of a surgical procedure to ensure none are left inside a wound or the thoracic cavity. All swabs must have a radiopaque marker strip to enable their visualization on a radiograph

Mayo bowl and bulb syringe

A sterile bowl for saline is always useful because exposed tissues should be kept moistened during surgery. This is particularly important when large flaps are raised for repair of tissue defects in the oral cavity (e.g. palate surgery, reconstruction of the nasal vestibule). Smaller bulb syringes or large catheters attached to a syringe can also be used to flush the nasal passages of animals with small nostrils. Moistened gauze swabs are less traumatic than dry swabs. Lavage often improves visibility during dissection, and cold lavage can provide excellent atraumatic haemostasis. Thorough lavage of contaminated or dirty surgical sites with a bulb syringe is mandatory. Warm saline is recommended when lavaging the thoracic cavity. This is less likely to disturb normal cardiac rhythm and is a useful method of treating mild hypothermia in anaesthetized patients. A stainless steel Mayo bowl is practical because it is autoclavable. Alternatively, plastic bowls may be used if gas sterilization is available.

Suction

Suction is mandatory for thoracic surgery to allow lavage and removal of fluid and blood from the chest. A Poole suction tip (Figure 1.14) is large and has a smooth rounded tip and multiple openings, which makes it suitable for suctioning the thoracic cavity. Frasier suction tips (Figure 1.14) or disposable plastic suction tips with a single end hole are available for general surgery in a selection of sizes (5–12 Fr). Most of these have a decompression hole, which can be covered or uncovered, to regulate suction pressure at the tip. Fine suction tips for gently aspirating blood during dissection are very useful in head and neck surgery. A fine suction tip is essential when performing a bulla osteotomy to enable lavage of the middle ear.

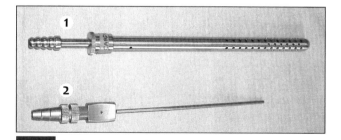

1.14 Suction tips. 1 = Poole; 2 = Frasier.

Drains

Commonly used drains in general surgery include the Penrose drain and various types of closed-system active drains. The latter have the advantage of being a sterile system, reducing the risk of iatrogenic infection, and are particularly useful for wounds in awkward locations that do not permit drainage via gravity. Oropharyngeal and sublingual foreign body penetration, severe lower lip avulsion and excessive iatrogenic dissection of tissue planes during mandibulectomies and removal of lymph nodes/salivary glands may sometimes warrant the use of surgical drains to allow the withdrawal of fluids and discharge from the wound. The use of a drain following routine total ear canal ablation and bulla osteotomy is controversial but it is recommended if a large amount of drainage is expected (see Chapter 5). A chest drain must be placed before the end of all thoracotomy procedures to enable lung re-expansion and allow removal of residual pleural fluid and air in the postoperative period (see Chapter 11).

Cotton-tipped applicators

These are sterile, long wooden handles with a cotton bud tip on one end. They are useful for atraumatically absorbing blood from delicate tissue or applying haemostatic agents to incision sites. When moistened they can be used as a gentle dissecting tool in friable tissue (e.g. separating parathyroid from thyroid tissue).

Dental units

Electrical and air-powered systems are available. Low-speed handpieces are used for polishing teeth, cutting bone and performing various other procedures. High-speed handpieces are primarily used for cutting holes in teeth for endodontic access, preparing dental defects for restoration, sectioning multi-rooted teeth into single-rooted crown–root segments in preparation for extraction, removing and shaping alveolar bone, and making precise cuts in bony structures during mandibulectomy and maxillectomy procedures. Various shapes, sizes and lengths of burrs are available (Reiter, 2013).

Headlamp and surgical loupe

Headlamps and surgical loupes are useful for surgery of the oral cavity and in small patients, to provide good illumination and adequate tissue magnification (Reiter, 2013).

Medical lasers

The carbon dioxide (CO_2) and diode lasers are the lasers most commonly marketed to veterinary surgeons (veterinarians). These lasers are used for incision, excision and ablation of soft tissues. The CO_2 and most solid-state diode lasers function through photothermal laser–tissue interaction. Water, haemoglobin, melanin and some proteins absorb varying wavelengths of laser light, resulting in tissue heating, necrosis and vaporization. Smoke evacuators are essential adjuncts to prevent inhalation of the laser plume.

CO_2 laser: CO_2 lasers (Figure 1.15) are used in nasal, oral and oropharyngeal surgery for precisely cutting or vaporizing soft tissue with haemostasis. The CO_2 wavelength is

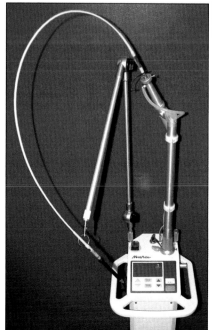

1.15 Nova Pulse CO_2 laser.
(Courtesy of Lumenis Inc.)

absorbed by the water content of oral tissues. The thermal necrosis zones of 100–300 µm at cut tissue edges are less deep than those of diode and other lasers. CO_2 lasers can be utilized for various soft tissue surgeries of the head, including gingivectomy and gingivoplasty, frenoplasty, ablation of stomatitis ulcers, marsupialization of sublingual sialoceles (ranulae), tonsillectomy and reduction of elongated soft palates, as well as various surgeries of the ears, nose, lips, cheeks, tongue and pharynx (Holt and Mann, 2002).

Diode laser: Diode lasers come as small compact units. They emit wavelengths that are easily transmitted through small flexible optical fibres, allowing use with most flexible and rigid endoscopes. Diode lasers penetrate deeply (1–2 mm) into most types of soft and hard tissue. Frequent water irrigation is used as a 'heat sink' to decrease thermal damage when using a diode laser in the oral cavity (Bellows, 2002).

Diathermy units

Diathermy (electrocoagulation) involves the application of a high-frequency current through tissue, which generates heat that coagulates and seals the bleeding vessel. This is in contrast to electrocautery, which is the application of a heated filament to tissue. Diathermy should only be used on arteries up to 1 mm in diameter and veins up to 2 mm in diameter. Diathermy is helpful in most head, neck and thoracic surgeries because it produces a blood-free field, which provides optimal visibility for accurate dissection and reduces surgical time. However, excessive or indiscriminate use of diathermy prolongs wound healing. Wound breakdown is of particular concern if electrosurgical equipment is used for incisions or for control of haemorrhage in tissues at sutured incision edges. Use of diathermy in the oral cavity and oropharynx is not recommended unless it is absolutely necessary. Monopolar or bipolar diathermy is available (Figure 1.16) and can be activated by either a hand or a foot switch.

Monopolar diathermy: The current flows from the handpiece through the animal to a ground plate. The small surface area of the handpiece concentrates the current density at the point of application to the tissue, resulting in electrocoagulation. The handpiece is usually touched to forceps that have been applied to the bleeding vessel. The larger surface area of the ground plate minimizes the current density, so that the rest of the animal's tissues are minimally affected. The ground plate must be placed in good contact with the patient to avoid thermoelectric burns. Monopolar diathermy can cut as well as coagulate tissue and works best in a relatively dry surgical field.

Bipolar diathermy: The tips of the handpiece are held about 1 mm apart so the current can flow from the tip of one handpiece, through the tissue being held, to the opposite tip. The risk of unintentional injury to surrounding tissues is greatly decreased. Bipolar diathermy is recommended when precise coagulation is required to reduce the risk of iatrogenic injury to important adjacent structures (e.g. the recurrent laryngeal nerves during neck surgery).

Vessel-sealing devices

Bipolar vessel-sealing devices and ultrasound-activated scalpels are now available from several manufacturers. They have the ability to induce heat to reliably seal vessels between 5 and 7 mm and may be particularly useful for resecting the pericardium and mediastinum either at open surgery or via thoracoscopic access to the chest.

Solutions for rinsing, antisepsis and storage

- **Dilute chlorhexidine gluconate:** A concentration of 0.12% is recommended for rinsing the mucosal surfaces of the oral cavity and oropharynx. Higher concentrations are to be avoided as they may cause epithelial desquamation and wound healing complications.
- **Povidone–iodine:** This may be applied with a swab to intact oral mucosal surfaces at a 10% concentration (diluted 10-fold if the mucosa is not intact) (Terpak and Verstraete, 2012).
- **Phosphate-buffered saline and lactated Ringer's solution:** These solutions were found to induce no significant fibroblast injury in an *in vitro* model (Buffa *et al.*, 1997). In comparison, normal saline was found to have cytotoxic effects on canine fibroblasts.
- **Hank's balanced salt solution:** A commercial tissue culture medium for temporary storage of avulsed teeth until they are reimplanted (Reiter, 2013).

Materials aiding in haemostasis

- **Cold lavage:** Lactated Ringer's solution placed in the freezer and then removed before the freezing point is reached may provide good haemostasis during maxillectomy and other surgical procedures that expose the nasal cavity.
- **Aluminium chloride:** This astringent produces tissue shrinkage and reduces minor haemorrhage. It may be added to cut surfaces following gingivoplasty or biopsy of gingival masses.
- **Bone wax:** This sterile beeswax-based compound can be used for haemostasis of cut bony surfaces following maxillectomies and mandibulectomies and excessive bleeding from, for instance, an alveolus, the mandibular or infraorbital canal or the retroglenoid foramen.
- **Oxidized regenerated cellulose:** Absorbable sterile mesh applied directly on to an area of bleeding.
- **Absorbable gelatin sponges:** These are derived from gelatin and are available as sheets (which may be cut into particles of appropriate size) or as a powder.
- **Microporous polysaccharide spheres:** Powder derived from potato starch, which when applied directly on to a bleeding site accelerates clot formation.

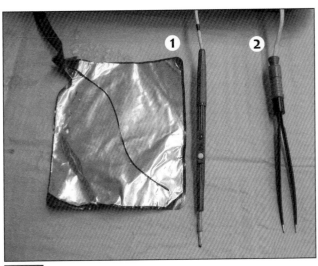

1.16 Diathermy equipment. 1 = monopolar; 2 = bipolar.

- **Microfibrillar collagen:** Obtained from bovine collagen and applied as a powder or sheet to act as a scaffold for clot formation.
- **Thrombin in a gelatin matrix:** This is indicated in surgical procedures (other than ophthalmic) as an adjunct to haemostasis when control of bleeding by ligature or conventional procedures is ineffective or impractical.
- **Cyanoacrylate tissue adhesives:** For closure of very minor wounds and to seal small bleeding sites.
- **Phenylephrine and lidocaine:** Phenylephrine is a vasoconstrictor with no beta-blocking action (fewer cardiac effects expected than with adrenaline (epinephrine), but hypertension and reflex bradycardia are still possible). Diffuse bleeding from nasal mucosa may respond to wound irrigation with a mixture (0.05–0.1 ml/kg in cats; 0.1–0.2 ml/kg in dogs) of 0.25 ml phenylephrine (1%) and 50 ml lidocaine (2%) (Reiter, 2013).

Postoperative care

Wounds of the head and neck are particularly vulnerable to self-trauma from rubbing and scratching, particularly during recovery. Many wounds of the head and neck cannot be bandaged satisfactorily without risking asphyxia, and some device to limit self-trauma (e.g. an Elizabethan collar) may be required. Adequate analgesia should be ensured in any animal showing self-trauma.

Chest bandages may help to protect a thoracotomy incision, but care should be taken to avoid placing them too tightly and restricting breathing. A bandage will also help to prevent the patient from dislodging a chest tube.

Particular care should be taken to avoid complications associated with thoracic drains. This includes:

- Ensuring that the drain is occluded at two sites (e.g. gate clamp and bung)
- Ensuring that the drain is attached to the patient (e.g. Chinese finger-trap friction suture)
- Ensuring that the patient cannot remove the drain (e.g. Elizabethan collar and bandage).

Daily inspection of the wound is important, particularly those classified as contaminated or dirty, or those where drains have been placed. Wound drains may be used in surgical procedures of the head and neck, either passive (e.g. a Penrose drain placed after sialoadenectomy for a salivary mucocele) or active (e.g. a suction drain placed after major oncological resection).

Principles of head, neck and thoracic surgery

Halsted's principles
- Asepsis and aseptic surgical technique
- Sharp anatomical dissection
- Atraumatic tissue handling and surgical technique
- Removal of devitalized tissue from the surgical wound
- Precise haemostasis with preservation of blood supply to tissues
- Accurate tissue apposition, minimizing tissue dead space but without excessive tension on tissues

---

Halsted's principles of surgery are at the heart of any successful soft tissue procedure. These principles are designed to reduce surgical morbidity and mortality, minimize patient discomfort, promote rapid wound healing, reduce surgical site infection and increase client satisfaction.

Timing of anaesthesia and surgery

Surgical procedures of the upper respiratory tract and thorax are best conducted at the beginning of the day's operating list. Careful observation is then possible throughout the remainder of the day for complications associated with the procedure, such as haemorrhage or oedema, that may cause airway obstruction. Similarly, many of the procedures are not suitable on an outpatient basis or where adequate 24-hour intensive care facilities are not available. Surgery of the external ear canal is generally contaminated or dirty and should be performed at the end of the day's list.

Surgery may need to be performed on an emergency basis for patients that have suffered from marked haemorrhage, or those that are severely dyspnoeic or that cannot eat and drink voluntarily, as soon as the patient has been stabilized. Many disorders causing upper respiratory tract obstruction are exacerbated by high ambient temperatures. For patients with relatively minor signs, delaying the procedure until the weather is cooler may be of benefit. However, because of this environmental influence, many animals will present with acute exacerbations of their disease when the weather is warm, necessitating prompt intervention at that time.

Preparation of the surgeon and team

Some of the key differences between surgery of the head, neck and thorax and other aspects of soft tissue surgery are:

- The disease process may affect tissues that do not tolerate surgical manipulation well (e.g. postoperative swelling of the laryngeal mucosa)
- Failure of a suture line may have catastrophic consequences (pneumothorax following pulmonary lobectomy)
- The close proximity of important structures, principally nerves and vessels (e.g. facial nerve and external ear canal)
- The limited surgical access to some structures (e.g. soft palate).

Therefore, the potential for intraoperative and postoperative complications is relatively high. This tendency should be reduced by:

- A good anatomical knowledge of the region in question
- Knowledge of the disease process and how this may distort the regional anatomy
- A knowledge of the surgical procedure to be performed
- A plan for an alternative surgical procedure
- Gentle atraumatic surgical technique
- Meticulous attention to haemostasis
- Good-quality surgical instruments, appropriate for the purpose
- The ability to perform manipulations with minimal access, e.g. the ability to hand-tie knots in a cavity
- Careful use of diathermy adjacent to 'excitable cells' such as cardiomyocytes and neurons. Avoiding the use of cutting diathermy in procedures involving the lumen of the airway.

Preparation of the patient and aseptic technique

Clipping and surgical preparation of the surgical site are often postponed until after the patient has been anaesthetized. This may be because:

- The surgical site is inaccessible (e.g. oral approach to the larynx)
- The surgical site is painful (e.g. external ear canal in otitis externa)
- The patient is in a compromised state and further stress is to be avoided (e.g. pleural effusion).

Although strict adherence to the standard principles of aseptic technique is ideal, for surgeries involving the external ear canal and the conducting airways aseptic preparation of the surgical site is difficult or impossible. Rather than performing repeated lavage of the external ear canal or swabbing of the mucosal surfaces, it is better to accept that surgical procedures in these locations are likely to be clean-contaminated, contaminated or dirty procedures. Hence, perioperative antibiotics are indicated.

Perioperative antibiotic use should consist of a single intravenous bolus 30–60 minutes before the start of surgery. Further doses may be given depending on the duration of the procedure and the nature of the surgery, but patients with clean or clean-contaminated wounds will not require further prophylaxis. However, some patients will present with evidence of infection of a part of the airway, and in these cases antibiotic use is warranted on a therapeutic basis.

Most bacterial infections of the external ear canal involve Gram-positive *Staphylococcus* spp. and Gram-negative *Pseudomonas* spp. and *Proteus* spp. However, the patient presented for surgical management of ear disease is likely to have been treated with antibiotics topically or systemically, with resulting derangement of the normal flora, inhibition of some pathogenic species and overgrowth of resistant bacteria. Hence, bacterial culture and sensitivity testing may be the only way to identify the organisms. Suitable choices for empirical therapy include clavulanate-potentiated amoxicillin for Gram-positive organisms and a fluoroquinolone or gentamicin for Gram-negative organisms.

The oral cavity is populated primarily by Gram-positive aerobes and anaerobes. Suitable choices for antimicrobial prophylaxis include ampicillin, amoxicillin, clavulanate-potentiated amoxicillin or cefazolin. Similar recommendations are made for the oesophagus.

Streptococcus spp., *Escherichia coli*, *Pseudomonas* spp., *Klebsiella* spp. and *Bordetella bronchiseptica* are commonly isolated from the respiratory tracts of normal dogs. Ampicillin or clavulanate-potentiated amoxicillin are suitable choices for prophylaxis. Most canine respiratory tract infections are due to Gram-negative organisms and many are resistant to commonly used antibiotics. The choice of a therapeutic antibiotic should be determined by cytological examination and culture of specimens. Suitable empirical choices whilst waiting for these results are ampicillin, clavulanate-potentiated amoxicillin, trimethoprim/sulfadiazine and fluoroquinolones.

References and further reading

Baines S, Lipscombe V and Hutchinson T (2012) *BSAVA Manual of Canine and Feline Surgical Principles: A Foundation Manual*. BSAVA Publications, Gloucester

Bellows J (2002) Laser use in veterinary dentistry. *Veterinary Clinics of North America: Small Animal Practice* **32**, 673–692

Boothe H (2012) Instrumentation. In: *Veterinary Small Animal Surgery*, ed. K Tobias and S Johnston, pp. 152–163. Elsevier, St Louis

Buffa ES, Lubbe AM, Verstraete FJM *et al.* (1997) The effects of wound lavage solutions on canine fibroblasts: an *in vitro* study. *Veterinary Surgery* **26**, 460–466

Duke-Novakovski T, de Vries M and Seymour C (2016) *BSAVA Manual of Canine and Feline Anaesthesia and Analgesia, 3rd edn*. BSAVA Publications, Gloucester

Hedlund C and Taboada J (2002) *Clinical Atlas of Ear, Nose and Throat Diseases in Small Animals*. Schlutersche, Hannover

Holt TL and Mann FA (2002) Soft tissue application of lasers. *Veterinary Clinics of North America: Small Animal Practice* **32**, 569–599

LaBagnara J (1995) A review of absorbable suture materials in head and neck surgery and introduction of monocryl: a new absorbable suture. *Ear Nose and Throat Journal* **74**, 409–415

Lane JG (1982) *ENT and Oral Surgery of the Dog and Cat*. John Wright, Bristol

Luis-Fuentes V, Johnson LR and Dennis S (2010) *BSAVA Manual of Canine and Feline Cardiorespiratory Medicine, 2nd edn*. BSAVA Publications, Gloucester

Monnet E (2002) Cardiovascular monitoring. In: *The Veterinary ICU Book*, ed. WE Wingfield and MR Raffe, pp.266–280. Teton New Media, Jackson

Orton EC (1995) *Small Animal Thoracic Surgery*. Williams & Wilkins, Baltimore

Orton EC (2002) Respiratory system. In: *The Veterinary ICU Book*, ed. WE Wingfield and MR Raffe, pp.281–297. Teton New Media, Jackson

Reiter AM (2013) Equipment for oral surgery in small animals. *Veterinary Clinics of North America: Small Animal Practice* **43**, 587–608

Reiter AM (2014) Open wide: blindness in cats after the use of mouth gags. *The Veterinary Journal* **201**, 5–6

Reiter AM and Gracis M (2018) *BSAVA Manual of Canine and Feline Dentistry and Oral Surgery, 4th edn*. BSAVA Publications, Gloucester

Terpak CH and Verstraete FJM (2012) Instrumentation, patient positioning and aseptic technique. In: *Oral and Maxillofacial Surgery in Dogs and Cats*, ed. FJM Verstraete and MJ Lommer, pp. 55–68. WB Saunders, Philadelphia

Tobias KM and Johnston SA (2012) *Veterinary Surgery: Small Animal*. WB Saunders, St Louis

Verstraete FJM (1999) *Self-Assessment Color Review of Veterinary Dentistry*. Manson Publishing, London

Chapter 2

Emergency management of respiratory distress

Daniel Holden and Kenneth Drobatz

Introduction

Respiratory distress is a life-threatening clinical syndrome that should be dealt with immediately. The principles of the approach to these critically ill patients are the same whether it is a first-time patient presenting, an inpatient or the postoperative animal. Immediate oxygen supplementation, a thorough physical examination and evaluation of clinical history and signs, and empirical localization of the lesion can help guide therapy when definitive diagnostics cannot be obtained because of the critical nature of the patient. Once the patient is stable, definitive diagnostics can be obtained and specific therapy can be instituted. What is done in the initial approach to these animals can make the difference between life and death.

Initial assessment and stabilization

Patients with respiratory distress are usually easily identified:

- Standing (dogs) or sternal recumbency (cats)
- Abducted elbows
- Extended neck
- Tachypnoea
- Weakness
- Abnormal stridorous (laryngeal or tracheal) and/or stertorous (nasal/oropharyngeal) sounds
- Increased inspiratory and/or expiratory effort
- Abnormal abdominal wall motion
- Vigorous resistance to restraint.

Cats are much more adept than dogs at concealing signs of respiratory distress, and disease is often much more advanced on presentation in this species.

Initial assessment in a patient with severe respiratory distress is directed at assuring a patent airway and adequate ventilation. If the airway is not clear or the patient is not ventilating adequately, immediate attempts should be made to clear the airway and intubate the patient.

If a patent airway cannot be obtained through intubation, tracheotomy should be performed **IF** it will bypass the airway obstruction. It is extremely rare that an emergency tracheostomy has to be performed (see Operative Technique 2.1). In most instances, airway access can be achieved via orotracheal intubation and tracheostomy may then be performed in a more controlled manner.

Oxygen supplementation should be provided whilst assessing the airway. The goal is to allow for continued assessment of the patient and the provision of further therapy, without causing excessive patient distress. The authors' first choice is mask or flow-by oxygen delivery (see later). The work of breathing may cause the patient to consume more oxygen; breath-holding can rapidly decrease the animal's inspired oxygen concentration and can severely compromise some patients. Even struggling against restraint, the placement of an intravenous catheter, or positioning for radiography can be devastating in animals with respiratory compromise. Good clinical judgement is extremely important in weighing the advantages and disadvantages of any diagnostic or therapeutic procedure in these critically ill patients.

If possible, an intravenous catheter should be placed. This procedure allows collection of three capillary tubes of blood for an emergency database (packed cell volume (PCV), total solids (TS), dipstick blood urea nitrogen (BUN), blood glucose and a blood smear) and administration of intravenous emergency drugs or fluids.

Pathophysiology

Under normal physiological conditions, alveolar ventilation is primarily driven by changes in the partial pressure of carbon dioxide in arterial blood (P_aCO_2). Increases in carbon dioxide (hypercapnia) will stimulate ventilation, but hypoxaemia (decreased partial pressure of oxygen in arterial blood, P_aO_2) needs to be more profound before a stimulatory effect is achieved. Hypercapnic respiratory disease involves a failure of the neural and/or muscular component of the respiratory system, and is often associated with a decrease in ventilatory effort. Hypoxaemic respiratory disease involves failure of efficient alveolar oxygenation, usually due to pulmonary parenchymal or airway-related disorders, and is often associated with increased ventilatory effort.

Diagnostic approach

Signalment, history and physical examination often provide enough information to localize the respiratory lesion. Localization of the lesion can narrow down the differential diagnosis list and provide a basis for empirical therapy if the animal is not stable enough for more definitive diagnostics. The empirical localization of the respiratory lesion lends itself to an algorithmic approach (Figure 2.1). As with any algorithmic approach in medicine, exceptions exist, and the empirical determination of the lesion using the algorithm should also be influenced by clinical judgement and experience.

History

Once an animal's respiratory distress has been alleviated, a detailed history should be obtained. The duration and dynamics of the respiratory distress, and association with trauma, coughing (especially in cats), vomiting or other obvious complaints, may indicate the underlying nature of the problem. Unwitnessed trauma and access to toxins (especially rodenticides) are common and should be anticipated.

Observation

Observation of the respiratory pattern can sometimes help localize the lesion but is rarely definitive, since lesions in different parts of the respiratory tract can have similar patterns. An irregular respiratory rhythm is associated with brain or brainstem injury. Animals with abnormal respiratory rhythms secondary to brain injury have other obvious signs of brain dysfunction.

Dynamic obstructions result in resistance to airway flow during inspiration or expiration. Extrathoracic dynamic airway obstructions (e.g. laryngeal paralysis) cause inspiratory difficulty, whilst intrathoracic dynamic airway obstructions (e.g. intrathoracic tracheal collapse or feline asthma) cause expiratory difficulty.

Disorders involving the upper airway commonly cause loud stertorous (rostral to the larynx) or stridorous (larynx and caudally) respiration. Noise in one phase of the respiratory cycle suggests a dynamic obstruction (such as laryngeal paralysis); noise that persists throughout the cycle suggests a fixed obstruction (mass, foreign body). Exaggerated respiratory effort with a normal to slow respiratory rate and paradoxical abdominal motion are also features of large airway disease.

Pleural space disorders commonly cause fast, shallow respiration with increased inspiratory effort and paradoxical abdominal motion (particularly with longstanding pleural effusions). Exaggerated respiratory effort with little actual airflow is also a hallmark of pleural space disease.

Fast, shallow respiration with paradoxical abdominal motion can also occur because of poor lung compliance as a result of pulmonary parenchymal disease. However, pulmonary parenchymal disease has also been associated with slow, laboured respiration and hyperpnoea, often with marked inspiratory and expiratory effort. Disorders involving the small airways commonly cause hyperpnoea with end-expiratory abdominal effort due to gas trapping in the small airways. Coughing may also be a feature of small airway disease, especially in cats.

It is important to remember that these categories and clinical signs are not exclusive.

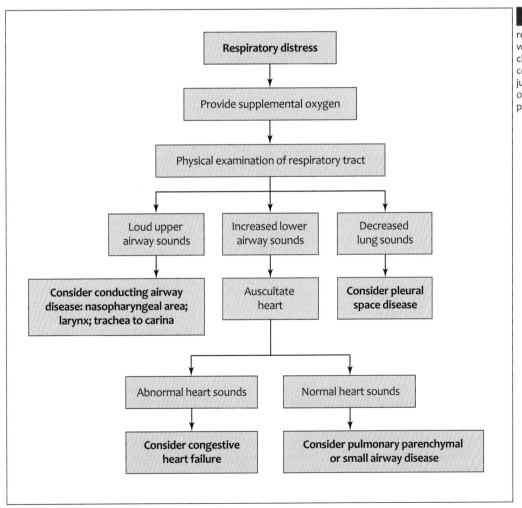

2.1 Algorithm for localization of the respiratory lesion in animals with respiratory distress. This chart should be used in conjunction with clinical judgement and experience to optimize assessment of the patient.

Auscultation

The essential goal of auscultation is to answer three questions:

- Are breath sounds present over the left and right lung fields?
- Are the breath sounds the same over the left and right lung fields?
- If the breath sounds are not the same over the left and right lung fields, how are they different (e.g. diminished, bronchial, presence of adventitious sounds)?

Because of variation in patient size and conformation, the easiest approach is to divide the thoracic wall into grid squares and auscultate each in turn. A good stethoscope (preferably with a paediatric chestpiece) and a quiet environment are essential for accurate and meaningful auscultation. Sounds on one side should be compared with those heard on the contralateral side, during both inspiration and expiration. The patient's hair can be moistened to limit misinterpretation of hair sounds as adventitious lung sounds.

Normal lung sounds can be defined as follows:

- Bronchial sounds are heard directly over the trachea and major bronchi during inspiration and expiration. They are loud and high pitched, with a pause between inspiration and expiration. The duration of the inspiratory sound is slightly shorter than that of the expiratory sound
- Bronchovesicular sounds are heard over the major bronchi and are softer and lower pitched than bronchial sounds. They are heard equally during inspiration and expiration
- Vesicular sounds are heard over all areas of the chest distal to the central airways. They have a softer intensity and are heard throughout all of inspiration and only the first third of expiration.

Absence or reduction of lung and/or heart sounds on auscultation is indicative of pleural space disease, with air, fluid or (in the case of diaphragmatic rupture) abdominal viscera separating the heart and lungs from the chest wall. Careful bilateral auscultation is important to determine any asymmetry in distribution, and diagnostic thoracocentesis is usually indicated.

Abnormal lung sounds can be most easily classified as wheezes or crackles.

- Wheezing results from airway narrowing and subsequent increases in airflow through the segment. A high-pitched wheeze is usually associated with tighter obstruction, whereas a low-pitched wheeze usually indicates less obstruction. Wheezes are generated in large bronchi and are musical sounds with a constant pitch, more often heard during expiration. They are commonly associated with small airway disease, bronchitis and feline asthma. A wheeze on inspiration usually comes from the extrathoracic airways; the sound heard when there is severe narrowing is known as stridor.
- Crackles are intermittent crackling or bubbling sounds of short duration, heard most commonly during inspiration. They are associated with both restrictive and obstructive disease. Early inspiratory crackles are a common feature of small airway disease, whereas late or end-inspiratory crackles can occur with atelectasis, pneumonia, pulmonary fibrosis or

congestive heart failure. Crackles occurring during both inspiration and expiration are a feature of chronic bronchitis or bronchiectasis. Coarse crackles are due to movement of secretions in the large upper airways and can be heard at the patient's mouth.

External examination and palpation

Examination should be thorough but as stress-free as possible. Careful palpation of the external nasal cavity, pharynx, larynx, neck and ribs should be performed and chest wall movement with respiration should be noted if this has not already been done. Mucous membranes and capillary refill should also be assessed. Cyanosis is always a late sign in respiratory disease and may not be evident in patients with severe anaemia or poor perfusion.

Radiography

A detailed discussion of cervical and thoracic radiography is outside the scope of this chapter. Although cervical and thoracic radiography is undoubtedly an invaluable tool for the assessment of respiratory disease, the necessary chemical or physical restraint required to produce an image of diagnostic quality may be counterproductive or even life-threatening. Sufficient information to allow the patient to be stabilized can usually be gained from the history, physical examination and initial laboratory investigations. If pleural space disease is suspected, thoracocentesis may prove therapeutic as well as being diagnostic.

Ultrasonography

Ultrasound examination in the investigation of non-cardiac thoracic disease is now a well-established tool. A detailed discussion is beyond the scope of this chapter, but the concept of TFAST (thoracic focused assessment with sonography in trauma, triage and tracking) examinations in patients with respiratory distress is well described. Examination is rapid, safe, non-invasive and allows prompt detection and monitoring of pneumothorax, pleural effusion, chest wall injury and pulmonary contusions or other pathology (Lisciandro, 2014).

Pulse oximetry

Saturation of arterial haemoglobin with oxygen can be more accurately monitored by pulse oximetry. This is an extremely useful non-invasive method for assessing and monitoring dyspnoeic patients. However, it has a number of limitations that must be understood if the information provided by the pulse oximeter is not to be misinterpreted.

Pulse oximetry works by comparing the absorption by haemoglobin of two different wavelengths of light passed through an extremity. The degree of absorption changes with the percentage of haemoglobin that is saturated with oxygen. A value of S_aO_2 (arterial haemoglobin oxygen saturation) is determined from the ratio of the absorption of the energy at the two wavelengths. Pulse oximeters generally display pulse rate and S_aO_2. A beep may sound to indicate pulse rate, with the pitch varying with changes in S_aO_2. A good estimation of the oxygen saturation of haemoglobin is provided. However, it should be realized, from the sigmoid shape of the oxyhaemoglobin dissociation curve, that although S_aO_2 varies in a fairly linear way with P_aO_2 at low partial pressures, the slope flattens at higher partial pressures. Therefore, S_aO_2 will be reasonably high (>90%) unless P_aO_2 is as low as about 60 mmHg. When using a pulse oximeter, therefore, unless it is reading an S_aO_2 in the high 90s, it is impossible to know whether P_aO_2 is at a safe level or whether the animal is about to desaturate.

Pulse oximeters do not provide any information on arterial blood pressure. As long as the pulse pressure is >20 mmHg, pulse oximeters are able to determine a pulse rate. It should also be noted that pulse oximeters amplify the signal they receive; therefore, the flashing lights vary with the signal received and not with arterial blood pressure.

Transmission probes can be placed over unpigmented hairless skin or mucous membranes. Useful sites include the tongue, toe web, ear pinnae, vulva and prepuce. Probes designed to wrap around a toenail are very useful, as they are much less susceptible to movement artefact. Reflection probes (which have the photodetector next to the light-emitting diodes) do not need two skin or mucous membrane surfaces. Therefore, they can be placed at sites such as in the rectum. However, this type of probe has been associated with problems of inaccuracy. Movement, such as shivering, also greatly reduces accuracy, although newer probes can overcome this.

Carboxyhaemoglobin (COHb) produces a falsely high reading of S_aO_2, because pulse oximeters measure COHb as fully oxygenated haemoglobin. Therefore, pulse oximetry cannot be used to monitor S_aO_2 in animals that may have been exposed to carbon monoxide. Methaemoglobinaemia can cause pulse oximeters to indicate low oxygen saturation.

Tissues such as cats' tongues or ear pinnae may be too thin for the probes (designed for human paediatric fingers) to measure. This can be compensated for by placing a folded paper towel around the tissue between the probes.

Blood gas analysis

If blood gas analysis is to be performed for assessment of respiratory disorders, an anaerobically drawn arterial sample is essential. This may be taken from the metatarsal, radial, auricular or femoral artery. Arterial stabs are painful and excessive bleeding is possible; the procedure is contraindicated in patients with evidence of bleeding disorders. Rapid (within 2 minutes) analysis is vital to ensure accurate results; if a delay is inevitable, the sample should be stored on ice.

Venous blood can be used for acid–base analysis, but it should be remembered that pH will be slightly lower and pCO_2 (partial pressure of carbon dioxide dissolved in plasma) slightly higher as long as perfusion is adequate. The pO_2 (partial pressure of oxygen dissolved in plasma) may also give valuable clues to the patient's underlying disease process. Reference values are shown in Figure 2.2.

The partial pressure of oxygen in arterial blood (P_aO_2) is essentially an indicator of the adequacy and efficacy of gas exchange in the lung. It is not an indicator of tissue oxygen delivery, nor of blood oxygen content. P_aO_2 represents the oxygen physically dissolved in the plasma; this is generally a little less than 2% of the total oxygen content of the blood. P_aO_2 can only really be evaluated relative to P_AO_2 (partial pressure of oxygen in the alveolus), which can be calculated from the alveolar gas equation:

$$P_AO_2 = F_iO_2 (PB - 47) - 1.2 (P_aCO_2)$$

Where F_iO_2 = the fractional inspired oxygen concentration (if the patient is on room air (21% O_2), $F_iO_2 = 0.21$) and PB = atmospheric pressure (usually 760 mmHg). The equation assumes that the patient's respiratory quotient (RQ) is 0.8 and that $P_ACO_2 = P_aCO_2$ (for the vast majority of cases this is true).

Parameter	Dog	Cat
pH	7.36–7.42	7.24–7.40
pO_2 (mmHg)	85–95	84–96
pCO_2 (mmHg)	29–42	29–42
[HCO_3^-] (mmol/l)	17–24	17–24
S_aO_2 (%)	97–100	97–100
TCO_2 (mmol/l)	19–26	19–26
Hb (g/l)	120–180	90–150

2.2 Normal reference values for arterial blood gas analysis when breathing room air (F_iO_2 = 0.21 at sea level). F_iO_2 = fractional inspired oxygen concentration; Hb = haemoglobin; pCO_2 = partial pressure of carbon dioxide dissolved in plasma; pO_2 = partial pressure of oxygen dissolved in plasma; S_aO_2 = arterial haemoglobin oxygen saturation; TCO_2 = total carbon dioxide.

Knowing the P_aO_2 and P_AO_2 allows calculation of the alveolar–arterial oxygen difference, or $P_{(A-a)}O_2$. This is useful because, in conjunction with other clinical information, it allows the cause of the hypoxia to be determined further (Figure 2.3). Normal $P_{(A-a)}O_2$ should be <20 mmHg on room air. The value increases as F_iO_2 increases. As a very rough guide, P_aO_2 (mmHg) should be approximately 4–5 times the inspired O_2 percentage.

Causes of low P_aO_2	Effect on $P_{(A-a)}O_2$
Cardiac/pulmonary right-to-left shunt	Increased
Decreased F_iO_2 (e.g. altitude, gas supply failure)	Normal
Ventilation–perfusion imbalance (e.g. pulmonary thromboembolism, general anaesthesia)	Increased
Hypoventilation (e.g. CNS trauma/disease, neuromuscular disease)	Normal
Diffusion impairment (e.g. pulmonary fibrosis, congestive heart failure)	Increased

2.3 Causes of low arterial oxygen partial pressure (P_aO_2) and the effect on alveolar–arterial oxygen difference ($P_{(A-a)}O_2$). CNS = central nervous system; F_iO_2 = fractional inspired oxygen concentration.

Oxygen saturation and oxygen content

Ninety-eight percent of all oxygen in the blood is bound to haemoglobin; this does not exert a pressure at the oxygen electrode. Neither S_aO_2 nor P_aO_2 indicates the oxygen content of arterial blood (C_aO_2).

$$C_aO_2 = ([Hb] \times 1.34 \times S_aO_2) + (0.003 \times P_aO_2)$$

(Note: 1.34 ml O_2 can bind to 1 g of haemoglobin; 0.003 mEq/l/mmHg is the solubility coefficient of oxygen in plasma.) It is generally accepted that 50 g/l of deoxygenated haemoglobin is required to produce clinically evident cyanosis. It is also possible for P_aO_2 to be normal and C_aO_2 to be grossly abnormal, as in severe anaemia or in the presence of abnormal haemoglobins.

Diseases associated with respiratory distress

Diseases of the conducting airway

Diseases of the conducting airway (pharynx, larynx or trachea) causing respiratory distress are associated with loud respiratory sounds heard without the stethoscope. Problems in these areas include oedema, infection, foreign bodies, neoplasia, neuromuscular disorders and degenerative diseases. An animal with loud upper airway sounds has to be considered to have upper airway disease until proven otherwise. This does not preclude respiratory lesions elsewhere in the tract and these areas should be investigated as well (e.g. aspiration pneumonia secondary to laryngeal paralysis).

The two most common abnormalities are laryngeal paralysis and collapsing trachea. Laryngeal paralysis occurs more commonly in large-breed dogs; collapsing trachea is more common in small-breed dogs. Both conditions represent dynamic airway lesions in which the collapse varies with the respiratory cycle. Brachycephalic upper airway syndrome is a common cause for respiratory stress (see Chapter 6). Loud upper airway sounds including stridor and stertor can be heard depending on the extent and severity of the condition. Also depending on the severity of the condition, the respiratory pattern and sounds can be consistent with a fixed or dynamic obstruction (more commonly consistent with extrathoracic dynamic obstruction). The harder the animal breathes, the more severe the obstruction; the more severe the obstruction, the more hypoxic the animal and the greater the respiratory drive; and so the vicious cycle progresses. Heat generated by the respiratory muscles, combined with the inability to move gas in and out of the pulmonary system, can result in high body temperature. This also contributes to further demand on the respiratory system.

It is important to break the cycle. Oxygen should be given immediately. This will help slow the respiratory cycle but is usually inadequate as a standalone therapy. Sedation with acepromazine maleate (30–50 μg/kg i.v. or i.m. or butorphanol 0.2–0.4 mg/kg i.v. or i.m.) will help calm the animal and slow ventilation. If the animal's temperature is high (>41°C), spraying water on the hair coat and blowing a fan over the body will expedite cooling. This three-pronged approach generally results in stabilization of the respiratory system within 30–60 minutes and the animal can be weaned off oxygen supplementation. Some patients may benefit from anti-inflammatory doses of corticosteroids because of laryngeal or tracheal inflammation and oedema.

It is extremely rare that emergency laryngeal surgery is required in patients with laryngeal paralysis; the above medical therapy is generally quite effective. If a patient is in acute distress and there is concern about imminent collapse, anaesthesia and intubation will relieve the distress immediately if laryngeal paralysis is the cause. It should be remembered that waking patients (from anaesthesia) with dynamic upper airway obstruction is extremely difficult. The excitement phase of recovery causes dynamic airway pressure changes, resulting in collapse of the affected area of the pulmonary tree, starting the vicious cycle again.

Heart disease

If an animal with respiratory distress has increased lower airway sounds or breath sounds and an auscultable cardiac abnormality, such as a loud heart murmur or a persistent arrhythmia, cardiac disease must be considered as a cause of the respiratory distress. Empirical therapy for cardiac disease should be administered if further diagnostics cannot be pursued. In animals with mild to moderate heart failure, furosemide (2 mg/kg i.v. or i.m. in dogs; 1 mg/kg i.v. or i.m. in cats) should be administered. In severely affected animals, these doses can be doubled. Furosemide therapy combined with oxygen supplementation is often successful in stabilizing animals with mild to moderate congestive heart failure on an emergency basis. In severely affected dogs, nitroprusside (an arterial and venous vasodilator) can also be used, beginning at a constant rate infusion of 1 μg/kg/min and slowly increasing the rate every 15 minutes whilst monitoring blood pressure (nitroprusside is a very potent vasodilator and may cause severe hypotension). Unfortunately, nitroprusside is not readily available any more in the USA. In most dogs, the effective dose is usually 5–10 μg/kg/min. Dogs with dilated cardiomyopathy may also benefit from a positive inotrope such as dobutamine (5–10 μg/kg/min). If used judiciously, these drugs are very effective in relieving respiratory distress in dogs with severe pulmonary oedema secondary to heart failure (particularly dilated cardiomyopathy). Once stable, the heart disease can be characterized fully and tailored therapy can be instituted.

Pulmonary parenchymal disease

Increased lower airway sounds or pulmonary crackles indicate small airway or pulmonary parenchymal abnormalities. These sounds may be due to oedema (cardiogenic or non-cardiogenic), haemorrhage, infection or infiltrative processes. Some of the more common causes of pulmonary parenchymal disease (in the authors' experience) are:

- Pulmonary oedema (cardiogenic or non-cardiogenic)
- Haemorrhage (trauma, anticoagulant rodenticide)
- Pulmonary thromboembolism (PTE)
- Feline asthma
- Pneumonia (aspiration)
- Pulmonary contusion
- Smoke or toxin inhalation
- Acute respiratory distress syndrome (ARDS).

The absence of audible cardiac abnormalities in the face of increased lower airway sounds strongly suggests pulmonary parenchymal disease or lower airway disease rather than congestive heart failure. The location of these sounds may help in the diagnosis. For example, a cranioventral distribution or right middle lung lobe distribution makes aspiration pneumonia a likely possibility, whilst a caudal dorsal distribution suggests neurogenic pulmonary oedema. These findings are not always consistent and, despite the animal's instability, thoracic radiographs are often necessary to characterize the disease so that empirical therapy can be instituted. A thorough clinical history, thoracic radiographs, blood tests, tracheal wash, bronchoscopy or even lung biopsy may be required to diagnose the problem definitively so that appropriate therapy can be applied, but often the radiographic distribution of pulmonary infiltrates, appearance of the heart, physical examination and clinical history can point towards a diagnosis.

Non-cardiogenic pulmonary oedema

This is oedema not due to cardiac disease, and encompasses nearly all the pulmonary parenchymal types of diseases. Neurogenic pulmonary oedema is a specific type of non-cardiogenic pulmonary oedema secondary to a brain insult. The four most common brain insults are head trauma, electrocution, seizures and upper airway obstruction. Neurogenic pulmonary oedema is characterized by an acute onset (typically within minutes) of respiratory abnormalities after one of the four listed insults. The degree of pulmonary oedema can vary from mild to severe, involving all lung fields. The typical pattern is interstitial to alveolar, with the distribution initially starting in the caudodorsal area. The treatment for this condition is supportive, with oxygen supplementation and diuretics (furosemide 2–4 mg/kg i.v. q6–8h). Animals with upper airway obstruction or head trauma tend to be more severely affected by pulmonary oedema than those with seizures or those that have been electrocuted. Some animals require positive pressure ventilation and synthetic colloid support because of the severity of the pulmonary oedema and the massive loss of high-protein fluid into the lungs; these animals have a poor prognosis and usually die. Most animals with neurogenic pulmonary oedema have either substantially improved or have died from respiratory compromise within 48 hours of the inciting event.

Haemorrhage

Spontaneous pulmonary haemorrhage is most commonly due to intoxication with a rodenticide anticoagulant or to thrombocytopenia. Supportive care, with oxygen supplementation and specific treatment of the underlying cause, is the only option available to treat this problem. Infection with *Angiostrongylus vasorum* should be also be considered in dogs with haemoptysis and respiratory distress.

Pulmonary thromboembolism

PTE can result in relatively mild to extreme respiratory distress. It is often associated with diseases such as hyperadrenocorticism, immune-mediated haemolytic anaemia, protein-losing nephropathy or chronic high-dose corticosteroid administration. Ante-mortem definitive diagnosis can usually only be achieved by pulmonary angiography or contrast computed tomography, tools that are not readily accessible to most veterinary surgeons (veterinarians) in practice. Therefore, the diagnosis is most commonly arrived at using the medical history, recognition of concurrent diseases or drug therapies that are commonly associated with PTE, a history of sudden onset of respiratory abnormalities, and thoracic radiography. Radiographs vary from almost normal to showing a patchy interstitial or alveolar pattern and/or mild pleural effusion. PTE should be considered in dogs with severe respiratory distress (not due to upper airway disease) that have normal-appearing thoracic radiographs. Treatment for PTE is primarily supportive, with oxygen supplementation, heparin therapy and specific therapy for the associated cause. Thrombolytic therapy can be used but the authors have had limited experience with this treatment.

Feline asthma

Feline asthma is an airway hypersensitivity condition in cats that results in bronchoconstriction, pulmonary air trapping and increased respiratory secretions. The degree of respiratory distress can be mild to life-threatening. Many owners describe their cat as retching or coughing, and some incorrectly think that their cat is vomiting. Most cats have a prolonged expiratory phase with end-expiratory wheezes heard on auscultation. Rarely, a cat will present with a 'barrel' chest secondary to severe airway trapping. In this instance, airway sounds cannot be auscultated because the animal is moving so little air. Emergency therapy for cats with asthma and respiratory distress includes oxygen supplementation, corticosteroids (dexamethasone sodium phosphate 0.2 mg/kg i.v. or i.m.) and terbutaline (0.01 mg/kg i.m. or s.c.). The authors have also used inhaled corticosteroids and bronchodilators in some cats. Improvement in respiratory rate and effort is usually noted within 30–60 minutes after terbutaline injection or inhalation therapy.

Aspiration pneumonia

Aspiration pneumonia is a relatively common cause of respiratory distress in animals that are vomiting and recumbent. This is primarily diagnosed based on the radiographic appearance of interstitial/alveolar infiltrates in the cranioventral and right middle lung lobe areas, as well as tracheal wash cytology and culture. Treatment includes oxygen supplementation, nebulization and coupage, maintenance of hydration, broad-spectrum antibiotics (ideally based on culture and sensitivity testing) and mild exercise (walking) if possible. In addition, diagnostics and therapy should also be directed at the underlying cause of the vomiting or regurgitation.

Pulmonary contusion

Pulmonary contusions vary from mild to severe, causing mild to severe respiratory distress. Increased lower airway sounds and/or crackles are often heard on auscultation. Some dogs with severe contusions will have a soft cough at presentation and some may show haemoptysis. Pulmonary contusions tend to worsen over the first 12 hours. In addition, radiographic signs will lag behind clinical signs by several hours. Treatment for pulmonary contusions is primarily supportive, with oxygen supplementation and judicious fluid therapy (only if resuscitation with fluids for other problems is necessary, e.g. hypovolaemia). Respiratory signs tend to start improving after about 36–48 hours in most cases.

Smoke inhalation

Smoke inhalation is a relatively rare problem. In large cities, smoke inhalation tends to occur in the colder months of the year, when the majority of house fires occur. Affected animals present with a wide range of physiological compromise. Most have only minor respiratory signs or ocular irritation but some may have severe respiratory and neurological compromise that can result in death. Respiratory signs occur as a result of swelling of the upper airways from direct heat injury, as well as bronchoconstriction and pulmonary inflammation due to chemical and particulate irritation of the lower airways and alveoli. Radiographic changes seen in dogs and cats with smoke inhalation vary, and include bronchiolar, interstitial and alveolar patterns. Rarely, a collapsed lung lobe may occur as result of bronchial obstruction from mucosal swelling, sloughing and debris. Treatment for smoke inhalation is primarily supportive, with oxygen supplementation, bronchodilators and maintenance of hydration (whilst avoiding overhydration), with nebulization and coupage if the lower airways are found to be affected.

Acute respiratory distress syndrome

ARDS is recognized in dogs and cats. It is an inflammatory condition of the lungs, resulting in severe respiratory compromise with hypoxaemia and decreased pulmonary compliance. It is characterized clinically by bilateral pulmonary infiltrates (on thoracic radiography) and hypoxaemia with normal heart function. Therefore, clinically, any of the non-cardiogenic pulmonary conditions could be classified as ARDS, but there are also certain histological characteristics that are recognized. ARDS can be an end-stage process secondary to almost any inflammatory condition within the lungs or any inflammatory condition remote from the lungs, such as pancreatitis, sepsis and trauma. Treatment is primarily supportive whilt the associated cause is treated.

Pleural space disorders

Pleural effusion, pneumothorax and diaphragmatic hernia are the most common pleural space disorders associated with respiratory distress. The clinical signs of pleural space disease are a result of the underlying disease process and the restriction of lung expansion. The latter is typically manifested by short and shallow respirations and decreased lung sounds on auscultation. In the authors' experience, pleural effusion is the most common of the three.

Pleural effusion

There are a variety of causes of pleural effusion (see Chapter 12). The diagnosis of the underlying cause of pleural effusion can be narrowed down and usually definitively determined by analysis of the pleural effusion (see the BSAVA Manual of Canine and Feline Clinical Pathology).

Pneumothorax

Pneumothorax (see Chapter 12) is the second most common pleural space disorder and is typically categorized by aetiology, i.e. spontaneous (non-traumatic) or traumatic. Spontaneous pneumothorax most commonly occurs in large-breed dogs and is usually secondary to a pulmonary parenchymal abnormality, such as a bulla, bleb or abscess. These patients often present in severe respiratory distress, with bilaterally diminished respiratory sounds dorsally. A large amount of air is often obtained during thoracocentesis. Both sides of the thorax should be aspirated. Air should be removed until a negative result is obtained. If a negative result cannot be obtained, then chest tubes should be placed and a constant vacuum applied.

Tension pneumothorax occurs when air continues to accumulate in the pleural space due to a one-way valve effect at the leak. Air continues to accumulate, causing intrapleural pressures greater than atmospheric, resulting in progressive atelectasis, interference with venous return and poor cardiac output. Immediate relief of the pneumothorax is required. A small intercostal incision into the pleural space may rapidly relieve the pneumothorax. After removal of the air, the incision should be sealed with a sterile dressing, and close monitoring for reoccurrence of the pneumothorax should be instituted. Chest tube placement is usually required in patients where a negative pressure cannot be achieved during thoracocentesis or when large amounts of air repeatedly accumulate.

Diaphragmatic rupture

Rupture of the diaphragm (see Chapter 17) is most commonly caused by blunt trauma. The respiratory signs are usually a result of restricted expansion of the lungs, although underlying pulmonary contusions may contribute. A diagnosis can be achieved by thoracic radiography, upper gastrointestinal positive contrast radiography, abdominal ultrasonography or intraperitoneal positive contrast imaging. Surgery is the definitive therapy.

Thoracic wall disorders

The two most common thoracic wall disorders are rib fractures and flail chest. Fractured ribs are relatively easily diagnosed by radiographic evaluation, but can be missed if the index of suspicion is not kept high. The respiratory signs are more typically a result of the underlying pulmonary contusion and pain rather than the mechanical dysfunction of the chest wall. For this reason, management is typically medical through oxygen supplementation, pain management and judicious fluid therapy, if the latter is required for other reasons.

Prolonged oxygen therapy

Enclosed techniques

With enclosed techniques, oxygen is pumped into a contained area over the head or muzzle of the animal. Most oxygen masks are made of transparent plastic, through which the animal can be observed. Several methods have been described by which increased inspired concentrations of oxygen can be achieved, including placement of a plastic bag over the head into which oxygen is pumped, and the use of an Elizabethan collar with plastic wrap covering the front. Advantages of these systems include their relative ease of use and rapid placement in emergency situations. Depending on flow rates and tightness of fit, very high oxygen concentrations can be achieved whilst access to the rest of the patient is still possible. Severely dyspnoeic or very mobile patients may, however, not tolerate these systems, and build-up of excessive heat and carbon dioxide due to excessive dead space as well as accumulated moisture, and water in panting dogs, can limit their usefulness or even lead to respiratory acidosis.

Nasal tube

For administration of oxygen by nasal tube, a rubber urinary catheter or soft polythene nasal feeding tube is commonly used. Catheters may vary in size from 5 to 10 Fr, depending on the size of the animal.

The catheter is measured from the nares to the medial canthus of the eye, and marked with a small piece of tape. Following desensitization of the nostril, the lubricated catheter is inserted gently into the nostril in a ventromedial direction and advanced to the marker. Once the catheter is in place, it is bent around and placed under the alar fold of the nostril, and sutured or glued in place on the side of the face (Figure 2.4). For the most secure placement, a suture should be placed as close to the nasal–cutaneous junction as possible. The nasal catheter is attached to an oxygen delivery system, with flow rates of 100–200 ml/kg/min.

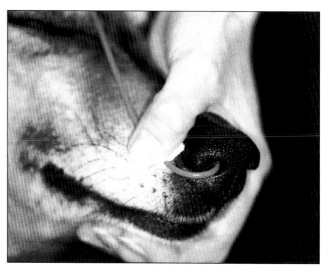

2.4 Nasal oxygen can be provided through a catheter inserted into one nostril to a premeasured length.
(Reproduced from the BSAVA Manual of Canine and Feline Emergency and Critical Care, 3rd edn)

In very dyspnoeic animals, bilateral nasal oxygen lines can be used. Some animals can be best managed using human bilateral nasal 'prongs' that penetrate only 1 cm or less into the nasal cavity (Figure 2.5). Inspired oxygen concentrations of 30–50% can easily be achieved using this type of system. If the nasal catheter is guided further into the nasopharynx under sedation, oxygen concentrations of up to 80% may be achieved in some animals.

A nasal catheter is easy to place and is well tolerated by most patients. It also allows patient mobility and permits examination of the animal without discontinuing therapy. Some animals, however, will not tolerate the nasal line, and inspired oxygen concentrations may not be high enough for very dyspnoeic animals, particularly if they are mouth breathing. It is also not a useful technique in brachycephalic animals or patients with facial disease or pain.

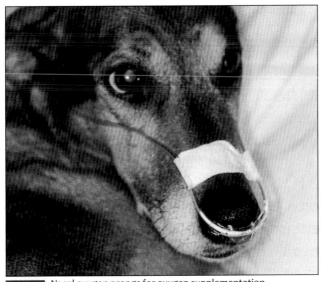

2.5 Nasal oxygen prongs for oxygen supplementation.
(Reproduced from the BSAVA Manual of Canine and Feline Emergency and Critical Care, 3rd edn)

Transtracheal oxygen

For administration of transtracheal oxygen, a catheter is placed transcutaneously into the trachea, and oxygen is insufflated directly into the airway. For placement of a tracheal catheter, a small patch of skin on the ventral midline of the neck is clipped and scrubbed. Lidocaine is used to provide local anaesthesia. A through-the-needle catheter is placed into the airway using the same method as may be used for a transtracheal wash. The catheter is secured in place with glue, sutures or tape, and humidified oxygen is administered via a delivery system at rates of 50–100 ml/kg/min. Higher oxygen concentrations can be achieved in the airway using this technique because there is less mixing with inhaled room air.

Transtracheal oxygen administration is a useful technique in patients with upper airway obstructive disease. It is usually well tolerated and will withstand moderate patient movement. However, it is invasive, and dislodgement or kinking of the catheter can occur. Oxygen must be humidified if it is delivered directly into the trachea, to prevent desiccation of the tracheal epithelium.

Oxygen cages and incubators

Oxygen cages are now widely available to the veterinary market. As well as providing a higher concentration of inspired oxygen, a good oxygen cage should also allow control of internal cage temperature and humidity. An oxygen cage should be capable of reaching oxygen concentrations >80% for use with severely dyspnoeic animals. Poor-quality oxygen cages will reach concentrations of only about 50–60%.

Oxygen cages and incubators can be invaluable for severely dyspnoeic cats, where the ability to administer a high oxygen concentration non-invasively is essential (Figure 2.6). Oxygen cages can be expensive to purchase and potentially wasteful of oxygen, since each time the door is opened the oxygen inside is lost. This is less of an issue with incubators, many of which have access ports.

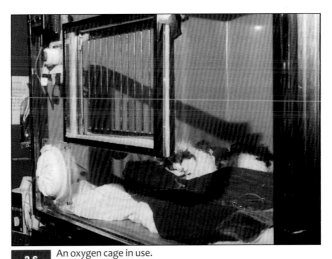

2.6 An oxygen cage in use.
(Reproduced from the BSAVA Manual of Canine and Feline Emergency and Critical Care, 2nd edn)

Intubation and ventilation

Orotracheal intubation and ventilatory support may be required if respiratory failure is already present or is predicted on the basis of the condition of the patient. Anaesthesia, intubation and positive pressure ventilation may be required to allow vital diagnostic tests, such as radiography, to be performed, especially in animals that are in extreme distress and not responding to non-specific therapy. Dyspnoeic patients should only be anaesthetized and ventilated as a last resort, to support respiratory function whilst diagnostic tests are performed and definitive therapy is pursued.

References and further reading

Lisciandro GR (2014) The Thoracic FAST3 (TFAST3) exam. In: *Focused Ultrasound Techniques for the Small Animal Clinician*, ed. GR Lisciandro, pp. 140–165. Wiley-Blackwell, Indianapolis

Villiers E and Ristic J (2016) *BSAVA Manual of Canine and Feline Clinical Pathology, 3rd edn*. BSAVA Publications, Gloucester

Waddell L and King L (2007) General approach to dyspnoea. In: *BSAVA Manual of Canine and Feline Emergency and Critical Care, 2nd edn*, ed. L King and A Boag, pp. 85–113. BSAVA Publications, Gloucester

Waddell L and King L (2018) General approach to respiratory distress. In: *BSAVA Manual of Canine and Feline Emergency and Critical Care, 3rd edn*, ed. L King and A Boag, pp. 93–122. BSAVA Publications, Gloucester

OPERATIVE TECHNIQUE 2.1

Emergency tracheotomy

PATIENT PREPARATION AND POSITIONING

Dorsal recumbency, with support under the neck, and the forelegs secured on either side of the thorax. The ventral neck should be clipped and aseptically prepared if time allows.

ASSISTANT

Ideally.

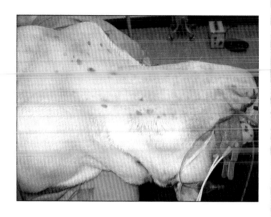

ADDITIONAL INSTRUMENTS

Tracheostomy tube (no larger than 75% of the diameter of the trachea). Two or three different sizes should be readily available.

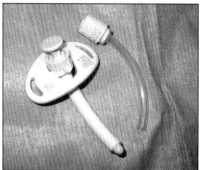

For routine airway maintenance, a non-cuffed tube with an inner cannula, with an outer diameter no greater than 75% of the luminal diameter of the trachea, should be used.

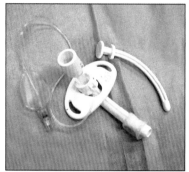

For maintenance of anaesthesia or prolonged mechanical ventilation, a tube with an inner cannula and a high-volume low-pressure cuff is more appropriate.

SURGICAL TECHNIQUE

Approach

The larynx and trachea should be palpated and then an approximately 7 cm (length depends on the size of the animal) skin incision made, running caudally from the larynx.

Surgical manipulations

1 Separate the sternohyoideus muscles at the midline and pull laterally. The trachea is visualized.

2 Place stay sutures around the tracheal rings just cranial and caudal to the proposed annular ligament incision. These stay sutures allow stabilization of the trachea when changing the tracheostomy tube.

3 Make an incision in one of the annular ligaments between the third and fifth tracheal rings. The incision of the annular ligament should not extend more than 50% of the diameter of the trachea.

4 Place the tube and secure it by tying cotton umbilical tape around each side of the tube flange and then tying the ends together behind the animal's neck.

Closure

The skin and subcutaneous tissue should be partially closed from each end of the incision.

→ **OPERATIVE TECHNIQUE 2.1 CONTINUED**

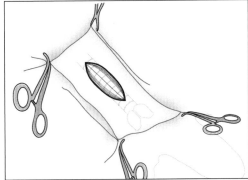

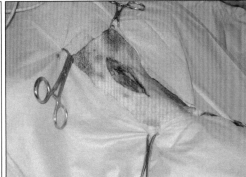

Skin incision and incision between thyohyoid muscle bellies.

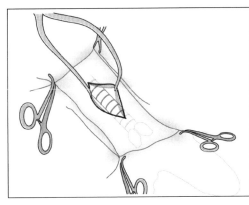

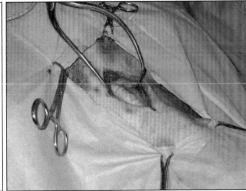

Incision between the sternohyoid muscle bellies. Gelpi retractors help to expose the trachea.

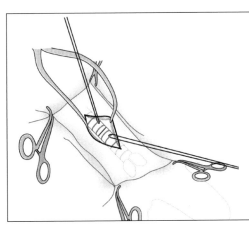

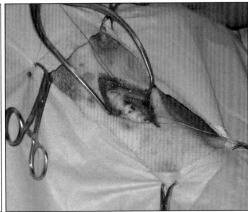

Stay sutures have been placed either side of the proposed annular ligament incision.

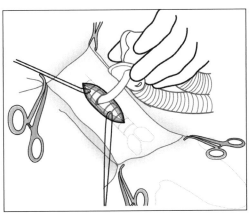

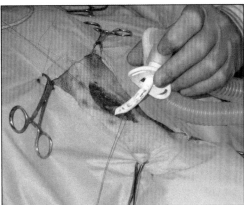

The annular ligament incision is made big enough (but not greater than half way around the circumference of the trachea) to permit gentle placement of the tracheostomy tube.

→ **OPERATIVE TECHNIQUE 2.1 CONTINUED**

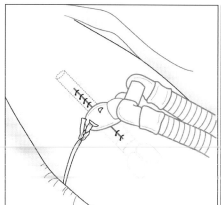
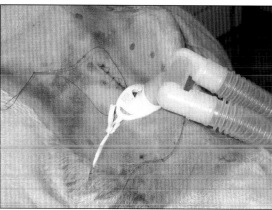

The tube is secured and skin sutures placed.

Tracheostomy tube care

The tracheostomy tube bypasses the normal warming and humidification mechanisms and creates airway inflammation that is superimposed on the inflammation associated with its placement. Dedicated care is essential to prevent potentially fatal occlusion of the tube by exudates and airway mucus.

Inner cannula cleaning

The inner cannula should be removed for cleaning whenever an increased noise or effort associated with breathing is noticed, or every 2 hours initially. The cannula should be cleaned thoroughly using warm water, dried and replaced.

Humidification

If the inner cannula is found repeatedly to be full of tenacious mucus and exudate, either periods of nebulized air should be provided for the animal to breathe or 0.1 ml/kg sterile saline should be instilled into the tube every 2 hours (the latter may induce transient coughing).

Suction

This is not a benign procedure and should be done sparingly. Repeated suctioning of the airway can cause 'desaturation' of the patient's haemoglobin with oxygen and exacerbate airway inflammation. It is more commonly needed in smaller dogs and cats. The patient should be preoxygenated for approximately 10 breaths prior to suctioning. The catheter should be introduced aseptically into the tube and suction applied for **no more than 15 seconds** whilst gently rotating the suction tube. Suction should be performed at least four times a day. Some coughing, retching or gagging may be seen during suctioning. Ideally a sterile catheter should be used each time, but if this is not possible the catheter should be flushed with sterile saline and changed daily.

Wound management

The tracheostomy wound should be inspected daily and cleaned with sterile saline and swabs as necessary.

Tube changes

If the above measures do not relieve breathing difficulty, the whole tube should be changed; this should **not** be done in the absence of a clinician or of facilities for endotracheal intubation and administration of oxygen. The patient is preoxygenated and the trachea stabilized using the stay sutures, applying gentle traction away from the wound. The old tube is removed and a new one inserted rapidly.

Chapter 3

Surgery of the oral cavity and oropharynx

Alexander M. Reiter and Mark M. Smith

Introduction

Surgery of the oral cavity and oropharynx is required to treat neoplasia, traumatic and congenital lesions, and diseases affecting the lips and salivary glands. These problems are addressed in this chapter. The reader is referred to the *BSAVA Manual of Canine and Feline Dentistry and Oral Surgery* for complementary information on the surgical treatment of small animal dental and oral surgical diseases.

Oral tumours

Oral tumours are common in dogs and cats. They may be of dental or non-dental origin. In dogs, periodontal ligament tumours, malignant melanoma and squamous cell carcinoma (SCC) are most commonly diagnosed. In cats, the predominant tumours are SCC and fibrosarcoma (Harvey and Emily, 1993).

Predisposing factors include patient age, sex, breed, size and pigmentation of oral mucosa. Geriatric patients are generally predisposed; however, fibrosarcoma has been reported to occur more frequently in young, large-breed dogs. Viral papillomatosis and undifferentiated malignancies may also be included in the differential diagnosis for young dogs with oral masses. Papillary SCC, previously thought to be a tumour in young dogs, is now considered to be a very well differentiated form of SCC whose occurrence is not dependent on age. Male dogs have been reported to be at higher risk for malignant melanoma and fibrosarcoma.

Breeds with an increased risk for oral neoplasia, irrespective of type, include German Shepherd Dogs, Short-haired Pointers, Weimaraners, Golden Retrievers, Boxers and Cocker Spaniels. Large-breed dogs have a higher incidence of fibrosarcoma and non-tonsillar SCC, whilst smaller breeds have a higher incidence of malignant melanoma and tonsillar SCC. Dogs with heavily pigmented oral mucosae are predisposed to malignant melanoma (Harvey and Emily, 1993).

Clinical signs

Clinical signs associated with oral neoplasms depend on size and location:

- Food prehension may be abnormal
- Secondary traumatic ulceration may occur in animals with larger neoplasms
- Inability to swallow or associated pain may result in drooling

- Saliva may be blood-tinged in animals with ulcerated lesions
- There may be increased plaque accumulation and this, in addition to necrosis of tumour tissue, may result in halitosis.

Diagnosis and staging

The diagnosis is based on histopathological examination. Advances in the development and application of immuno-histochemical techniques in veterinary medicine may provide methods for early detection of malignant neoplasms (Stromberg *et al.*, 1995; Gamblin *et al.*, 1997; Oliver *et al.*, 1997; Ramos-Vara *et al.*, 2000). Staging of the disease should be considered as an active investigative process to be performed in concert with the diagnostic evaluation.

A complete blood count, biochemistry profile and urinalysis should be reviewed to determine organ abnormalities related to metastatic or concurrent disease, which would alter the anaesthetic protocol or preclude the use of general anaesthesia. Thoracic radiography or computed tomography (CT) is used to evaluate metastasis to the lung.

The size of the neoplasm is more accurately assessed after administration of general anaesthesia. Radiography, CT or magnetic resonance imaging (MRI) of the head can be performed during anaesthesia to provide information on the extent of local tissue invasion. Regional lymph node enlargement indicates either metastasis or reactivity related to oral inflammation. Regardless of size, lymph nodes should be evaluated by fine-needle aspiration (NB: false-negative results are possible) or excisional biopsy. A surgical approach was developed to provide exposure for excisional biopsy of ipsilateral parotid, mandibular and medial retropharyngeal lymph nodes through a single incision (Smith, 1995). A negative lymph node biopsy does not preclude the possibility of regional metastasis, which may occur along the perineural or vascular routes, or metastasis to other less accessible lymph nodes.

Many oral neoplasms are detected late in the disease process owing to their location deep in the oral cavity. Consequently, oral malignancies have usually progressed to at least stage II disease at the time of diagnosis. Higher staged malignant tumours are associated with a poorer prognosis.

Biopsy

Biopsy is indicated for all oral masses, unexplained lesions and autoimmune diseases with oral manifestation. The biopsy sample should always be taken from a location that can be incorporated in a definitive resection. The accuracy of diagnosis increases with increasing volume of tissue submitted, but so does the risk of biopsy-induced tissue contamination. If the biopsy results do not correlate with the clinical findings, a deeper and larger biopsy specimen should be obtained.

The systematic examination of a primary tumour, regional lymph nodes and any distant metastasis – the so-called TNM (tumour, node, metastasis) system – provides a method of describing the clinical extent (staging) of a malignancy and is an essential prerequisite for rational treatment of oral tumours (Arzi and Verstraete, 2012).

Obtaining and examining a biopsy specimen allows the clinician to establish the diagnosis, formulate a treatment regimen and give the owner an accurate prognosis.

Sampling for cytology: Cytological samples can be obtained from awake or sedated patients. The two most obvious examples of oral lesions that can be diagnosed cytologically are SCC and eosinophilic granuloma.

- **Fine-needle sampling ('woodpecker method') and fine-needle aspiration:** Fine-needle techniques have some value for oral lesions. Cytological examination of lymph node aspirates may be adequate for diagnosing metastatic melanoma and SCC but is less satisfactory for other oral tumours (Herring *et al.*, 2002).
- **Impression smears:** Smears obtained from the surface of an ulcerated tumour often have low diagnostic value, as imprints may harvest only bacteria and superficial inflammatory cells and not the underlying tumour cells. Impression smears may be of greater value if taken from the cut surface of a tumour.
- **Scrapings:** Cytological examination of oral tissues can be useful if the sample is scraped from cut tissue surfaces. This technique may also be suitable for firm ulcerated lesions that are unlikely to exfoliate well using fine-needle techniques.

Sampling for histology: Surgical biopsy under general anaesthesia and microscopic examination of a formalin-fixed specimen provide a more accurate diagnosis than cytological sampling techniques. Electrosurgical/radio-surgical equipment, laser and other tissue-damaging techniques should be avoided so as not to obscure a diagnosis. Areas of superficial necrosis should be avoided so that the sample contains deeper, viable tissue. It is rarely satisfactory to snip a small piece from the most protuberant area, even though it is tempting to do so in the consulting room as a means of avoiding anaesthesia and expediting the diagnostic process. Multiple samples are preferred, as a single sample may not be representative. Haemostasis is achieved by digital pressure. Continuously bleeding biopsy sites and sampling locations in more deeply invading and pharyngeal tumours should be sutured with a pattern (cruciate or mattress) that promotes compression.

For adequate fixation, the biopsy sample is placed in 10% buffered formalin at 1 part tissue to 10 parts fixative (White, 2003a). For diagnosis of suspected autoimmune disorders by direct immunofluorescence, a specimen should be obtained from the most active area of disease, ideally with an intact epithelial vesicle, and should include adjacent grossly normal epithelium. The sample is placed in Michel's preservative instead of formalin (Harvey and Emily, 1993).

- **Grab sampling instruments:** Straight alligator or oval/round cup forceps are used for less accessible pharyngeal tumours. Rongeurs are very useful for obtaining samples from firm or bony tissue.

- **Core sampling instruments:** These are used for superficial masses or for those masses that can be palpated well enough to be stabilized during biopsy, and also for lymph nodes.
- **Disposable punch biopsy instruments:** Because lesions may be hidden beneath a layer of normal tissue, open-ended skin biopsy punches are useful for obtaining deep samples (Figure 3.1).
- **Incisional biopsy:** This is performed using a scalpel blade to obtain a wedge of tissue. Incisional biopsy should not be performed in areas of ulceration, necrosis or inflammation, as the tissue obtained may not be representative of the actual lesion.
- **Excisional biopsy:** The biopsy procedure may be curative as well as diagnostic. Keeping in mind that the first attempt at surgical resection of a malignancy has the best chance for cure, excisional biopsy may be indicated for smaller masses and lymph nodes that can easily be excised *en bloc*.

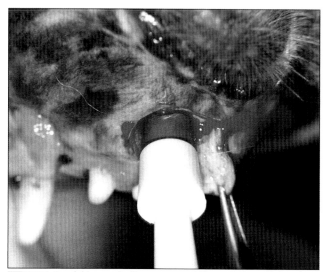

3.1 Punch biopsy of a fibrosarcoma at the rostral maxilla in a dog. Two previous biopsies had indicated a peripheral odontogenic fibroma. A small mucoperiosteal flap was created to obtain a deeper tissue sample.

Benign neoplasms
Canine viral papillomatosis

Papillomas appear on the oral mucosa as pale, smooth elevations that develop a rough surface early in the disease process. Older lesions of 3–4 weeks' duration usually have deep and closely packed fronds. Lesions observed during regression appear shrivelled and dark grey. Complete regression may take several weeks but typically leaves no scar. Papillomas that interfere with prehension, mastication and swallowing should be removed. Azithromycin seemed to have an accelerating effect on the regression of papillomas in dogs in one study (Yağci *et al.*, 2008).

Odontogenic tumours

These tumours are often located in the gingiva near the incisor, canine or premolar teeth, or the mandibular first molar.

- Peripheral odontogenic fibromas (previously called fibromatous and ossifying epulides) are pedunculated, non-ulcerating and non-invasive masses (Figure 3.2), containing varying amounts of bone, osteoid, dentinoid or cementum-like tissue.

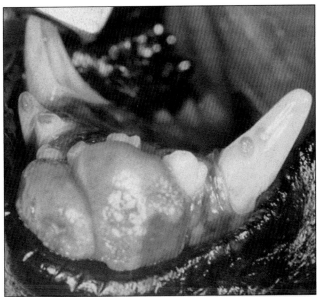

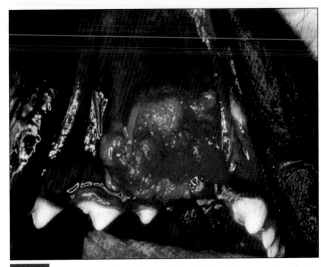

3.2 Peripheral odontogenic fibroma of the mandibular incisor area in a dog.

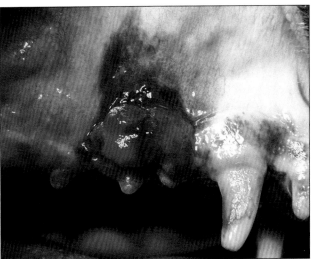

3.3 Right maxillary malignant melanoma in a dog. Note the extension of tumour tissue into alveolar and buccal mucosa.

- Acanthomatous ameloblastoma has characteristics of malignancy, including local invasiveness and bone destruction. However, it does not metastasize and is therefore considered to be benign (Gardner, 1995).
- Odontomas are not true tumours but rather a conglomerate of disorganized normal tissue cells. The mass may be composed of enamel, dentin, cementum and small tooth-like structures. Lesions with characteristics resembling normal teeth are considered to be compound, whereas complex odontomas have a more disorganized arrangement.
- Less common odontogenic tumours include amyloid-producing odontogenic tumours and feline inductive odontogenic tumours.

Other tumours

Other benign tumours include plasmacytomas, giant cell granulomas, osteomas and lipomas.

Malignant neoplasms

Malignant melanoma

These tumours grow rapidly and are characterized by early invasion of gingiva and bone. Metastasis to regional lymph nodes occurs early in the disease process. The lung is the most common site for visceral metastasis. Malignant melanomas (Figure 3.3) are dome-shaped or sessile, with varying amounts of pigmentation ranging from black and brown through mottled to non-pigmented. Although a minority of oral melanocytic lesions may be benign, all suspected melanomas should be considered malignant pending microscopic evaluation. Melanomas of the mucocutaneous junction are invariably malignant.

Squamous cell carcinoma

SCCs may project from oral soft tissues but more commonly present as ulcerated lesions, frequently involving the gingiva in dogs (Figure 3.4) and the sublingual tissue and root of the tongue in cats (Soltero-Rivera et al., 2014). Other sites include buccal and labial mucosa, tonsillar crypts and the body of the tongue. SCC destroys mucosa

3.4 Squamous cell carcinoma of the right maxillary area in a dog.

and submucosa and frequently invades muscle and bone. Metastasis to regional lymph nodes is common, whilst visceral metastasis to the lungs may occur late in the disease process.

Fibrosarcoma

These occur in similar locations to SCCs, with a greater frequency along the maxillary dental arch between the canine and fourth premolar teeth and on the hard palate. The neoplasm is firm and smooth, with nodules that may become ulcerated (Figure 3.5). Fibrosarcomas are invasive, and recurrence following local excision is common. Early regional lymphatic and visceral metastasis is unusual. Some fibrosarcomas appear benign on histological examination but show malignant behaviour clinically and on diagnostic imaging (i.e. histologically 'low-grade' but biologically 'high-grade') and thus require similar treatment to other fibrosarcomas (Ciekot et al., 1994).

Other tumours

Other malignant neoplasms include malignant peripheral nerve sheath tumours, osteosarcomas, multilobular tumours of bone, mast cell tumours, lymphosarcomas and undifferentiated tumours.

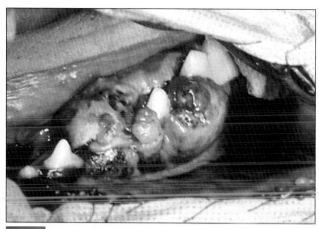

3.5 Fibrosarcoma of the left mandible in a dog.

Surgical management

Animals with no radiographic signs of distant metastasis are considered for aggressive therapy. The concept of complete local excision of the tumour, followed by (or concurrent with) chemotherapy and/or immunotherapy, has achieved marked acceptance in human oncological therapy and is being applied in veterinary medicine. This multimodal treatment is usually well tolerated by dogs and cats, leaving conservative management for only the more debilitated and/or geriatric patients. Such treatment plans are best designed and executed at specialist centres that have expertise in all the required disciplines (Marconato *et al.*, 2013).

The goal of surgery is curative resection, cytoreduction or palliation. The ideal surgical procedure is one that offers the greatest possibility of cure, restores or maintains function and has an acceptable cosmetic result. Benign neoplasms which do not involve bone are excised surgically. For malignant neoplasms, a 2 cm margin of tumour-free tissue is recommended, often necessitating ostectomy as part of the operative procedure.

Neoplasms with radiographic evidence of local bone metastasis require surgical procedures including extensive maxillectomy (see Operative Technique 3.1) and total mandibulectomy (see Operative Technique 3.2) (White, 2003b). These procedures maximize the removal of the entire bony component of the neoplastic process. Segmental procedures resulting in partial maxillectomy or mandibulectomy without intraoperative frozen section analysis of tissue margins risk incomplete resection due to intrabone perineural and microvascular metastatic routes. This is of particular importance for mandibular lesions, in which case total mandibulectomy may be preferred to partial or segmental mandibulectomy, as cosmesis and function are acceptable despite a greater degree of resection.

Prognosis

Oral malignancies often have a guarded to poor prognosis, which may be affected by size of the lesion, age of the patient and species.

Younger dogs with SCC rostral to the second premolars have a better prognosis than older dogs and those with neoplasms in other locations. Cats with SCC have a shorter tumour-free interval than dogs, regardless of the type of treatment. The most positive prognosis for oral SCC in dogs is attained when both surgery and radiation therapy are combined. Treatment of SCC of the root of the tongue in cats is strictly palliative.

Malignant melanoma may be resected locally with tumour-free margins. However, regional or distant metastasis is common. Tumour-free margins for fibrosarcoma are more difficult to achieve, making local recurrence likely. Low-grade mandibular osteosarcomas in dogs tend to be associated with a longer survival time than long-bone osteosarcomas.

Cheek and lip

Chewing lesions

Chewing lesions may result from chronic self-induced trauma to the sublingual mucosa or the labial and buccal mucosa along bite planes. Usually, no treatment is required. Surgical resection is indicated for excessive hyperplastic tissue that continues to be traumatized.

Lacerations

Initial wound management includes debridement and copious lavage. Lacerations are sutured with separate layers for apposition of the mucosa and skin. Delayed primary closure is indicated when the wound is grossly contaminated, purulent, extensively devitalized, oedematous or inflamed, and is performed 3–5 days after injury.

Lip avulsion

Avulsion injuries of the lips may occur after a traffic accident or a fall from a high-rise building (cat), when the lip is inadvertently stepped on by someone or when the animal is grasped and lifted at its snout by another animal (dog). These injuries are more common in cats than in dogs, and the lower lip is more often affected (Figure 3.6).

The wound should be gently debrided and rinsed. The lip is then replaced and kept in position with simple interrupted sutures in areas with enough soft tissue remaining, and with large horizontal mattress sutures that can be passed around tooth crowns. Reducing dead space is important. Subcutaneous tissue is attached ventrally to the intermandibular tissues and the mandibular symphysis with absorbable suture material. Plastic tubing can be used to form tension-relieving sutures. Surgical drains are rarely required (Reiter and Lewis, 2011; Reiter, 2012).

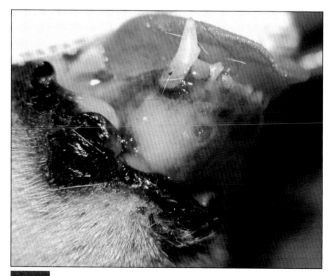

3.6 Lower lip avulsion in a kitten after motor vehicle trauma.

Necrosis

Extensive lacerations, avulsions, bite wounds, insect stings and thermal injuries can cause necrosis of lip and cheek tissue. If insufficient rostral skin is available to cover bare sites, advancement, rotation or transposition flaps can be harvested from the intermandibular or neck areas.

It may be necessary to incise the lip commissures to mobilize sufficiently large flaps. The donor area can be repaired easily by using the loose skin of the neck. If injury to the rostral upper lip has caused loss of one nostril, patency of both nasal passages can be achieved by creating a window into the rostral portion of the nasal septum. Alternatively, if sufficient tissue is present, a modified nasal rotation flap with incorporation of dorsal nasal planum tissue can be used for reconstruction of the nares (ter Haar et al., 2013).

Lip and cheek necrosis can result in stricture of the commissure and inability to open the mouth. This is corrected by incising the scar at the commissure, and closing the mucosa and skin in two layers to lengthen the commissure. Z-plasty techniques (Fowler, 1999) can also be attempted to resolve strictures due to excessive scar formation in the cheek tissue.

Cheilitis and dermatitis

An abnormal congenital lip-fold conformation is commonly seen in spaniels and setters and occasionally in other dog breeds. The indentation of the tissues laterally causes saliva and debris to collect on the skin of the lip. The result is a foul-smelling, chronic moist cheilitis and dermatitis. Conservative treatment (clipping the hair, frequently washing the lip-fold area with chlorhexidine solution or benzoyl peroxide shampoo, followed by application of a benzoyl peroxide gel, corticosteroid ointment or topical antibiotic) may be helpful. Severe cases are treated by resection of the folds.

Infection of the lip skin may also occur following partial or total mandibulectomy, as a result of constant lateral extrusion of the tongue. This can be corrected by rostral advancement of the lip commissure on the involved side (commissuroplasty). The mucocutaneous junction tissue of the upper and lower lips is resected to the level of the maxillary second premolars. The incised edges are sutured with separate layers for apposition of the mucosa and skin. A loose tape or fabric muzzle may be kept in place during the healing period to prevent dehiscence when the dog opens its mouth fully.

Inappropriate drooling

Heavy pendulous lower lips in large and giant-breed dogs may form a channel through which saliva flows directly on to the skin or hangs in ropes down to the floor. This can be treated by bilateral mandibulosublingual salivary duct ligation through a small incision in the sublingual mucosa, combined with resection of excessive lip tissue by making a V-shaped incision through the skin and mucosa. The two layers (mucosa and skin) are sutured separately.

Tight lip

Shar-Peis often have very tight lower lips due to insufficient depth to the lower rostral vestibule. This causes the lower lip to extend over the incisal edge of the incisor teeth, which can restrict the complete growth potential of the lower jaw and may result in malocclusion and difficulty

in mastication. Vestibuloplasty is designed to increase the depth of the vestibule, allowing the lower lip to swing free of the incisor teeth.

The incision is begun in the mucogingival junction caudal to the labial frenulum. A deep frenotomy is performed, avoiding the neurovascular structures that exit from the middle mental foramen. The incision is continued in the mucogingival junction around the mandibular incisors to the opposing labial frenulum, where the same procedure is performed. Once the lip has been fully dissected from the bone with a periosteal elevator, the periosteum is incised at the ventral border of the flap with a scalpel blade. The lip flap is sutured down and back on itself to the underlying tissues at several sites. The frenulum incisions are sutured in a similar manner. On completion, the lip will appear to dip ventrally at a steep angle, which is the desired result. A mucosal graft can be placed between the cut edges to prevent their healing together. Another option is to cut a piece of Penrose drain lengthwise to open it up, and then customize its shape to the defect created. The Penrose template is sutured to the edges of the defect circumferentially, and sutures are used at the depth of the defect to tack down the material to the underlying tissue. After the incised edges of the defect have sufficiently epithelialized, the Penrose template is removed.

Harelip

See Palate, below.

Tongue

Lacerations and avulsions

Injury to the tongue can be secondary to burns, external trauma, self-trauma during recovery from anaesthesia or seizures, foreign bodies, strangulation from elastic materials and frenulum laceration by 'string' foreign bodies. Clean lacerations are sutured with absorbable material. Jagged lacerations require careful conservative debridement before suturing. Treatment of irregular lacerations or avulsions includes irrigation of the affected areas with dilute chlorhexidine and nursing care to assist with feeding until the injured areas heal.

Trauma to salivary gland ducts in the sublingual tissues has been proposed as a cause of sublingual sialocele (ranula). If ducts are injured by acute trauma, ligation of transected ducts will result in transient glandular swelling, followed by atrophy.

Electric cord injury and other burns

This occurs most often in young animals. Neurogenic pulmonary oedema is an immediate life-threatening concern. It may take several days before the extent of local injury is clearly defined. Necrosis of the lips, cheeks, tongue and hard palate is common. More extensive burns cause necrosis of dental pulp tissue and incisive bones, maxillae, palatine bones or mandibles.

Initially, the patient is managed conservatively; injured tissues are left to necrose so that all the viable tissue is retained. Once the necrotic tissue is evident, surgical intervention may be initiated. If the injury resulted in osteonecrosis or oronasal fistula, further surgery is required.

When electric cord injuries include the tongue, tube feeding may be necessary for several days. Once the necrotic portion of the tongue has sloughed, the remaining stump is rapidly covered by epithelium. Loss of approximately one-third of the body of the tongue may be well tolerated in dogs. Animals compensate for greater amounts of tongue loss by sucking in liquid food or tossing boluses of food into the oropharynx. Sloughing of part of the tongue is more likely to be troublesome in cats; even though they can eat and drink, they may be unable to groom effectively (Lewis and Reiter, 2011).

Other thermal burns may be caused by eating overheated foods. Oral injury from direct ingestion of caustic agents is less likely to occur in cats than dogs because of their fastidious eating habits. Cats may get tongue burns when such agents are contacted during self-grooming. The lesions are typically acute-onset ulcers covered by necrotic debris. Initial therapy is copious lavage with saline, followed by conservative management.

Foreign bodies

Linear foreign bodies caught around the tongue can 'saw' their way into the lingual frenulum, causing a granulating mass similar in appearance to SCC or eosinophilic granuloma, both observed in this location in cats. Treatment is removal of the foreign body. Barbed objects or bone spicules may require incision along the object for removal and prevention of further damage. Glossitis may result from plant foreign material penetrating the dorsal lingual mucosa during self-grooming. Treatment requires scraping of the lingual mucosa to remove the particulate plant material.

Calcinosis circumscripta

Well defined mineralizations in the rostral portion of the tongue (Figure 3.7) are more common in young large-breed dogs. The cause of deposition of amorphous mineralized material in lingual tissue is unknown, although the rostral location and the young age of the patients suggest that mechanical trauma or chemical agents may be aetiological factors. Treatment involves resection of affected tissue and apposition of the incised edges with synthetic absorbable suture material.

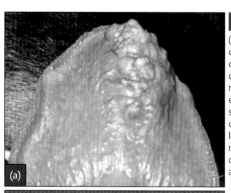
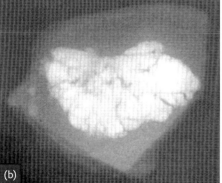

3.7 (a) Lingual calcinosis circumscripta in a dog. (b) A radiograph of the excised tissue showing a circumscribed lesion containing material with bone density that is arranged in lobules.

Neoplasia

Protuberant ulcerated lesions should always be investigated by biopsy before resection (or before euthanasia if the lesion appears to be too extensive for surgery or radiation therapy). Lingual eosinophilic granuloma, which is treated medically with good results, appears similar to an invading neoplasm in some cats and dogs. The most common malignant lingual tumour is SCC.

Tongue masses are resected with good results if the resection can be confined to the free rostral or the dorso-caudal portions. Partial surgical resection is likely to result in significant haemorrhage. Clamping the tongue caudal to the excision site with non-crushing tissue forceps greatly aids in controlling bleeding. Ideally, tongue tissue is removed as a wedge so that the mucosa can be apposed with synthetic absorbable sutures. Malignancies located deep in the root of the tongue or causing the tongue to be tied down to the adjacent soft tissues are not amenable to complete resection (Culp et al., 2013).

Other conditions

In dogs with ankyloglossia, a congenital anomaly characterized by fusion between the tongue and floor of the oral cavity ('tongue-tie'), frenuloplasty can be used to free the tongue (Temizsoylu and Avki, 2003).

Puppies born with macroglossia, individuals with an extremely long tongue (commonly seen in brachycephalic animals) and those that cannot retract it due to a neurological deficit may suffer from prehension difficulties, desiccation and ulceration of the tongue surface. Resection of the rostral portion of the tongue may be of benefit.

Palate

Congenital palate defects

In contrast to humans (where the upper lip is formed by maxillary and medial nasal processes), in dogs and cats the upper lip and primary palate are formed by midline fusion of the maxillary processes (Reiter and Holt, 2012). Lateral palatine processes move towards the midline and fuse with the nasal septum originating from the nasal process. This constitutes the secondary palate, which will ossify (hard palate), except in the caudal part where it will form the soft palate.

Defects of formation of the lip and palatal structures may be inherited or may result from an insult during fetal development (intrauterine trauma or stress). In most cases the cause is an intrauterine insult. Brachycephalic breeds are at higher risk.

Cleft lip

Congenital defects of the primary palate (cleft lip) appear as a lip defect only or as a defect of the lip and most rostral hard palate (Figure 3.8). They may be associated with abnormalities of the secondary palate. As in children, unilateral cleft lips in dogs are more commonly on the left side. Except for being externally visible, cleft lips rarely result in clinical signs beyond mild local rhinitis, and repair may be performed for aesthetic reasons. Surgical success depends on tension-free apposition of well vascularized tissue flaps positioned to separate the oral and nasal spaces. Attempts to close the defect by simple sliding procedures are rarely successful because there is no connective tissue bed to support the flaps (Harvey and Emily, 1993).

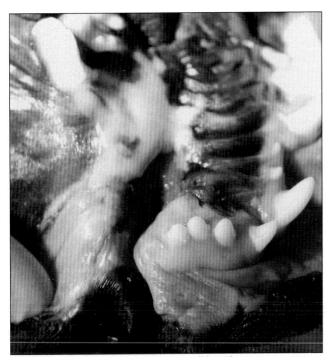

3.8 Cleft of the primary palate in a Bulldog. There are no rugae on the left side of the hard palate, indicating previous repair of a cleft of the secondary palate.

The most rostral palate and the floor of the nasal vestibule are reconstructed by creating flaps of both oral and nasal tissue or flaps that are harvested from oral tissue only. This is often complicated by the presence of teeth in the tissue, and removal of one or more incisors and also the canine tooth on the affected side will facilitate flap management. Successful repair is achieved by creating overlapping double flaps, followed by reconstructive cutaneous surgery to provide symmetry. These can be very challenging operations and require careful planning.

Cleft palate

Clefts of the secondary palate (cleft hard and/or soft palate) are more serious. They are almost always along the midline, and cleft hard palate is usually associated with a midline soft palate abnormality. Soft palate defects without hard palate defects may occur in the midline or can be unilateral. The prognosis for congenital hypoplasia or aplasia of the soft palate, as opposed to cleft soft palate, is poor, because restoration of a pharyngeal sphincteric ring and normal swallowing function may not be achieved despite careful surgical planning and meticulous technique.

Clinical signs and history associated with secondary palate defects include failure to create negative pressure for nursing, nasal discharge, coughing, gagging, sneezing, nasal reflux, tonsillitis, rhinitis, aspiration pneumonia, poor weight gain and general failure to thrive. The prognosis without surgical repair is guarded because of the risk of aspiration. Surgical correction is usually possible if the animal can survive and grow to a suitable size for anaesthesia and surgery. Management requires intensive nursing care by the owner, which includes transoral tube feeding to avoid aspiration pneumonia.

Most procedures for correction of congenital palate defects are performed on animals at 3–4 months of age (Harvey and Emily, 1993). A prolonged interval between diagnosis and an attempt at repair may result in a wider cleft as the animal grows, and also in compounded management problems, which are not desirable. Clefts of

the secondary palate are surgically repaired, using the overlapping flap or medially positioned flap (Langenbeck) technique (see Operative Technique 3.3). Owners should always be warned that multiple procedures may be required to close a cleft completely.

Acquired palate defects
Oronasal fistula

The most common cause of acquired palate defects is loss of upper jaw bone, associated with severe periodontal disease or tooth extraction. An acute oronasal fistula following tooth extraction (Figure 3.9) is diagnosed by direct visualization of the nasal cavity or observing nasal haemorrhage at the nares. Clinical signs of a chronic oronasal fistula include sneezing and ipsilateral nasal discharge. A defect at the rostral aspect of the maxillary dental arch that communicates with the nasal cavity noted during the oral examination confirms the diagnosis. Elevating and positioning a labial mucosa flap over the defect repairs the oronasal fistula (see Operative Technique 3.5).

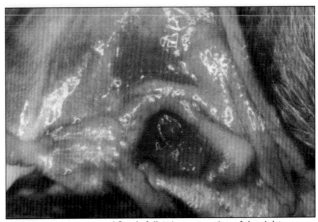

3.9 Acute oronasal fistula following extraction of the right maxillary canine tooth.

Other

Other causes of palate defects are: trauma (e.g. 'high-rise syndrome', electric cord and gunshot injuries, dog bites, foreign body penetration, pressure wounds); neoplasms; severe chronic infections; and surgical and radiation therapy (Bonner et al., 2012). Pressure necrosis is often secondary to malocclusion. In all cases, the cause of the defect must be removed prior to repair.

Techniques for palate surgery

The choice of technique will depend on the location and size of the defect and the amount of tissue available for flap procedures. Usually, there is considerable haemorrhage during palate surgery because of the rich blood supply to the tissues involved. Digital pressure is often sufficient to control bleeding.

Principles

- The best chance of success is with the first procedure.
- Avoid electrocoagulation for haemostasis.
- Make flaps larger than the defect they will cover.
- Retain blood supply to the flaps.
- Handle flaps as carefully as possible.

- Suture connective tissue surfaces or cut edges together.
- Provide a two-layer closure if practical.
- Do not locate suture lines over a void if possible.
- Avoid creating closure that is under tension.

Congenital defects

The overlapping flap technique is the preferred technique for congenital primary and secondary hard palate defects (Figure 3.10) and is described in Operative Technique 3.3. There is less tension on the suture line, the suture line is not located directly over the defect and the area of opposing connective tissue is larger, which results in a stronger scar. It provides more reliable results than the medially positioned flap technique, though for very narrow congenital or traumatic hard palate clefts, the medially positioned technique may be utilized.

The medially positioned flap technique is an alternative technique utilized for closure of midline hard palate defects. The technique is described in Operative Technique 3.3. If the relieving incisions are long and tend to gape, a lateral oronasal defect may result, particularly in narrow-nosed dogs. Another disadvantage of this technique is that rostral defects have a tendency to break down. For these reasons, the overlapping flap technique is preferred for repair of midline hard palate defects.

Congenital midline soft palate defects are corrected by making incisions along the medial margins of the defect to the level of the middle aspect or caudal end of the tonsils. The palatal tissue is separated with blunt-ended scissors to form a dorsal and a ventral flap on each side. The two dorsal and the two ventral flaps are sutured separately in a simple interrupted pattern to the midpoint or caudal end of the tonsils (Harvey and Emily, 1993).

Acquired defects

Trauma: Traumatic cleft of the hard palate associated with 'high-rise syndrome' in cats can be managed easily and effectively by approximating the displaced bony structures with digital pressure, followed by suturing of the torn palatal soft tissues in a simple interrupted or mattress pattern.

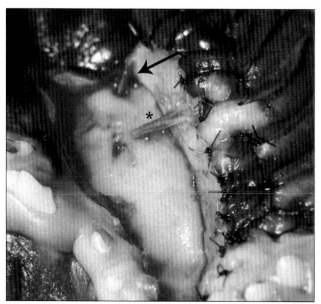

3.10 Cleft of the secondary hard palate in a Bulldog repaired using the overlapping double flap technique. The larger major palatine artery (∗) and smaller accessory palatine artery (arrowed) are attached to the overlapped flap.

The benefit of this initial management outweighs the risk inherent in leaving this injury to heal by second intention, although this may be sufficient in many cases. If the separation is extensive, with involvement of the maxillae and palatine bones, inter-quadrant fixation may be required to re-establish proper occlusion (Figure 3.11) (Reiter and Lewis, 2011).

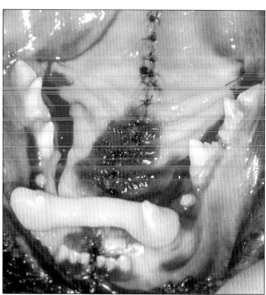

3.11 Traumatic cleft palate in a cat repaired with medially positioned double flaps. An inter-arcade fixation was necessary to reduce bone separation, and bilateral relieving incisions were made to accommodate the flaps.

Split palatal U-flap: This technique is useful for large caudal defects. The original technique described the creation of a large U-shaped mucoperiosteal flap rostral to the defect; an incision was then made along the midline of the flap to create two flaps of equal size. An alternative (see Operative Technique 3.4) is to create one flap slightly longer and another slightly shorter in length (Reiter and Smith, 2005).

Oronasal fistula repair: For large rostral defects following the extraction of teeth, a labial-based flap can be formed and sutured across the defect (see Operative Technique 3.5). Alternatively, a two-layer flap technique may be used. The first flap must provide an epithelial surface for the nasal cavity. The connective tissue surface of the first flap lies in the oral cavity. The second flap is designed to cover the connective tissue surface of the first flap and also provides an epithelial surface for the oral cavity. Synthetic absorbable sutures are placed in a simple interrupted pattern.

Other techniques: An alternative for repair of defects in the mid-portion of the hard palate is the use of a tongue flap that is later amputated and left attached to the palate. Another alternative is to create a permanent or removable silicone or acrylic obturator (Harvey and Emily, 1993).

Oropharynx

Trauma

Animal bites or foreign bodies may result in penetrating wounds of the oral cavity and oropharynx. Foreign body penetration can cause deep, contaminated wounds to the sides and root of the tongue, suborbital area, tonsillar crypts or pharyngeal walls.

Initial wound management includes control of haemorrhage without compromising the blood supply to the damaged area. Most traumatic wounds are contaminated, and early efforts should be made to reduce further contamination. Particulate debris is removed by gentle lavage with saline or dilute chlorhexidine solution. Larger fragments embedded in a wound are removed manually during surgical wound exploration.

Dog owners are often unaware of a problem until the animal shows clinical signs and is taken to the veterinary surgeon (veterinarian). A history of chewing wooden objects may be reported. Older penetrating injuries are serious and require surgical exploration, cleansing and, if appropriate, suturing. Finding a foreign body that has penetrated deep into the tissues can be challenging despite the support of advanced imaging techniques.

Foreign body impaction, including stick injuries, may lead to abscess formation in suborbital, submandibular and retropharyngeal tissues. Abscesses must be lanced and explored, and the foreign body removed. Excision of necrotic tissue is essential to promote early granulation. Surgical drains are useful for severely contaminated wounds (Lewis and Reiter, 2011).

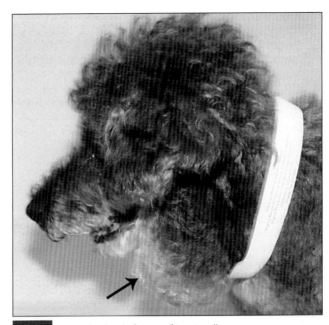

3.12 Cervical sialocele (arrowed) in a Poodle.

Salivary glands

Neoplasia

Neoplasia of the salivary glands is uncommon. Spaniel breeds, Poodles and Siamese cats may be predisposed. The prevalence of salivary gland neoplasia in cats is almost twice that in dogs, with the mandibular salivary gland most commonly affected. In dogs, the parotid and mandibular salivary glands are most often affected (Hammer et al., 2001).

Tumour type

Multiple tumour types affecting the salivary glands have been described, including mucoepidermoid tumours, SCC, malignant mixed tumours, adenoid cystic carcinoma, acinic cell carcinoma, adenocarcinoma, undifferentiated carcinoma and sarcoma. Adenocarcinoma is the most common neoplasm affecting the salivary glands in dogs and cats and is locally infiltrative, with frequent metastasis to regional lymph nodes and lungs. Cats have a more advanced stage of disease at the time of diagnosis when compared with dogs (Hammer et al., 2001).

Management

Salivary gland neoplasia should be staged according to the TNM system to generate an appropriate prognosis and treatment plan. Thoracic radiography and biopsy of the neoplasm and nearest regional lymph nodes provide necessary information.

Total surgical excision of malignant neoplasms is difficult because of their invasive characteristics and the intricate neurological and vascular anatomy of the salivary gland region. Therefore, local treatment should include radiotherapy, with or without surgical intervention to debulk the neoplasm.

Sialocele

Sialocele (Figure 3.12) is the most commonly recognized clinical disease of the salivary glands in dogs. A sialocele is an accumulation of saliva in the subcutaneous or submucosal tissue and the consequent tissue reaction to saliva. They have a non-epithelial, non-secretory lining, consisting primarily of fibroblasts and capillaries (Smith and Reiter, 2015).

Sialoceles occur most often in dogs aged 2–4 years and more frequently in German Shepherd Dogs and Miniature Poodles. Trauma has been proposed as the cause of sialoceles because of the activity of young dogs and the documented damage to the salivary gland–duct complex associated with sialoceles. The inability to induce sialoceles by trauma in healthy dogs suggests the possibility of a developmental predisposition in affected animals.

The sublingual gland is the most common salivary gland associated with sialocele. Sialography indicates that the sialocele origin most often occurs in the rostral portion (that portion of the sublingual gland superimposed on the mandible) of the sublingual gland–duct complex. Regardless of the location of the origin, a sialocele often forms near the intermandibular area (cervical sialocele). Other locations include the pharynx (pharyngeal sialocele) and associated with a sublingual or mandibular gland–duct defect in the sublingual area (sublingual sialocele or ranula).

Clinical signs

The clinical signs depend on the location of the sialocele.

- A cervical sialocele is initially acutely painful, due to the inflammatory response. Cessation of the inflammatory response results in a marked decrease in size of the mass. A decreased inflammatory response allows for the more common presenting history of a slowly enlarging or intermittently large, fluid-filled, non-painful mass.
- Blood-tinged saliva secondary to trauma caused by eating, abnormal prehension of food or reluctance to eat may be clinical signs associated with sublingual sialocele.
- The most common clinical signs associated with sialocele of the pharyngeal wall are respiratory distress and difficulty in swallowing secondary to partial obstruction of the pharynx.

- Zygomatic sialoceles are infrequently reported in dogs. The clinical signs of zygomatic sialocele and neoplasia are similar. A visible periorbital mass is usually the presenting clinical sign. Secondary ophthalmic signs depend on the location and size of the sialocele (e.g. exophthalmos). Additional signs, such as osteolytic changes of the zygomatic arch and enlargement of the mandibular lymph node, may accompany neoplasia originating in the zygomatic gland.

Diagnosis

The diagnosis is based on clinical signs, history and the results of paracentesis. Sialocele paracentesis reveals a stringy, sometimes blood-tinged, fluid with low cell numbers. Mucin and amylase analyses of the fluid are not reliable diagnostic procedures.

A chronic cervical sialocele may contain palpable firm nodules that are remnants of sloughed inflammatory tissue previously lining the sialocele. Sialoliths are concretions of calcium phosphate or calcium carbonate and may occur with a chronic sialocele. Physical examination and history usually denote the origin of the sialocele. Cervical sialoceles that appear on the midline usually shift to the originating side when the patient is placed in exact dorsal recumbency.

Sialography can be used to determine the affected side if observation and palpation are unsuccessful. Sialography is also a diagnostic aid when considering traumatic injury to one of the salivary glands, salivary neoplasia, fistulous tract of unknown origin or a foreign body in the head or neck. The disadvantages of sialography include the need for general anaesthesia and the difficulty associated with locating the duct opening(s).

Treatment

Surgical removal of the zygomatic gland is indicated for sialoceles of zygomatic gland origin. Various approaches have been used to treat cervical sialoceles. Sialocele drainage, removal of the sialocele only, and chemical cauterization have been reported. The basis for these therapies was the belief that a sialocele was a true cyst with a secretory lining. Recognition of the fact that a sialocele is a non-cystic reactive encapsulating structure has prompted surgical removal of the affected gland–duct complex.

The intimate anatomical association of the sublingual and mandibular salivary glands and their ducts requires resection of both structures by a lateral approach (see Operative Technique 3.6) if either of them is believed to be the origin of the sialocele. Although a ventral approach has been described (Marsh and Adin, 2013), the authors consider the lateral approach to provide better overall exposure for the procedure. Another technique for treating sialoceles involves marsupialization. However, resective surgery is preferred for pharyngeal sialoceles because life-threatening upper airway compromise and morbidity from swallowing dysfunction (e.g. aspiration pneumonia) are potential complications of conservative management or recurrence (Lewis and Reiter, 2011).

Postoperative care

Pain control

Regional nerve blocks (infraorbital, inferior alveolar and middle mental) and local infiltration are performed intra-operatively with longer-lasting local anaesthetics, such as 0.5% bupivacaine.

Postoperative pain control is achieved with methadone, oxymorphone, hydromorphone, butorphanol, buprenorphine, tramadol and transdermal fentanyl patches. Non-steroidal anti-inflammatory drugs can be used for pain management following less involved surgical procedures.

Antimicrobial therapy

Antibiotic treatment is usually not required after oral and oropharyngeal surgeries in the otherwise healthy patient. Broad-spectrum antibiotics (e.g. amoxicillin, clavulanate-potentiated amoxicillin, clindamycin, cefazolin, spiramycin/metronidazole) are given perioperatively to debilitated and immunosuppressed patients and those suffering from organ disease, endocrine disorders, cardiovascular disease, severely contaminated wounds and systemic infections.

Nutritional support

Oral intake may not be permitted during the first few hours following surgery (except in paediatric patients who are at risk of hypoglycaemia). Hydration may be maintained with intravenous fluids. Water is offered once the animal has recovered from anaesthesia. Soft food is offered 12–24 hours after surgery and maintained for about 2 weeks. Most dogs and cats will eat and drink even after major oral surgery. However, some animals may refuse any oral intake. The owner is then instructed in syringe feeding of a liquid, high-caloric diet. Rarely, naso-oesophageal, oesophageal or gastrostomy tubes are needed to bypass the oral cavity.

Wound management

Dilute chlorhexidine solution or gel is administered into the mouth for 1–2 weeks. A major complication after oral surgery is wound dehiscence, usually as a result of tension on suture lines or compromised vascularity of flaps. Elizabethan collars, tape muzzles, soft muzzles or other restraining devices may be used for some animals to prevent disruption of the surgical site. A re-examination is performed in 10–14 days for removal of skin sutures.

References and further reading

Arzi B and Verstraete FJM (2012) Clinical staging and biopsy of maxillofacial tumors. In: *Oral and Maxillofacial Surgery in Dogs and Cats*, ed. FJM Verstraete and MJ Lommer, pp. 373–486. Saunders Elsevier, Edinburgh

Bonner SE, Reiter AM and Lewis JR (2012) Orofacial manifestations of high-rise syndrome: a retrospective study of 84 cats (2000–2010). *Journal of Veterinary Dentistry* **29**, 10–18

Ciekot PA, Powers BE, Withrow SJ *et al.* (1994) Histologically low-grade, yet biologically high-grade, fibrosarcomas of the mandible and maxilla in dogs: 25 cases (1982–1991). *Journal of the American Veterinary Medical Association* **204**, 610–615

Culp WT, Ehrhart N, Withrow SJ *et al.* (2013) Results of surgical excision and evaluation of factors associated with survival time in dogs with lingual neoplasia: 97 cases (1995–2008). *Journal of the American Veterinary Medical Association* **242**, 1392–1397

Fowler D (2009) Tension relieving techniques and local skin flaps. In: *BSAVA Manual of Canine and Feline Wound Management*, ed. D Fowler and JM Williams, pp. 57–68. BSAVA Publications, Gloucester

Gamblin RM, Sagartz JE and Couto CG (1997) Overexpression of P53 tumor suppressor protein in spontaneously arising neoplasms of dogs. *American Journal of Veterinary Research* **58**, 857–863

Gardner DG (1995) Canine acanthomatous epulis. The only common spontaneous ameloblastoma in animals. *Oral Surgery, Oral Medicine, Oral Pathology, Oral Radiology and Endodontics* **79**, 612–615

Hammer A, Getzy D, Ogilvie G *et al.* (2001) Salivary gland neoplasia in the dog and cat: survival times and prognostic factors. *Journal of the American Animal Hospital Association* **37**, 478–482

Harvey CH and Emily PP (1993) *Small Animal Dentistry*. Mosby Year Book, St Louis

Herring ES, Smith MM and Robertson JL (2002) Lymph node staging of oral and maxillofacial neoplasms in 31 dogs and cats. *Journal of Veterinary Dentistry* **19**, 122–126

Lewis JR and Reiter AM (2011) Trauma-associated soft tissue injury to the head and neck. In: *Manual of Trauma Management in the Dog and Cat, 1st edn*, ed. K Drobatz, MW Beal and RS Syring, pp. 279–292. Wiley-Blackwell, Ames

Marconato L, Buchholz J, Keller M *et al.* (2013) Multimodal therapeutic approach and interdisciplinary challenge for the treatment of unresectable head and neck squamous cell carcinoma in six cats: a pilot study. *Veterinary and Comparative Oncology* **11**, 101–112

Marsh A and Adin C (2013) Tunneling under the digastricus muscle increases salivary duct exposure and completeness of excision in mandibular and sublingual sialoadenectomy in dogs. *Veterinary Surgery* **42**, 238–242

Oliver JL, Wolfe LG, Lopez MK *et al.* (1997) Isolation and characterization of the canine melanoma antigen recognized by the murine monoclonal antibody IBF9 and its distribution in cultured canine melanoma cell lines. *American Journal of Veterinary Research* **58**, 46–52

Ramos-Vara JA, Beissenherz ME, Miller MA *et al.* (2000) Retrospective study of 338 canine oral melanomas with clinical, histologic, and immunohistochemical review of 129 cases. *Veterinary Pathology* **37**, 597–608

Reiter AM and Gracis M (2018) *BSAVA Manual of Canine and Feline Dentistry and Oral Surgery, 4th edn*. BSAVA Publications, Gloucester

Reiter AM (2012) Dental and oral diseases. In: *The Cat: Clinical Medicine and Management, 1st edn*, ed. SE Little, pp. 329–370. Saunders, St Louis

Reiter AM and Holt D (2012) Palate surgery. In: *Veterinary Surgery: Small Animal, 1st edn*, ed. KM Tobias and SA Johnston, pp. 1707–1717. Elsevier, St Louis

Reiter AM and Lewis JR (2011) Trauma-associated musculoskeletal injuries of the head. In: *Manual of Trauma Management in the Dog and Cat, 1st edn*, ed. K Drobatz, MW Beal and RS Syring, pp. 255–278. Wiley-Blackwell, Ames

Reiter AM and Smith MM (2005) The oral cavity and oropharynx. In: *BSAVA Manual of Canine and Feline Head, Neck and Thoracic Surgery, 1st edn*, ed. DJ Brockman and DE Holt, pp. 25–43. BSAVA Publications, Gloucester

Smith MM (1995) Surgical approach for lymph node staging of oral and maxillofacial neoplasms in dogs. *Journal of the American Animal Hospital Association* **31**, 514–518

Smith MM and Reiter AM (2015) Salivary gland disorders. In: *Clinical Veterinary Advisor, 3rd edn*, ed. E Cote, pp. 916–919. Mosby, St Louis

Soltero-Rivera MM, Krick EL, Reiter AM *et al.* (2014) Prevalence of regional and distant metastasis in cats with advanced oral squamous cell carcinoma: 49 cases (2005–2011). *Journal of Feline Medicine and Surgery* **16**, 164–169

Stromberg PC, Schumm DE, Webb TE, Ward H and Couto CG (1995) Evaluation of oncofetal protein-related mRNA transport activity as a potential early cancer marker in dogs with malignant neoplasms. *American Journal of Veterinary Research* **56**, 1559–1563

Temizsoylu MD and Avki S (2003) Complete ventral ankyloglossia in three related dogs. *Journal of the American Veterinary Medical Association* **223**, 1443–1445

ter Haar G, Buiks SC and Kirpensteijn J (2013) Cosmetic reconstruction for a nasal plane and rostral nasal skin defect using a modified nasal rotation flap in a dog. *Veterinary Surgery* **42**, 176–179

White RAS (2003a) Core, incisional and excisional biopsy. In: *BSAVA Manual of Canine and Feline Oncology, 2nd edn*, ed. JM Dobson and BDX Lascelles, pp. 38–40. BSAVA Publications, Gloucester

White RAS (2003b) Tumours of the oropharynx. In: *BSAVA Manual of Canine and Feline Oncology, 2nd edn*, ed. JM Dobson and BDX Lascelles, pp. 206–213. BSAVA Publications, Gloucester

Yağci BB, Ural K, Ocal N *et al.* (2008) Azithromycin therapy of papillomatosis in dogs: a prospective, randomized, double-blinded, placebo-controlled clinical trial. *Veterinary Dermatology* **19**, 194–198

OPERATIVE TECHNIQUE 3.1

Partial rostral maxillectomy

PATIENT POSITIONING

Lateral recumbency.

ASSISTANT

Optional.

ADDITIONAL INSTRUMENTS

Periosteal elevator; osteotome and mallet (or other bone-cutting equipment).

SURGICAL TECHNIQUE

Approach

The labial mucosa is incised at least 1 cm from the lesion.

Surgical manipulations

1 Use a periosteal elevator to elevate the mucosa from its attachment on the incisive bone and maxilla. The infraorbital artery, vein and nerve exit the infraorbital canal and should be avoided unless wide resection requires their division and ligation.

2 Incise the palatal mucosa and elevate the mucoperiosteum. Ligate the major palatine artery if the resection approaches the major palatine foramen.

3 Perform maxillectomy using power saws, dental burrs or an osteotome and mallet; resection of the incisive bone and/or maxilla exposes the nasal cavity.

4 Perform local turbinectomy if the neoplasm is in contact with or invading adjacent turbinates.

5 Interference of the ipsilateral canine tooth with lip function may necessitate crown reduction and vital pulp therapy, or extraction.

→ **OPERATIVE TECHNIQUE 3.1 CONTINUED**

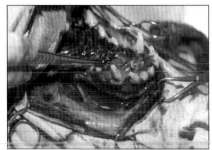

Maxillectomy with an osteotome and mallet.

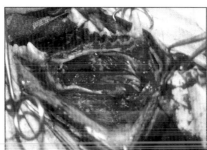

Resection of the premaxilla and/or maxilla exposes the nasal cavity.

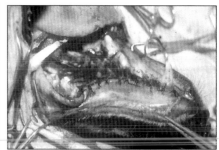

A single-layer, buccal mucosal closure is performed.

Closure

The labial mucosa is undermined to allow tension-free apposition of the flap to the palatal mucosa. A single-layer, mucosal closure is performed using synthetic absorbable suture material in a simple interrupted or vertical mattress pattern.

> **PRACTICAL TIP**
>
> Tension-free closure is imperative to avoid wound dehiscence and subsequent oronasal fistula. Failure of second-intention healing for partial wound dehiscence requires utilization of oronasal fistula repair techniques

POSTOPERATIVE CARE

Feed soft food for 2 weeks.

OPERATIVE TECHNIQUE 3.2

Total mandibulectomy

PATIENT POSITIONING

Lateral recumbency.

ASSISTANT

Optional.

ADDITIONAL INSTRUMENTS

Periosteal elevator; osteotome and mallet.

SURGICAL TECHNIQUE

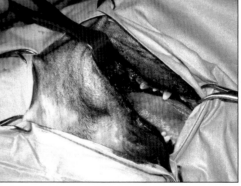

The dog is positioned in lateral recumbency. Exposure of the caudal mandible can be enhanced by retraction of the labial commissures.

Approach

The oral mucosa is incised labially/buccally (or with skin) and lingually from the mandibular symphysis to the ramus of the mandible, at least 2 cm peripheral to the neoplasm.

Surgical manipulations

1 Elevate the buccinator muscle from the body of the mandible using a periosteal elevator.

2 Elevate the masseter muscle from the masseteric fossa of the mandibular ramus in a similar fashion.

3 Perform mandibular symphyseal osteotomy using a scalpel blade (possible in the cat) or an osteotome and mallet.

4 Displace the mandible laterally to allow elevation of the mylohyoid muscle medially and digastricus muscle caudoventrally. Full-thickness incision of the lip commissure may be performed to gain additional exposure of the caudal operative field. →

→ OPERATIVE TECHNIQUE 3.2 CONTINUED

5 Ligate the inferior alveolar artery and vein and transect them near the mandibular foramen.

6 Transect the inferior alveolar nerve.

7 Elevate the masseter, temporal and medial pterygoid muscles from the caudal body and ramus of the mandible, to expose the temporomandibular joint (TMJ).

8 Disarticulate the TMJ to complete the total mandibulectomy.

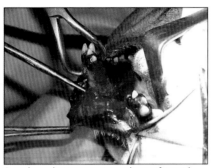

Symphyseal osteotomy must be performed early in the procedure to enhance surgical exposure of the medial mandible and associated structures. A large Backhaus towel clamp or bone-holding forceps will facilitate manipulation of the mandible.

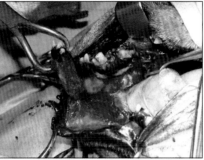

The mandible is displaced laterally and the labial incision is continued, the mylohyoid and digastricus muscles divided and the mandibular alveolar artery, vein and nerve identified and divided.

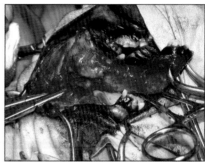

The masseter temporalis and medial pterygoid muscles are removed from the lateral mandible and coronoid process to expose the temporomandibular joint.

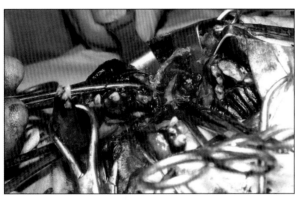

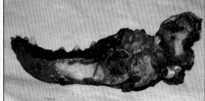

Disarticulate the temporomandibular joint and remove the final attachments of the temporalis muscle to the dorsal mandibular coronoid process to complete the mandibulectomy.

PRACTICAL TIP

A commissuroplasty will prevent lateral tongue displacement as a postoperative complication. The treatment for mucosal ulceration related to the remaining contralateral mandibular canine tooth contacting the hard palate is crown reduction and vital pulp therapy

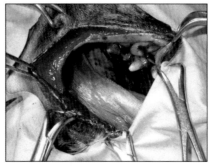

Commissuroplasty can minimize lateral tongue displacement as a complication of this procedure and is essential for brachycephalic dogs.

Closure

The oral mucosa is apposed using synthetic absorbable suture material in a simple interrupted pattern. Incised skin is closed with non-absorbable suture material in a simple interrupted pattern.

POSTOPERATIVE CARE

Feed soft food for 2 weeks.

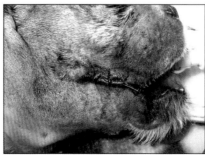

Oral mucosa is closed with synthetic absorbable suture material and the skin with non-absorbable suture material.

OPERATIVE TECHNIQUE 3.3

Cleft palate repair

Dorsal recumbency. The head is positioned so that the palate is parallel to the table. The mouth is taped open to permit optimal visualization during surgery.

ASSISTANT

Optional.

ADDITIONAL INSTRUMENTS

Periosteal elevator.

SURGICAL TECHNIQUE: OVERLAPPING FLAP TECHNIQUE

Approach

Incisions are made in the mucoperiosteum to the bone at the medial margin of the hard palate defect on one side, forming flap B, and along the dental margin about 2 mm away from the gingiva and to the rostral and caudal margins of the defect on the other side, forming flap A.

Surgical manipulations: hard palate repair

1   Elevate the flaps with a periosteal elevator, flap A laterally and flap B medially. Take care not to transect the major palatine artery, which exits the palatine shelf of the maxillary bone 0.5–1 cm medial to the maxillary fourth premolar. When the artery is identified, further careful dissection close to it will release it from surrounding tissue, and it will readily stretch to accommodate the rotation of the flap.

2   Fold flap A on itself, turn it and suture it under flap B, so that connective tissue surfaces are in contact.

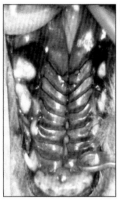
Hard palate defect.

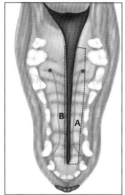
Incisions are made in the mucoperiosteum of the hard palate.

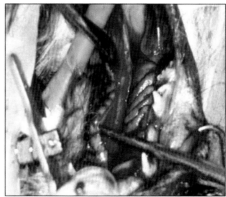
Elevating flap B.

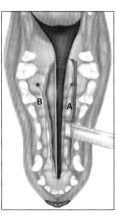
Elevating flap A.

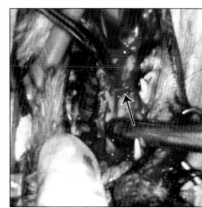
Elevating flap A. Note the major palatine artery (arrowed) attached to the flap.

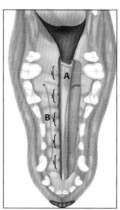
Flap A is turned on itself and sutured under flap B so that connective tissue surfaces are in contact.

→ **OPERATIVE TECHNIQUE 3.3 CONTINUED**

Closure

Synthetic absorbable sutures are placed in a horizontal mattress pattern. Granulation and epithelialization of exposed tissues are generally completed in 3–4 weeks.

Surgical manipulations: soft palate repair

1 Make incisions along the medial margins of the defect to the level of the caudal end of the tonsils.

2 Separate the palatal tissue with blunt-ended scissors to form a dorsal and a ventral flap on each side.

3 Suture the two dorsal and two ventral flaps separately in a simple interrupted pattern to the midpoint or caudal end of the tonsils.

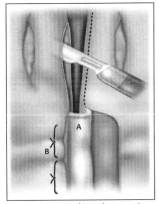
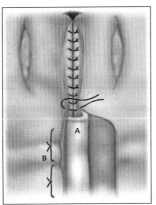
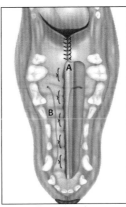
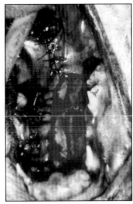

Incisions are made at the margins of the soft palate defect.

Dorsal and ventral flaps are sutured separately.

Both defects closed.

Appearance at end of operation.

SURGICAL TECHNIQUE: MEDIALLY POSITIONED FLAP TECHNIQUE

Approach

Incisions are made at the medial edges of the hard palate defect.

Surgical manipulations

1 Undermine the mucoperiosteum with a periosteal elevator laterally.

2 Slide the flaps together and suture them over the defect with synthetic absorbable material. To avoid tension on the suture line, relieving incisions about 2 mm away from the gingiva on one or both sides may be necessary so that the flaps can be moved medially into apposition.

Closure

The exposed bone next to the teeth is left to granulate and epithelialize.

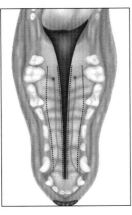
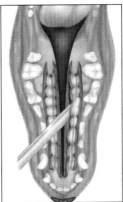
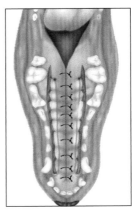

Incisions are made at the medial edges of the hard palate defect. Relieving incisions 2 mm away from the gingiva are often necessary for accommodation of the flaps.

Undermining the mucoperiosteum.

The flaps are slid together and sutured over the defect.

POSTOPERATIVE CARE

Soft food for 2 weeks.

OPERATIVE TECHNIQUE 3.4

Split palatal U-flap technique

PATIENT POSITIONING

Dorsal recumbency. The head is positioned so that the palate is parallel to the table. The mouth is taped open to permit optimal visualization during surgery.

ASSISTANT

Optional.

ADDITIONAL INSTRUMENTS

Periosteal elevator.

SURGICAL TECHNIQUE

Approach

The epithelial margins of the defect are debrided with a No. 15 scalpel blade. Then the mucoperiosteum of the hard palate is incised, creating two flaps of unequal length rostral to the defect, separated from each other in the midline.

Surgical manipulations

1   Raise the mucoperiosteal flaps A and B with a periosteal elevator. The transected major palatine arteries at the rostral extent of the flaps may require ligation. Caudal elevation of the flaps must be performed with caution as the palatine arteries are the only major blood supply to the flaps.

2   Rotate the shorter flap (B) through 90 degrees and transpose it to cover the defect.

3   Suture the medial aspect of flap B to the caudal aspect of the palatal defect, and the tip of the flap to the lateral aspect of the palatal defect, using synthetic absorbable material.

4   Rotate the longer flap (A) through 90 degrees and transpose it rostral to flap B.

5   Suture the medial aspect of flap A to the edge of flap B.

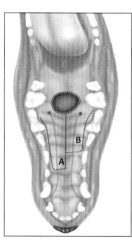

The margins of the defect are debrided, and two flaps of unequal length are created rostral to the defect.

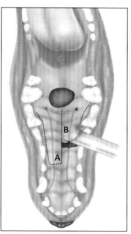

The mucoperiosteal flaps are raised with a periosteal elevator.

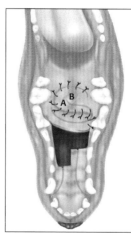

The shorter flap (B) is rotated through 90 degrees and sutured over the defect. The longer flap (A) is rotated through 90 degrees and sutured to the edge of flap B.

Closure

The denuded rostral aspect of the palate from which the flaps were harvested is left to heal by secondary intention.

POSTOPERATIVE CARE

Soft food for 2 weeks.

PRACTICAL TIP

Leaving a short strip of connective tissue in the midline allows the underside of the longer flap (A) to be sutured to the bone, thus reducing excessive gaping of the flap and potential food entrapment in this area

OPERATIVE TECHNIQUE 3.5

Oronasal fistula repair

Lateral recumbency.

Not required.

Iris forceps; curved iris scissors; periosteal elevator.

Approach

The alveolar and buccal mucosa is incised using a No. 15 scalpel blade.

Surgical manipulations

1 Elevate a full-thickness buccal flap using a periosteal elevator.

2 Incise the periosteal attachment at the base of the flap with a scalpel blade.

3 Use blunt submucosal dissection with small scissors to mobilize the flap.

4 Advance the flap to cover the defect.

PRACTICAL TIP

The flap should cover the defect without tension before suturing. The primary reason for dehiscence is excess tension due to insufficient flap mobilization prior to closure

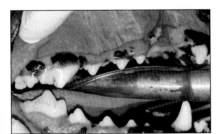 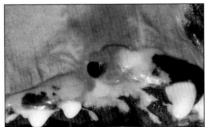 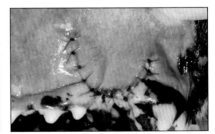

Chronic oronasal fistula in the area of a missing right maxillary canine tooth in a dog.	Appearance of the oronasal fistula once the debris and hair have been removed.	A labial mucosal flap has been sutured to the hard palate mucosa.

Closure

The flap is sutured to hard palate mucosa and adjoining alveolar and buccal mucosa using an absorbable suture material in a simple interrupted pattern.

Soft food for 2 weeks.

OPERATIVE TECHNIQUE 3.6

Mandibular and sublingual salivary gland resection (lateral approach)

Lateral recumbency. The patient's neck is rotated contralaterally and extended over an elevated padded area (rolled towel); the mandible is secured to the operating table with adhesive tape.

ASSISTANT

Optional.

SURGICAL TECHNIQUE

Approach

A curvilinear skin incision is made from the bifurcation of the external jugular vein to the caudoventral aspect of the mandibular body. The subcutaneous tissue and platysma are incised. The parotidoauricular muscle is divided to expose glandular, venous and neurological structures.

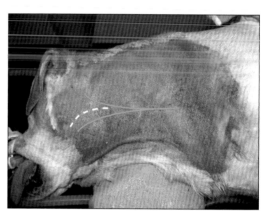

Position of curvilinear incision (white dotted line) from the bifurcation of the external jugular vein (shown in blue) to the caudoventral aspect of the mandibular body.

Surgical manipulations

1 Identify the mandibular salivary gland between the maxillary and linguofacial veins.

2 Incise the gland capsule and grasp the parenchyma with tissue forceps to provide caudal traction.

3 Incise the fascia between the masseter and digastricus muscles, allowing digital and sharp dissection of connective tissue attachments to expose the entire mandibular salivary gland and the contiguous sublingual gland complex. The end point for dissection is visualization of the lingual nerve that courses laterally over the sublingual gland complex.

4 Ligate the gland–duct complex and divide just caudal to the lingual nerve. The digastricus muscle may obscure the surgeon's view rostrally, necessitating either increased caudal retraction on the mandibular and sublingual gland complex or manoeuvring the complex under the digastricus muscle and floor of the sialocele to allow further rostral dissection. Myotomy of the digastricus muscle can be performed to aid complete visualization of the gland–duct complex and the location of the defect causing the sialocele.

5 Incise the sialocele and drain it to facilitate tissue manipulation around the digastricus muscle.

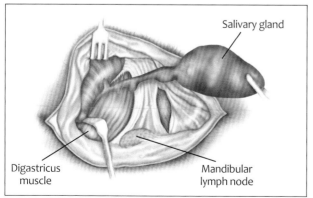

The mandibular salivary gland and the contiguous sublingual gland complex course between the masseter and digastricus muscles. Dissection is performed carefully rostral to the digastricus muscle in order to visualize the lingual nerve.

PRACTICAL TIP

The gland–duct defect causing the sialocele rarely occurs rostral to the lingual nerve. If the lingual nerve is not visualized, dissection may continue to the oral mucosa. The surgeon should make every effort to isolate the origin of the defect, verifying that the correct side has been operated upon. Failure to identify the defect indicates that the sialocele may have originated from the contralateral gland–duct complex. Bilateral resection of the mandibular and sublingual gland–duct complex is not associated with xerostomia

→ **OPERATIVE TECHNIQUE 3.6 CONTINUED**

Closure

Incised digastricus muscle is apposed with mattress sutures of synthetic absorbable material. Subcutaneous tissues are apposed with a similar material in a simple interrupted pattern. This is followed by skin closure using non-absorbable suture material in a simple interrupted pattern.

POSTOPERATIVE CARE

Penrose drains are placed through the sialocele and maintained for 1–3 days to allow drainage.

Chapter 4

Surgery of the nose and nasopharynx

Gert ter Haar and Cheryl S. Hedlund

Investigation of nasal discharge

Nasal disease in dogs and cats is relatively common. Sneezing, reverse sneezing and unilateral or bilateral nasal discharge (from mucopurulent to frank blood: epistaxis) are indicators of nasal disease. Nasal discharge is a cardinal sign of disease and is often the impetus for clients to seek veterinary attention, but other signs can predominate (Figure 4.1). The aetiology, treatment, and prognosis vary widely among patients with nasal disease. In a study of 42 dogs with chronic persistent nasal discharge, neoplasia was the most common cause (33%), followed by inflammatory rhinitis (24%), periodontal disease (10%), fungal rhinitis (7%) and foreign body reaction (7%) (Tasker et al., 1999). Adenocarcinoma was the most common nasal tumour diagnosed. The type of nasal discharge does not appear to predict aetiology (Bissett et al., 2007). Seventy-eight percent of 176 dogs in the latter study had local disease, with a similar distribution (neoplasia 39%, trauma 37%, idiopathic rhinitis 22% and periapical abscess 2%). Twenty-two percent of dogs with epistaxis suffered from systemic disease (thrombocytopenia 48%, thrombocytopathia 28%, coagulopathy 12%, hypertension 0.08% and vasculitis 0.04%) (Bissett et al., 2007). Chronic inflammatory or idiopathic lymphoplasmacytic rhinitis was diagnosed in 37 dogs with no identified cause in another study, suggesting that this may be a specific contributor to chronic nasal disease in dogs (Windsor et al., 2004); however, every effort should be made to exclude other causes before settling for this diagnosis.

In a study of 37 dogs with a primary nasopharyngeal condition, 54% had a neoplastic process, 11% had non-infectious inflammatory disease and the remainder had foreign bodies, benign cystic structures or cryptococcosis (Hunt et al., 2002). Studies in cats with nasal disease have shown that nasal neoplasia (39–49%) and chronic rhinitis (23–35%) are far more common than nasopharyngeal stenosis, polyps or trauma (Allen et al., 1999; Henderson et al., 2004; Demko and Cohn, 2007). Cats with neoplasia are older than other cats with nasal disease, and are more

likely to be dyspnoeic and have haemorrhagic and/or unilateral nasal disease than other cats with chronic rhinitis (Henderson et al., 2004). Lymphosarcoma is the most common tumour in cats. Viral infection with or without secondary bacterial infection is an extremely common cause of nasal disease and discharge in young cats. Lymphoplasmacytic rhinitis, foreign body, mycotic rhinitis, nasopharyngeal polyps and periapical tooth abscessation are less common causes of nasal disease in cats.

The animal's age, environment and history may provide clues to the aetiology of nasal discharge. Congenital abnormalities, viral infections or polyps are common in young animals, whereas older animals are more prone to neoplastic disease. Older small-breed dogs are more prone to the development of acquired oronasal fistulas from tooth root abscesses. Certain parasitic infections, such as Pneumonyssoides caninum (nasal mite), are reported in very specific areas (Scandinavian countries: Movassaghi and Mohri, 1998; Gunnarsson et al., 2004). Hunting dogs often inhale foreign bodies, whilst urban pets or show dogs and cats may be more likely to inhale a toxin or be exposed to an infectious agent.

The duration of the problem may not be apparent to the owners because fastidious animals often continuously remove the nasal discharge. The owner should be questioned regarding whether the nasal discharge occurred acutely or had a chronic onset, has changed in volume or character over time, if there were other clinical signs and the animal's response to any medications.

Physical examination

Careful physical examination of the dog or cat with nasal discharge is important (Schmiedt and Creevy, 2012). Sneezing may or may not be present. Reverse sneezing is a violent paroxysmal inspiratory effort made in an attempt to move material from the nasopharynx to the oropharynx and may accompany caudal nasal or nasopharyngeal disease (Venker-van Haagen, 2005). The animal may paw at the face or nose because of discomfort or to remove discharge. Facial deformity may be present if there is swelling or bony destruction from neoplasia, cryptococcosis in cats or occasionally severe dental disease. Facial symmetry should be carefully assessed, and ocular retropulsion should be performed to evaluate the retrobulbar space. Cats with nasal disease have clinical findings similar to those in dogs but may also have concurrent vomiting (69%) (Demko and Cohn, 2007).

- Nasal discharge – mucoid, mucopurulent, haemorrhagic, serous
- Sneezing or reverse sneezing
- Facial deformity
- Pawing at the face or nose
- Planum ulceration or depigmentation
- Airway obstruction – stridor, stertor, open-mouth breathing

4.1 Frequent clinical signs associated with nasal disease.

Upper airway obstruction occurs more commonly with nasopharyngeal disease than with nasal disease alone. Open-mouth breathing usually relieves airway obstruction, although some cats with nasopharyngeal polyps can have severe respiratory difficulty despite open-mouth breathing. Nasal obstruction may occur in brachycephalic breeds that have contact between intranasal structures due to aberrant conchae and mucosal thickening, septal deviation or nasopharyngeal turbinate protrusion (Schuenemann and Oechtering 2012, 2014b; Grosso *et al.*, 2015). Auscultation of the upper airway may reveal stridor or stertor. Stertor is an inspiratory snorting noise associated with (naso)pharyngeal disease. Stridor is a high-pitched wheeze that occurs during inspiration and is associated with diseases of the larynx and cervical trachea. Airway noise (or lack thereof) may be prominent on a particular side of the nasal cavity or localized caudally to the nasopharynx or larynx. Holding a cool glass slide to the nostrils and observing for bilaterally symmetrical condensation can confirm differential movement of air through the nares. Auscultation of the lower airway may reveal crackles and wheezes suggesting pulmonary disease.

Characterization of the nasal discharge may help determine its cause. Purulent discharge is common because many primary diseases of the nasal cavity allow secondary bacterial infection. Discharge that is serous, haemorrhagic, mucoid or contains food may also be observed; discharge can have multiple characteristics. Discharge may be unilateral or bilateral; nasal diseases may start on one side and progress to involving both. Determination of the original side of the discharge and changes in the character of discharge over time may be helpful in determining the cause of discharge, but the type of discharge is not pathognomonic for any condition.

Unilateral nasal discharge suggests local rather than systemic disease, although approximately half of the cases with systemic disease can have unilateral discharge (Bissett *et al.*, 2007). Unilateral serohaemorrhagic nasal discharge with peracute onset of clinical signs, if left untreated and later shows an intermittent response to antibiotics, suggests the presence of a foreign body (Figure 4.2). Dental disease can also cause unilateral nasal discharge, and periodontal disease should be ruled out during an oral examination.

Fractured or worn teeth should be evaluated by dental radiographs or computed tomography (CT) for secondary abscessation. Osteomyelitis, bony sequestra, oronasal fistula or intranasal tooth displacement are other forms of dental disease that may cause unilateral nasal discharge.

Bilateral nasal discharge is commonly seen with infections or advanced disease. In cats it can be caused by infectious agents, especially viral rhinitis, with or without secondary bacterial infection. Infectious agents sometimes cause unilateral rather than bilateral nasal disease. *Aspergillus fumigatus* is the most common cause of nasal fungal disease in dogs. Cryptococcosis, blastomycosis, penicilliosis and rhinosporidiosis are other causes of fungal rhinitis. Parasitic rhinitis (*P. caninum*) is rare and usually manifests with reverse sneezing only, but can cause bilateral nasal discharge in dogs. Inflammatory diseases such as allergy or inflammatory polyps may also cause bilateral nasal discharge.

Bilateral nasal discharge is also associated with some systemic diseases. Severe pneumonia may cause a mucopurulent discharge. Hyperadrenocorticism and disorders of coagulation can cause a haemorrhagic nasal discharge, whilst dental disease or palatal defects may also lead to bilateral nasal discharge that is usually purulent (Venker-van Haagen, 2005).

Congenital disorders can cause nasal discharge and are usually diagnosed in young animals. Cleft palate will cause nasal discharge of food, often milk, at a very early age, and is often accompanied by aspiration pneumonia (Reiter and Holt, 2012). Primary ciliary dyskinesia, the result of a defect in the formation and function of cilia (Merveille *et al.*, 2014), will cause a serous nasal discharge, unless a secondary bacterial infection exists. This condition is relatively uncommon and is associated with a host of other signs (situs inversus, hydrocephalus, sterility, recurrent pneumonia). Choanal atresia is a rare condition in which a thin persistent membrane partially or completely occludes one or both choanae (Willard and Radlinsky, 1999). A similar condition, called nasopharyngeal stenosis, can occur with formation of scar tissue occluding the nasopharynx secondary to an inflammatory process such as bacterial or viral rhinotracheitis, trauma or possibly following nasopharyngeal reflux under general anaesthesia (Mitten, 1988; De Lorenzi *et al.*, 2015).

Diagnostics

The diagnostic evaluation should be guided by clinical observations (Figure 4.3). Evaluation of regional lymph nodes is an important part of the physical examination. The lymph nodes should be evaluated by fine-needle

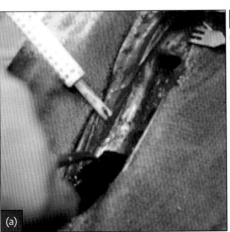

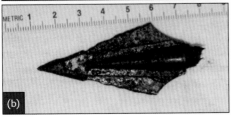

4.2 (a) An arrowhead lodged in the nasal cavity of a dog that caused signs of chronic mucopurulent rhinitis is removed during a dorsal rhinotomy. (b) Close-up of the arrowhead.

High-yield diagnostics
• Diagnostic imaging: radiographs, CT, MRI
• Rhinoscopy
• Biopsy

Low-yield diagnostics
• CBC
• Serum chemistry
• Urinalysis
• Cultures: bacterial and fungal
• Coagulation profile
• Fungal serology
• Nasal cytology

4.3 Many diagnostics performed whilst working up chronic nasal disease do not lead to a specific diagnosis but provide general health status information. CBC = complete blood count; CT = computed tomography; MRI = magnetic resonance imaging.

aspiration if they are enlarged or if there is suspicion of neoplastic disease. Cytological evaluation of these aspirates often provides diagnostic information. A complete blood count, serum chemistry profile and urinalysis, whilst not commonly diagnostic of a particular disorder, should be performed to assess general health. The complete blood count may reveal thrombocytopenia, anaemia or changes consistent with inflammation or infection. Hypercalcaemia has been associated with nasal adenocarcinoma, and increased serum alkaline phosphatase (ALP), may accompany bony destruction (ALP may also be elevated if associated with hyperadrenocorticism). A coagulation profile (including prothrombin time (PT) and activated partial thromboplastin time (aPTT)) should be performed prior to nasal surgery. For animals that have epistaxis as a prominent feature of their disease, it is crucial to identify any underlying or consequent perturbations of the clotting system by assessing platelet numbers and performing functional tests of primary and secondary haemostasis such as buccal mucosal bleeding time, PT and aPTT, or a test of 'global' haemostasis such as thrombo-elastography, prior to any procedures such as biopsy or surgery.

Fungal or bacterial culture of discharge is rarely helpful. Cultures of nasal swabs will yield normal flora and fail to differentiate between normal, non-pathological colonization and active infection. Primary nasal bacterial infection is very rarely (if ever) observed clinically. There is usually a primary aetiology such as a viral infection, foreign body, devitalized tissue or neoplasm allowing secondary infection. Most animals with upper respiratory bacterial infections secondary to viral disease will respond to broad-spectrum antibiotic therapy.

Fungal serology is often of little benefit. Determination of an antibody titre at a given time may only indicate exposure to the fungus. Fungal organisms that cause nasal disease are ubiquitous in the environment, and exposure is not indicative of disease. However, paired serological samples may assist in diagnosis. A latex agglutination test for cryptococcal capsular antigen has proven to be valuable for the diagnosis of cryptococcosis.

Cytological evaluation of a smear of the discharge itself may be a useful diagnostic tool, although imprinting a slide with a tissue sample or using a small brush to obtain an intranasal sample may provide a more accurate diagnosis. Feline nasal cryptococcosis can be diagnosed by cytological evaluation of nasal flushes. Imprint cytology has been shown to identify the histological tumour type correctly more often than brush cytology (Clercx *et al.*, 1996). If appropriate samples can be obtained, fungal or neoplastic disease can often be diagnosed cytologically. Functional tests to quantify nasal airflow are not routinely performed in veterinary practice, although subjective qualitative assessment of nasal airflow can be helpful. Nasal resistance and transnasal pressure can be determined using rhinomanometry to detect nasal obstructions (Wiestner *et al.*, 2007). However, the procedure can be difficult and time consuming.

Selective biopsy
• Rhinoscopy – biopsy via scope port or biopsy instrument placed alongside the scope
• Ultrasonography, CT or MRI – biopsy instrument placed with guidance

Non-selective biopsy
• Transnasal biopsy – cup forceps, alligator forceps or plastic tubing
• Hydropulsion – occlude nares and flush forcefully

4.4 Nasal biopsy techniques can be used in conjunction with diagnostic imaging or rhinoscopic visualization, or specimens may be obtained non-selectively by other techniques. It is important to protect the airway, collect specimens from the nasopharynx and lavage fluid, and to expect haemorrhage. CT = computed tomography; MRI = magnetic resonance imaging.

Diagnostic imaging

Results of various imaging techniques are often vital to the diagnosis of nasal diseases. Radiography, CT and MRI techniques can be performed. All imaging should be done under general anaesthesia and performed prior to rhinoscopy or biopsy. Several radiographic views are needed to assess the nasal cavity completely because of the complex anatomy of the nose and skull. Radiographic views should include lateral, ventrodorsal (VD) open mouth (best for evaluating the cribriform plate), intraoral dorsoventral (DV) occlusal and rostrocaudal (frontal sinus). Interpretation of the radiographic images is based on subtle changes; therefore, it is important to obtain high-quality radiographs (Figure 4.5).

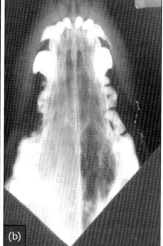

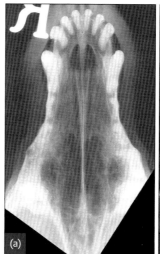

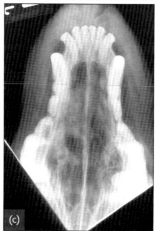

4.5 Intraoral dorsoventral radiographs of the nasal cavity. (a) Normal middle-aged dolichocephalic dog. (b) A 10-year-old Border Collie with a nasal carcinoma. (c) A 2-year-old Labrador Retriever with bilateral fungal rhinitis.

Diagnosis of diseases of the nose and nasal cavities primarily relies upon diagnostic imaging (radiography, CT, magnetic resonance imaging (MRI)) and endoscopy (rhinoscopy, nasopharyngoscopy) (Figure 4.4), and inspection of the oral cavity with dental probing, and should be executed in this order

> **WARNING**
>
> Neoplastic, fungal and inflammatory nasal diseases all share similar radiographic features

The radiographic appearance of nasal tumours will change with the duration of the lesion and the histological type of the tumour. Plain radiography is not a highly sensitive diagnostic method for identification of the cause of nasal diseases, especially in cases of early or less aggressive neoplasia (Saunders *et al.*, 2004; Pownder *et al.*, 2006; Johnson and Wisner, 2007). Conchal deviation or destruction, and destruction of the nasal septum, vomer bone, palatine bone, frontal bone or maxillary bone are suggestive of neoplasia. The presence of bony lysis often indicates a poor prognosis. In cats, a unilateral aggressive lesion that results in lysis of lateral nasal bones, turbinate destruction or loss of teeth is more likely to be a neoplasm, whereas a bilaterally symmetrical lesion is suggestive of chronic rhinitis (Mukaratirwa *et al.*, 2001; Johnson and Wisner, 2007). Neoplasia may also cause increased soft tissue opacity both within and outside the confines of the nasal cavity, indicating tumour extension beyond the limits of the nasal cavity. Increased opacity of the frontal sinus may result from primary disease or may be secondary to an obstructive rhinitis and subsequent accumulation of mucus.

In general, fungal disease causes destruction of the turbinates, decreasing radiographic density or creating increased lucency within the nasal cavity or nasal bones, often with a characteristic 'punctate' appearance (see Figure 4.5), whereas neoplastic disease will typically cause a uniform increased soft tissue opacity along with bony lysis. Most pathological fungal diseases (aspergillosis, blastomycosis, penicilliosis) cause destructive rhinitis. Destruction of the bony nasal septum is uncommon except in advanced fungal disease (Russo *et al.*, 2000; Saunders *et al.*, 2004; Karnik *et al.*, 2009). Cryptococcosis will cause a hyperplastic rhinitis and bony destruction is, therefore, not observed frequently with this condition.

Foreign bodies may or may not be visible on radiographic images, depending on the composition of the material. Changes observed on nasal radiographs in animals with nasal foreign bodies depend in large part on the chronicity of the problem. The only change observed early in the course of the disease may be increased soft tissue opacity, whereas bony destruction secondary to intense inflammation may be observed if the foreign body has been present for some time.

CT or MRI is superior to radiographs for distinguishing neoplasia from infection (Lefebvre *et al.*, 2005; Drees *et al.*, 2009; Kuehn, 2014) (Figure 4.6). These imaging modalities are superior because they more effectively differentiate soft tissue structures and provide a three-dimensional image. In a study of 80 dogs, nasal CT was over 90% accurate for differentiation of neoplasia, fungal rhinitis and foreign body rhinitis (Saunders and Van Bree, 2003). CT imaging is also essential for planning radiotherapy treatment of nasal tumours. In a study of 78 dogs examined by MRI, lack of a mass effect was associated with inflammatory disease whilst, in those with a mass effect, vomer bone lysis, cribriform plate erosion, paranasal bone destruction and mass invasion of the sphenoid sinus or nasopharynx were associated with neoplasia (Miles *et al.*, 2008).

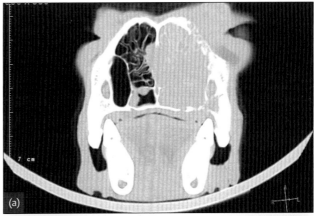

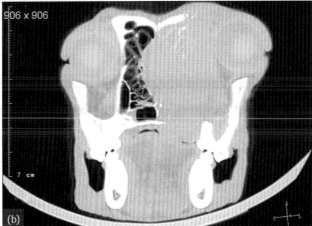

4.6 Computed tomographic (CT) images of the nasal cavity of a dog with nasal carcinoma: (a) at the level of the second premolar; (b) at the level of the cribriform plate. The left nasal cavity is filled with soft tissue, the tumour extends through the nasal septum and there is destruction of the palatine, maxillary, frontal and turbinate bones. Exophthalmos is evident.
(Courtesy of C Lamb)

Rhinoscopy

Endoscopic examination (rhinoscopy) may be very helpful in both diagnosing and treating nasal disease (Figure 4.7). The examination should be performed under general anaesthesia with a cuffed endotracheal tube in place. Protection of the airway is critical to prevent aspiration of mucus, blood and debris. The pharynx should be packed with gauze prior to the start of the examination, and debris and fluid should be suctioned from the pharynx prior to extubation.

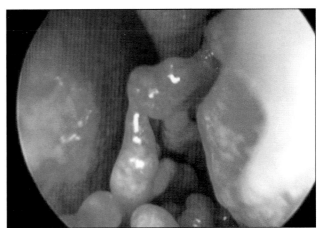

4.7 Rhinoscopic view from the left abnormal common meatus of the branched maxilloturbinates, obtained using a rigid endoscope.

Endoscopic examination of the choana and nasopharynx is performed initially, because this is easy, rapid, unlikely to cause iatrogenic trauma and subsequent bleeding, and may provide a diagnostic sample (Willard and Radlinsky, 1999; McCarthy, 2005; Johnson et al., 2006). Examination is most easily performed with a retroflexed endoscope but a rigid telescope with a 120-degree lens may also be used. Diagnosis of choanal atresia, nasopharyngeal stenosis, caudal pharyngeal mass lesions, aberrant turbinates or foreign bodies is possible.

Anterior rhinoscopy can be performed with a flexible endoscope or rigid telescope (5 mm in large dogs; 2–3 mm in cats and small dogs) (Willard and Radlinsky, 1999; McCarthy, 2005; Johnson et al., 2006). Suction during an endoscopic examination is essential to clear blood and tissue debris from the visual field. Flushing is recommended by some authors; sterile saline is instilled from caudal to rostral using a Foley catheter passed over the soft palate or from rostral to caudal by delivery of the solution through the endoscope. Diagnostic samples may be collected from the flush.

Guided by imaging-derived localization of abnormalities, the nasal passages should be assessed in a logical and standard manner during rhinoscopy. The nasal meati should be assessed for loss of turbinates or inflammatory or neoplastic growth, inflammation and the presence of foreign bodies.

Turbinate atrophy, with fungal plaques covering chronically inflamed mucosa, is often visible rhinoscopically in animals with *Aspergillus* spp. infections. The plaques usually appear as small flattened greenish-white structures that adhere to the nasal mucosa, and these plaques may be mistaken for foreign bodies. If aspergillosis is suspected but not identified, sinusoscopy or trephination has been found to be useful in identifying frontal sinus involvement (Johnson et al., 2006). Fungal 'balls' or granulomas, especially those caused by cryptococcosis, may also be found in the nasopharynx (Hunt et al., 2002). Some veterinary surgeons (veterinarians) recommend rhinoscopic debridement of fungal material prior to antifungal treatment.

Nasal biopsy

Nasal tumours usually result in an obvious mass protruding into one of the meati and can appear as pink, yellow-greyish or purple abnormal, often friable tissue that bleeds easily. Inflammatory masses and polyps, fungal granulomas and tumours cannot always be differentiated on the basis of radiographic and gross endoscopic appearance, hence nasal biopsy is always indicated to obtain tissue samples for histopathological analysis. For dogs with a documented bleeding tendency or clinico-pathologically documented deficiency in coagulation or platelet function, blood typing and crossmatching (if appropriate) should be performed prior to the biopsy of nasal disease. The location of the biopsy should be determined from previous imaging studies and rhinoscopy. The results of these studies should be available for evaluation during the biopsy procedure and multiple samples should be taken from the area of interest. The most reliable way of taking representative samples is using rhinoscopic guidance with cup forceps introduced into the nasal cavity alongside the endoscope. Cup forceps that are passed through the working channel of flexible endoscopes often result in tiny biopsy samples and false-negative results.

> **WARNING**
>
> Nasal biopsy using any technique will result in haemorrhage that can be severe. Identification of coagulopathies prior to nasal biopsy is essential

Alternatively, non-endoscopically guided transnasal biopsy can be used to obtain diagnostic samples. This is the fastest and easiest technique, but false-negative results are possible. The distance to the medial canthus of the eye is noted and marked on the biopsy instrument. Biopsy instruments should not be inserted past this point, to prevent iatrogenic damage to the cribriform plate and brain. Cup biopsy forceps or alligator forceps can be used to grasp tissue blindly; alternatively, a piece of hard plastic tubing or catheter cover cut at an angle can be forced into the nostril and the mass. The tube may be connected to a large syringe to provide suction or used alone. The biopsy sample will be retained within the tube. The tube should be redirected and advanced several times to obtain multiple samples.

Flushing after the biopsy procedure can be used to remove any tissue fragments left behind and to gather more tissue samples. A bulb syringe is used to instil the flushing solution with pressure into the nostril. For cats, a small bulb syringe or a 10 ml syringe can be used. Samples are collected in a gauze sponge placed within the pharynx. Flushing may also be performed regardless of whether or not a lesion is found endoscopically because flushing can dislodge occult foreign bodies or provide samples from unobserved lesions.

Flushing can also be used as the sole biopsy technique. This is more successful if done using hydropulsion after a mass has been confirmed using a rhinoscope (Ashbaugh et al., 2011). To perform nasal hydropulsion, one nostril is digitally occluded and a 20–60 ml regular luer tip syringe filled with sterile saline is inserted into the contralateral nostril. Prior to forcefully infusing the saline, a towel is placed under the nose, the endotracheal tube cuff is checked for proper inflation and a Poole suction tip is placed at the opening to the oesophagus. Twenty to sixty millilitres of saline is then rapidly injected under pressure (<2 seconds). The procedure is repeated (2–3 times) until no additional tissue can be dislodged, then the entire nasal cavity is re-evaluated via rhinoscopy. Tissue is collected from the towel, oral cavity and nasopharynx. Thorough suctioning of the oropharynx, proximal oesophagus, larynx and the proximal trachea around the endotracheal tube is performed. Using this technique, diagnostic samples were dislodged from the nasal cavity in 90% of dogs and cats (37 of 41) with nasal tumours (Ashbaugh et al., 2011). Additionally, immediate relief of nasal obstruction was noted in some patients. Minor expected postoperative complications include sneezing, reverse sneezing and mild epistaxis.

> **PRACTICAL TIP**
>
> Always flush the nasal cavity after biopsy, even if no lesion was identified

Endoscopic biopsy should be performed at the end of an examination because the field of view is often obscured by haemorrhage after the biopsy procedure.

CT, MRI or ultrasonography can also be used to guide a biopsy procedure. These techniques require general anaesthesia, special equipment and a thorough knowledge of the imaging modality and pertinent anatomy. Biopsy instruments can be directed through the nares, through the soft palate or laterally through areas of bony destruction. If initial attempts at biopsy fail to provide a definitive diagnosis, an open biopsy (rhinotomy) should be considered.

A thorough oral examination with dental probing guided by imaging results should be performed under general anaesthesia in cases where chronic rhinitis is found with no obvious abnormalities on rhinoscopy. Abnormalities such as oronasal fistulae and cleft palate may be identified during visual and digital examination of the palate and nasopharynx. Probing of periapical alveolar pockets of especially the canine teeth is essential in diagnosing oronasal fistulation, even in cases where there are no apparent dental abnormalities. Mass lesions in the nasopharynx can be sampled either using endoscopic biopsy forceps or following rostral traction on the soft palate to expose the mass. In addition, fine-needle aspirates can be obtained by probing through the soft palate into the suspected mass. Alternatively, it may be necessary to incise the soft palate on the midline to biopsy or remove masses from the nasopharynx. Closure is performed in two or three layers with small-gauge (1–2 metric (3/0–5/0 USP)) absorbable suture material in a continuous pattern to avoid placement of excessive knots in the tissues.

Surgical techniques

Rhinotomy

Indications for rhinotomy include biopsy, debridement of necrotic tissue, exploration for chronic nasal discharge with unknown aetiology, removal of nasal foreign bodies, cytoreduction of nasal masses (as discussed previously) and flushing mucus or fungal balls. Most surgeons prefer a dorsal approach to the nasal cavity and paranasal sinuses, because of enhanced accessibility to the cribriform plate and frontal sinuses, but ventral rhinotomy may be indicated in selected patients with focal abnormalities in the ventral meatus, choana and/or nasopharynx. A lateral rhinotomy is indicated in those instances where access is only required to the rostral part of the nasal cavity (nasal vestibule) (Hedlund, 1998, 2007; ter Haar and Hampel, 2015).

Haemorrhage should be anticipated when performing a rhinotomy. Efficient surgical technique is paramount to reduce blood loss. The more rapidly and efficiently the surgery is performed, the less likely it is that haemorrhage will become a major problem. Electrocautery should be used judiciously, especially if a ventral rhinotomy is being performed. Compression can be applied to the operative field with sponges or laparotomy pads to control haemorrhage during surgery. When working caudally the rostral nasal cavity is packed, and vice versa. Flushing with cold saline or diluted (1:100,000) adrenaline (epinephrine) will cause local vasoconstriction and reduce surface bleeding. This dilution of adrenaline rarely causes systemic effects, unless an overwhelming volume is used; however, the patient should be carefully monitored for development of cardiac arrhythmias. Bone wax can be used to occlude intraosseous haemorrhage. If the sphenopalatine arteries can be identified and ligated, haemorrhage can be reduced. Performing temporary occlusion of the carotid arteries prior to rhinotomy may minimize haemorrhage and improve visualization during turbinectomy (Hedlund *et al.*, 1983). If temporary carotid artery occlusion has not been performed preoperatively and severe haemorrhage occurs,

temporary unilateral or bilateral occlusion of the common carotid artery can be performed following rhinotomy to reduce blood loss.

If haemorrhage persists after turbinectomy, the nasal cavity can be packed with sterile moistened umbilical tape prior to closure. The packing should exit the nostril and be secured to the skin with suture. Nasal packing is usually left in place for 24 hours. Removal of packing material can usually be done in an awake or sedated animal, and the material should be removed rapidly to minimize discomfort to the patient.

Dorsal rhinotomy

This is the most common approach to the nasal cavity. The technique provides unilateral or bilateral access to the nasal cavity and can be extended caudally to expose the frontal sinuses (see Operative Technique 4.1). A unilateral dorsal rhinotomy can also be performed more laterally if indicated.

A dorsal midline incision is made through the skin and periosteum from just above the level of the eyes to the nasal cartilages, and the periosteum is reflected laterally over the nasal bone. The limits of a bone flap are identified, and the bone flap is removed with rongeurs, an oscillating saw, air-powered burr or an osteotome. There appears to be no increase in complications or reduction in cosmesis when the bone flap is not replaced. If the bone flap is going to be returned following surgery, osteotome bone cuts are recommended because there is little loss of bone, and the flap returns to a near normal position. If the flap is to be replaced after surgery, it is hinged on its most rostral attachment to the cartilage. Complete removal of the bone is especially useful in cats and small dogs because the flap is quite small. If radiation therapy will be performed after surgery, removal of the bone flap is recommended. The flap is often devitalized by the radiation and may have to be removed during a second surgery.

Following exposure, the nasal cavity is gently explored. If the turbinates are damaged they are usually removed. Biopsy specimens and samples for culture are taken as needed, and haemorrhage is controlled as discussed previously. If the bone flap is replaced, small holes are drilled in the four corners of the flap and the corresponding areas of the skull, and surgical steel wire or heavy non-absorbable suture material is used to attach the flap. The periosteum and subcutaneous tissues are closed with small (1–1.5 metric (4/0–5/0 USP)) absorbable suture material in a continuous pattern, and the skin is closed routinely.

Postoperative haemorrhage is a relatively common complication. The haemorrhage is usually mild to moderate and should resolve if coagulation function is normal. Ice packing of the muzzle may facilitate vasoconstriction and reduce haemorrhage as well as provide some analgesia. In rare cases where the haemorrhage is severe or prolonged, the animal may need to be returned to surgery to pack the nasal cavity. Subcutaneous emphysema is another possible complication following surgery, but is rare if proper airflow through the nasal passages is restored during surgery and the periosteum is tightly sutured. There is little consequence of this complication, but it requires several weeks to resolve completely. As mentioned earlier, persistent nasal discharge is common after rhinotomy, especially if the turbinates were removed.

Ventral rhinotomy

A ventral approach for rhinotomy has also been described (Holmberg *et al.*, 1989). Advantages of ventral rhinotomy include potentially improved cosmesis, a lower risk of sub-cutaneous emphysema and better exposure to the caudal ventral nasal cavity and nasopharynx. This approach is not recommended if exposure of the frontal sinuses is required. The animal is placed in dorsal recumbency with the mandible taped open or with a mouth gag in place. A midline incision is made through the oral mucosa and the mucoperi-osteum of the palatine bone, and the mucoperiosteum is reflected bilaterally. Stay sutures are placed in the mucoperi-osteum to aid in retraction and improve exposure. The caudolateral limits of the dissection are the major palatine arteries, which are identified and preserved. The incision can be extended caudally to include the soft palate if increased exposure of the nasopharynx is required. The palatine bone is removed with an air burr or rongeurs; no effort is made to save or replace the bone flap. The wound is closed in two layers using absorbable suture material in a simple inter-rupted or continuous pattern. A soft, pliable suture material is used in the oral cavity to minimize lingual irritation.

Postoperative considerations specific for this tech-nique include a need to protect the mucosal incision during the healing process. The animal is fed soft food for 1 month and not allowed access to chew toys, bones or sticks. The incision should be inspected weekly for 2–3 weeks to ensure proper healing. If this procedure is per-formed on a growing dog, growth deformities are possible (Holmberg et al., 1989).

Other approaches

An alveolar mucosal rhinotomy approach has been des-cribed to remove a dorsally displaced canine tooth (Priddy et al., 2001). This approach is performed through the oral cavity and provides a narrow window into the most rostral aspect of the nasal cavity. Limited lateral rhinotomies have also been described in combination with maxillectomy for tumour removal. A proper lateral rhinotomy was described by Hedlund (1998, 2007), which gives access to the nasal vestibule and rostral nasal cavity (Figure 4.8). When com-bined with elevation of the central planum as described by Pavletic (2010), the approach allows access to the entire rostral nasal septum for removal of septal tumours such as squamous cell carcinoma (ter Haar and Hampel, 2015).

With the dog positioned in sternal recumbency, the nasal planum is first elevated as a dorsally based U-flap. This exposes the very rostral nasal septum, after which a lateral rhinotomy is performed on the ipsilateral side to the nasal septal mass. This requires incising the skin from the angle of the rhinarium to the nasomaxillary notch, and subsequently transecting the maxillary cartilage between the dorsal and ventral parietal cartilages (Hedlund, 1998; ter Haar and Hampel, 2015). The nasal vestibule is thus completely exposed (Figure 4.8b), and full-thickness resection of a rostral nasal septal mass can be performed. The lateral rhinotomy incision is closed in three layers by suturing the nasal cartilages back into place first, followed by routine closure of the subcutaneous tissues and skin. The nasal planum U-flap is then sutured back into its anatomical position (ter Haar and Hampel, 2015).

Rhinoscopic turbinectomy can also be performed, to remove aberrant nasal turbinates and when intraconchal and septoconchal contact occurs, causing nasal obstruc-tion in brachycephalic dogs (Oechtering et al., 2007a, 2007b). The technique is performed by introducing the 0.4 mm fibre of a diode laser (980 nm) into the nasal cavity through the working channel of a 2.7 mm rigid telescope. The abnormal turbinates are dissected from their origin with the laser power setting at 4 W and extracted from

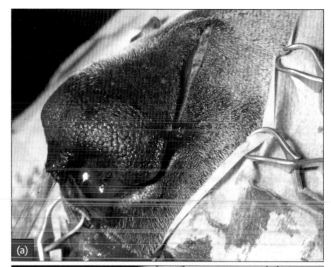

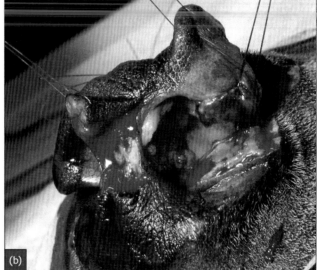

4.8 Lateral rhinotomy. (a) The most rostral aspect of the nasal planum is preserved by creating a U-shaped flap to access the most rostral part of the nasal vestibule. (b) A lateral rhinotomy incision is shown, which will allow for complete exposure of the nasal vestibule.

the nasal cavity with small grasping forceps. The procedure is time consuming, intra- and postoperative haemorrhage is relatively common and some conchal regrowth is expected (Schuenemann and Oechtering, 2014a and b).

Postoperative care

Immediately after surgery of the nasal cavity, the pharynx should be suctioned and cleaned of debris prior to extu-bation. Extubation should be performed with the cuff of the endotracheal tube partially inflated to help clear the proximal airway and decrease the chance of aspiration pneumonia postoperatively. Increased respiratory noise, rate and effort along with poor oxygenation, coughing, hyperthermia, lethargy and anorexia are signs of aspiration pneumonia that can occur after nasal surgery. Thoracic radiographs are indicated for patients with pulmonary signs following nasal surgery. Samples for cytological examin-ation and microbial culture and sensitivity testing can be obtained with a transtracheal, endotracheal or tracheo-bronchial wash. Aggressive medical therapy and supportive care are indicated for patients with aspiration pneumonia. Antibiotic therapy should be guided by the results of micro-bial culture and antibiotic sensitivity testing of material retrieved by tracheal wash.

If substantial haemorrhage has occurred intraoperatively, fluid replacement therapy should be continued until the deficit is restored and the animal is eating and drinking independently. Blood products should be used as needed. Analgesia is continued until the animal is subjectively comfortable (usually within 3–5 days). Oral or transdermal opioid analgesics or non-steroidal anti-inflammatory drugs are usually provided during this time.

Nasal planum resection and reconstruction

Resection of the nasal planum is indicated when neoplasia involves this area, after extensive trauma and sometimes for fungal disease. Nasal planum resection alone, or in conjunction with the premaxilla, is performed depending on the location and tumour type (Kirpensteijn *et al.*, 1994; Gallegos *et al.*, 2007). The original technique for nasal planum amputation was described by Withrow and Straw (1990), and it remains the easiest technique for resection of nasal planum tumours in cats. The postoperative appearance of the animal is not always acceptable to the owners.

With the animal positioned in sternal recumbency, the surgical area is carefully palpated to estimate tumour extension into adjacent tissue. The nasal planum is completely removed with a 360-degree skin incision made with a scalpel. The incision is made so that it transects the underlying turbinates. The cartilage of the nasal plane and the turbinates should be cut with an incision angled at about 45 degrees to the hard palate (Withrow and Straw, 1990). Haemorrhage can be controlled by direct pressure. A purse-string suture of 2 or 3 metric (3/0 or 2/0 USP) absorbable or non-absorbable suture material is placed through the skin around the incision to cover the exposed nasal conchae partly with skin. The new nasal orifice is closed to approximately 1 cm in diameter (Withrow and Straw, 1990).

Alternatively, for a more cosmetic result, an advancement flap can be created from the dorsal aspect of the nose to reconstruct the dorsal wound. Laterally, the exposed turbinate cartilage can be denuded from the overlying mucosa and sutured to the lateral cartilage. The wound is further closed using interrupted sutures from the skin to the remaining planum cartilage. If wider margins are required, complete nosectomy with premaxillectomy may be required (Figure 4.9). Postoperative care consists of an Elizabethan collar, broad-spectrum antibiotics for 1 week and analgesia for 3 days.

For lateralized (nostril) granulomatous/fungal or malignant lesions where the central planum can be preserved, cosmetic reconstruction of the nostril is possible using a unilateral nasal rotation flap incorporating dorsal nasal plane tissue, with excision of Burow's triangles (ter Haar *et al.*, 2013). Larger defects will inevitably cause some facial distortion, but can be closed with a facial artery axial pattern flap or buccal advancement/rotation flaps (Buiks and ter Haar, 2012).

Specific conditions

Nasal aspergillosis

Aspergillus fumigatus is a ubiquitous saprophyte found in mouldy hay, wood chips, rotting vegetation and compost. This fungus easily becomes airborne and, therefore, is easily inhaled. Dogs with nasal aspergillosis usually do not have malignant or immunosuppressive diseases and are generally in good health, and although some have been demonstrated to have T- and B-cell dysfunction, it is unclear whether this represents the cause or the effect of the disease. *A. fumigatus* has been shown to cause lymphocyte transformation in T and B cells *in vitro* (Sharp *et al.*, 1991a, 1991b, 1993; Peeters *et al.*, 2005). In contrast to dogs, cats have been more commonly reported to suffer from disseminated aspergillosis associated with an immunosuppressive disease or condition (Tomsa *et al.*, 2003). More recently, feline upper respiratory tract aspergillosis has been reported more frequently, often in association with nasal infections (Wilkinson *et al.*, 1982; Kano *et al.*, 2008; Barachetti *et al.*, 2009; Furrow and Groman, 2009; Karnik *et al.*, 2009; Giordano *et al.*, 2010; Smith and Hoffman, 2010; Barrs *et al.*, 2012; Declercq *et al.*, 2012; Kano *et al.*, 2013; Barrs *et al*; 2014; Barrs and Talbot, 2014). The disease occurs over a wide geographical range, including Australia, the USA, the UK, mainland Europe and Japan. Two anatomical forms have been reported: sino-nasal and sino-orbital aspergillosis (Barrs *et al.*, 2012; Barrs and Talbot, 2014). The environmental saprophytic fungi that cause these infections are most commonly from the *A. fumigatus* complex, including *A. fumigatus* and *A. felis* (Kano *et al.*, 2008, 2013; Barrs *et al.*, 2012; Kano *et al.*, 2013; Whitney *et al.*, 2013; Barrs and Talbot, 2014). Diagnosis of nasal aspergillosis in both dogs and cats is based on imaging, rhinoscopic (Figure 4.10), cytological and histopathological findings.

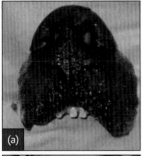
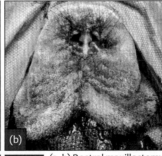
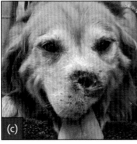

4.9 (a, b) Rostral maxillectomy with nasal planum resection was performed for an invasive squamous cell carcinoma. (c) Owners should be aware and accepting of their pet's altered appearance prior to selecting this treatment option.

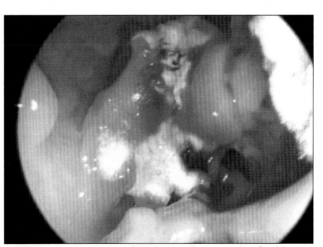

4.10 Rhinoscopic view of nasal aspergillosis; atrophy of turbinates with severe inflammation of the mucosal lining of remnant turbinates is visible, with macroscopically identifiable fungal growth.

Following diagnosis of nasal aspergillosis, topical antifungal treatment is indicated. Systemic antifungal therapy requires prolonged treatment (2–3 months), has poor efficacy and is not recommended as the sole form of treatment (Peeters *et al.*, 2005; Sissener *et al.*, 2006; Billen *et al.*, 2010). Systemic therapy has been used as part of a combination protocol for cases that do not respond to topical treatment alone. Topical antifungal therapy is considered the treatment of choice for nasal aspergillosis. Some authors recommend meticulous debridement of fungal plaques, fungal balls and necrotic tissue prior to topical antifungal therapy (Zonderland *et al.*, 2002). Topical medication can be instilled into the nasal cavity through an infusion catheter placed surgically into the frontal sinus or via catheters passed through the nares (Mathews *et al.*, 1996, 1998; Davidson *et al.*, 2005). Clotrimazole cream (20 g) instilled into each frontal sinus using a 10 Fr urinary catheter placed through a 3.2 mm Steinmann pin hole was shown to have excellent filling of the frontal sinuses and nasal cavity, based on CT scans (Burrow *et al.*, 2013).

Current evidence suggests that the two methods of treatment have equal efficacy, although the non-invasive technique has fewer complications (Richardson and Mathews, 1995; Mathews *et al.*, 1998). A non-invasive topical antifungal nasal infusion must be done under general anaesthesia (Figure 4.11). The patient is intubated and the pharynx is packed with moist gauze. A 24 Fr Foley catheter is placed through the mouth and over the soft palate so that the tip is facing rostrally. The balloon is inflated to occlude the nasopharynx. The caudal nasopharynx is subsequently further packed with gauze. Two 10 Fr infusion catheters are placed through the nostrils into the dorsal nasal meatus to the level of the medial canthus or guided rhinoscopically into the frontal sinus. A 12 Fr Foley catheter is inserted into each nostril and the balloons are inflated to occlude the nares. Alternatively, the distal end of an 18 Fr Foley catheter is cut with scissors, after which a urinary catheter is passed through the Foley catheter, to decrease leakage from the nostril site as a result of having two round catheters in place. The dog is put into dorsal recumbency, and 1 g of clotrimazole (some formulations of clotrimazole contain alcohol; these should be avoided) in 100 ml of polyethylene glycol 200 is infused into the nasal cavity through the infusion catheters. When fluid is noted within the lumen of the pharyngeal catheter, the infusion catheters are occluded and the dog is rotated to each lateral position for 15 minutes and left in dorsal and ventral recumbency for 15 minutes each, for a total infusion time of 1 hour. After treatment, the catheters are removed, and the pharynx is suctioned to remove fluid and debris.

The reported success rate of this procedure after one treatment is 86% (Mathews *et al.*, 1998; Davidson *et al.*, 2005), but large studies on long-term outcome using this technique are not available. Topical infusion of clotrimazole has been described in cats, with success (Tomsa *et al.*, 2003), although it has been suggested that topical enilconazole (either 1% or 2%) is more efficacious than clotrimazole (Zonderland *et al.*, 2002). Enilconazole is not available in the USA, however.

Follow-up rhinoscopy is strongly recommended 3–6 weeks after infusion to assess the response to therapy. The procedure may need to be repeated more than once depending on clinical signs and the results of follow-up rhinoscopy. Further improvements in topical treatment consist of the use of viscous antifungal creams for application in the frontal sinuses. Combined trephination, a short clotrimazole (1%) soak and application of clotrimazole (1%) cream to the frontal sinuses (10–20 g per sinus) led to a great reduction in the duration of the procedure and hospitalization and good success rates (50–86% clinical cure) (Sissener *et al.*, 2006; Sharman *et al.*, 2010). Depot therapy with bifonazole cream applied via per-endoscopic frontal sinus catheters has also been described and, in combination with debridement and enilconazole infusion, resulted in nearly 60% clinical cure (Billen *et al.*, 2010).

A report of successful treatment of mycotic rhinitis in three dogs was published that involved extensive surgical debridement and open wound management using a topical povidone–iodine dressing (Moore, 2003). The disadvantages of surgical rhinotomy include increased time, cost and morbidity, as well as disruption of the local blood supply, which may impede healing. There is no proven increase in efficacy with surgical rhinotomy and open debridement for fungal disease (White, 2006).

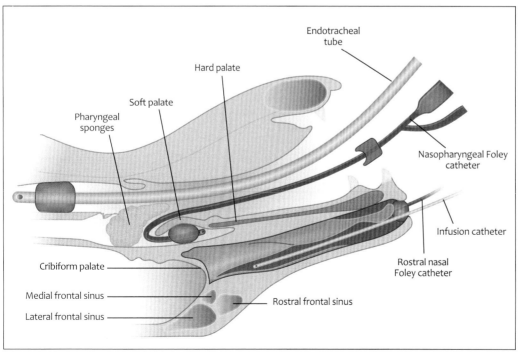

4.11 Placement of catheters for nasal and sinus infusion with clotrimazole. Endotracheal intubation with cuffing and packing the caudal pharyngeal area are mandatory to prevent aspiration of clotrimazole.

Chronic rhinitis/sinusitis in cats

The specific aetiology of chronic rhinitis and sinusitis in cats may vary. Viral infections (feline rhinotracheitis virus, feline calicivirus) are often initiating pathogens, although bacterial infections may also be involved. Sinusitis may be a primary problem. Viral, fungal, bacterial or lympho-plasmacytic sinusitis may be primary conditions or may occur secondary to obstructive nasal disease.

Cats with chronic rhinitis/sinusitis usually exhibit nasal discharge with variable degrees of sneezing, anorexia, gagging or vomiting. These clinical signs show a variable response to antibiotics or anti-inflammatory doses of steroids. The diagnosis is based on the results of biopsy, imaging studies (radiographs, CT, MRI) and rhinoscopy. Treatment of chronic rhinitis/sinusitis is based on the results of the biopsy and other diagnostic tests.

Surgery is not recommended as an initial treatment for chronic rhinitis unless a foreign body or a bony sequestrum is present, or if polypoid/granulomatous changes are thought to be significantly reducing airflow. Ethmoid conchal curettage and placement of an autogenous fat graft to fill the sinus has been described (Tomlinson and Schenck, 1975; Anderson, 1987); however, the authors do not recommend this technique. If an animal fails to respond to medical therapy or suffers from severe nasal congestion as a result of polypoid deformation of the mucosal lining of the turbinates, surgical exploration of the frontal sinus and nasal cavity and debridement of necrotic or diseased tissue should be considered.

Nasal neoplasia

Nasal neoplasia can be divided into neoplasia of the nasal planum or the rostral nasal septum and intranasal neoplasia. Neoplasia of the nasal planum is rare in the dog and more common in the cat. Squamous cell carcinoma (SCC) is the most common tumour of the planum and occurs secondary to effects of ultraviolet (UV) light on unpigmented skin (Withrow, 2013). The biological behaviour of SCC can vary from local disease to highly invasive carcinomas. The treatment of choice for SCC is nasal planum resection with or without radiation therapy (Holt et al., 1990; Cox et al., 1991). Reconstructive techniques performed during wound closure can improve the cosmetic outcome, but owners should be warned that perfect cosmesis is not usually possible. Preventive measures include tattooing a high-risk area of skin or avoidance of UV light (indoor housing). Primary SCC of the rostral nasal septum that is limited to the septum itself can be cured with full-thickness resection of the septum using a combined rostrolateral rhinotomy approach (ter Haar and Hampel, 2015).

Intranasal neoplasms include carcinomas (about 66%) and sarcomas (about 33%) (Turek and Lana, 2013). These tumours in general grow slowly, metastasize late in the course of disease and occur more commonly in older animals. Tumour type is generally not prognostic; however, the stage of tumour does relate to prognosis (Turek and Lana, 2013).

Treatment of intranasal tumours with cytoreductive surgery alone is not indicated. Cytoreductive surgery alone or prior to megavoltage radiation therapy fails to improve survival (MacEwen et al., 1977; Theon et al., 1993; Adams et al., 1998), but radiation therapy delivered using cobalt or a linear accelerator improves survival. A censored median survival time of 19 months was reported when nasal tumours were treated with an accelerated radiotherapy protocol using cobalt (Adams et al., 1998; Turek and Lana, 2013). Cytoreductive surgery performed after radiation therapy can improve survival; however, significant postoperative complications can occur. These are probably the result of radiation-induced poor tissue healing (Turek and Lana, 2013). Occasionally, surgical rhinotomy may be performed prior to radiation therapy to obtain a diagnostic biopsy sample.

Acute and late toxicities of radiotherapy have been reported. Acute toxicity develops during treatment and typically manifests as oral mucositis, keratoconjunctivitis and blepharitis, rhinitis and skin desquamation (Theon et al., 1993; Adams et al., 1998; Lawrence et al., 2010). These effects normally resolve within 2–8 weeks after treatment (McEntee, 2006). Late toxicity is more serious and potentially very detrimental to the patient. It develops months to years after treatment and is usually permanent. Late effects include cataracts, keratoconjunctivitis sicca, uveitis, retinal degeneration, brain necrosis, osteonecrosis and skin fibrosis (LaDue et al., 1999; Gieger et al., 2008; McEntee, 2006; Lawrence et al., 2010).

If surgery is performed on a nasal tumour before or after radiation therapy, the owners should be warned to expect life-long serous to mucoid nasal discharge postoperatively. There is also an increased risk of developing opportunistic fungal or bacterial infection after radiation therapy and surgery, owing to the damage to tissues and blood supply. These patients routinely receive broad-spectrum antibiotics for 3–4 months after surgery, and nasal infections in these patients are challenging to treat.

Stenotic nares

Stenotic nares are a congenital defect in the diameter of the nares causing pathological resistance to airflow during nasal breathing in brachycephalic dogs. This is a common component of the brachycephalic airway disease. In-creased mucosal contact points, nasopharyngeal turbinate protrusion, elongation of the soft palate, hypoplastic trachea, secondary eversion of the laryngeal saccules and laryngeal collapse are other components of this syndrome (Oechtering, 2010; Schuenemann and Oechtering, 2014a and b; Grosso et al., 2015). Stenotic nares are less common in cats, but may occur in brachycephalic cat breeds. Surgical correction of stenotic nares is described in Chapter 6.

Nasal dermoid sinus

A dermoid sinus (dermoid cyst, pilonidal sinus) is a congenital abnormality caused by incomplete separation of the ectodermal neural tube from the skin during embryological development. The condition is most commonly seen along the neck and back in the Rhodesian Ridgeback but has been reported in other breeds. Nasal dermoid sinuses have been reported in the American Cocker Spaniel, Springer Spaniel, Brittany Spaniel and Golden Retriever (Anderson and White, 2002). The diagnosis is suspected on the basis of a history of intermittent discharge from a small opening along the midline of the bridge of the nose at a junction between the nasal planum and the skin (nasal pit) (Figure 4.12). The tract may extend into the cranial vault. Infusion of contrast medium into the tract may help determine its caudal extent. Successful treatment requires complete excision of the tract and reconstruction of the defect.

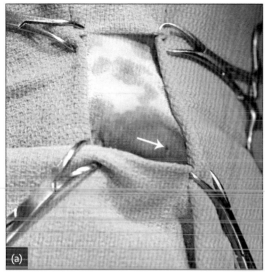

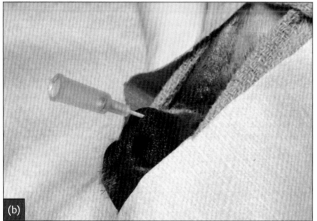

4.12 (a) The arrow points to a nasal pit in the nasal planum of this dog with nasal dermoid sinus. (b) A catheter has been placed in this dog's nasal dermoid sinus to help identify the tract during excision.

Choanal atresia and nasopharyngeal stenosis

Obstruction of the caudal choanae or nasopharynx can be congenital or secondary to severe inflammation or trauma. Inspiratory stertor and severe mucoid to mucopurulent nasal discharge are typical presenting signs. Attempts at relieving the obstruction often fail but have included resection of scar tissue, balloon dilation and stenting (Mitten, 1988; Coolman *et al.*, 1998; Novo and Kramek, 1999; Boswood *et al.*, 2003; Berent *et al.*, 2006, 2008). Use of balloon-expandable metallic stents has been the most effective means of treatment (Berent *et al.*, 2008) although, recently, 15 cats with acquired nasopharyngeal stenosis were reported to have been successfully treated by stenosis dilation followed by temporary stenting with a silicone stent (De Lorenzi *et al.*, 2015).

Nasopharyngeal polyps

Nasopharyngeal polyps are benign masses that have been diagnosed in dogs and cats but are more often found in cats. Cats with nasopharyngeal polyps may also have polyps in the middle ear or external ear canal. Clinical signs include nasal discharge, sneezing, laboured breathing, nasopharyngeal stridor, dysphagia and voice change. Signs of otitis externa and media are seen in animals with

ear canal involvement. Nasopharyngeal polyps can usually be removed through the oral cavity after retraction of the soft palate by applying traction. Ventral bulla osteotomy is recommended when polyps removed by traction–avulsion in this location recur (Pratschke, 2003; Donnelly and Tillson, 2004).

Nasopharyngeal polyps are approached through the oral cavity with the soft palate retracted rostrally, or by incising the soft palate when dealing with very small polyps. After retracting and applying digital pressure to the soft palate, the polyp is forced caudally so that it can be grasped as close to the opening of the Eustachian tube as possible with forceps (Allis or alligator forceps), and slow, steady traction with rotation is applied until the polyp avulses. It is unusual that a soft palate incision is required, but when necessary the palate is incised on the midline with the caudal tip left intact. Following polyp extraction, the soft palate edges are apposed in two layers. Histopathology of the polyp is necessary to rule out malignancy. Recurrence is not expected if removal is complete, and long-term complications are unexpected.

References and further reading

Adams WM, Miller PE, Vail DM, Forrest LJ and MacEwen EG (1998) An accelerated technique for irradiation of malignant canine nasal and paranasal sinus tumors. *Veterinary Radiology and Ultrasound* **39**, 475–481

Allen HS, Broussard J and Noone K (1999) Nasopharyngeal diseases in cats: a retrospective study of 53 cases (1991–1998). *Journal of the American Animal Hospital Association* **35**, 457–461

Anderson DM and White RAS (2002) Nasal dermoid sinus cysts in the dog. *Veterinary Surgery* **31**, 303–308

Anderson GI (1987) The treatment of chronic sinusitis in six cats by ethmoid conchal curettage and autogenous fat graft sinus ablation. *Veterinary Surgery* **16**, 131–134

Ashbaugh EA, McKiernan BC, Miller CJ and Powers B (2011) Nasal hydropulsion: a novel tumor biopsy technique. *Journal of the American Animal Hospital Association* **47**, 312–316

Barachetti L, Mortellaro CM, Di Giancamillo M *et al.* (2009) Bilateral orbital and nasal aspergillosis in a cat. *Veterinary Ophthalmology* **12**, 176–182

Barrs VR, Beatty JA, Dhand NK *et al.* (2014) Computed tomographic features of feline sino-nasal and sino-orbital aspergillosis. *Veterinary Journal* **201**, 215–222

Barrs VR, Halliday C, Martin P *et al.* (2012) Sinonasal and sino-orbital aspergillosis in 23 cats: aetiology, clinicopathological features and treatment outcomes. *Veterinary Journal* **191**, 58–64

Barrs VR and Talbot JJ (2014) Feline aspergillosis. *Veterinary Clinics of North America: Small Animal Practice* **44**, 51–73

Berent AC, Kinns J and Weisse C (2006) Balloon dilatation of nasopharyngeal stenosis in a dog. *Journal of the American Veterinary Medical Association* **229**, 385–388

Berent AC, Weisse C, Todd K, Rondeau MP and Reiter AM (2008) Use of a balloon-expandable metallic stent for treatment of nasopharyngeal stenosis in dogs and cats: six cases (2005–2007). *Journal of the American Veterinary Medical Association* **233**, 1432–1440

Billen F, Guieu L-V, Bernaerts F *et al.* (2010) Efficacy of intrasinusal administration of bifonazole cream alone or in combination with enilconazole irrigation in canine sino-nasal aspergillosis: 17 cases. *Canadian Veterinary Journal* **51**, 164–168

Bissett SA, Drobatz KJ, McKnight A and Degernes LA (2007) Prevalence, clinical features, and causes of epistaxis in dogs: 176 cases (1996–2001). *Journal of the American Veterinary Medical Association* **231**, 1843–1850

Boswood A, Lamb CR, Brockman DJ, Mantis P and Witt AL (2003) Balloon dilatation of nasopharyngeal stenosis in a cat. *Veterinary Radiology and Ultrasound* **44**, 53–55

Buiks SC and ter Haar G (2012) Reconstructive techniques of the facial area and head. In: *Reconstructive Surgery and Wound Management of the Dog and Cat*, ed. J Kirpensteijn and G ter Haar, pp. 95–116. Manson Publishing, London

Burrow R, Baker M, White L and McConnell JF (2013) Trephination of the frontal sinus and instillation of clotrimazole cream: a computed tomographic study in canine cadavers. *Veterinary Surgery* **42**, 322–328

Clercx C, Wallon J, Gilbert S, Snaps F and Coignoul F (1996) Imprint and brush cytology in the diagnosis of canine intranasal tumours. *Journal of Small Animal Practice* **37**, 423–427

Coolman BR, Marretta SM, McKiernan BC and Zachary JF (1998) Choanal atresia and secondary nasopharyngeal stenosis in a dog. *Journal of the American Animal Hospital Association* **34**, 497–501

Cox NR, Brawner WR and Powers RD (1991) Tumors of the nose and paranasal sinuses in cats: 32 cases with comparison to a national database (1977 through 1987). *Journal of the American Animal Hospital Association* **27**, 339–347

Davidson AP, Mathews KG and Koblik PD (2005) Diseases of the nose and nasal sinuses. In: *Textbook of Veterinary Internal Medicine: Diseases of the Dog and Cat, 6th edn*, ed. SJ Ettinger and EC Feldman, p. 1018. Saunders, Philadelphia

De Lorenzi D, Bertoncello D, Comastri S and Bottero E (2015) Treatment of acquired nasopharyngeal stenosis using a removable silicone stent. *Journal of Feline Medicine and Surgery* **17**, 117–124

Declercq J, Declercq L and Fincioen S (2012) Unilaterale sino-orbitale en subcutane aspergillose bij een kat. *Vlaams Diergeneeskundig Tijdschrift* **81**, 357–362

Demko JL and Cohn LA (2007) Chronic nasal discharge in cats: 75 cases (1993–2004). *Journal of the American Veterinary Medical Association* **230**, 1032–1037

Donnelly KE and Tillson DM (2004) Feline inflammatory polyps and ventral bulla osteotomy. *Compendium on Continuing Education for the Practicing Veterinarian* **26**, 446–454

Drees R, Forrest LJ and Chappell R (2009) Comparison of computed tomography and magnetic resonance imaging for the evaluation of canine intranasal neoplasia. *Journal of Small Animal Practice* **50**, 334–340

Furrow E and Groman RP (2009) Intranasal infusion of clotrimazole for the treatment of nasal aspergillosis in two cats. *Journal of the American Veterinary Medical Association* **235**, 1188–1193

Gallegos J, Schmiedt C and McAnulty JF (2007) Cosmetic rostral nasal reconstruction after nasal planum and premaxilla resection: technique and results in two dogs. *Veterinary Surgery* **36**, 669–674

Gieger T, Rassnick K, Siegel S *et al.* (2008) Palliation of clinical signs in 48 dogs with nasal carcinomas treated with coarse-fraction radiation therapy. *Journal of the American Animal Hospital Association* **44**, 116–123

Giordano C, Gianella P, Bo S *et al.* (2010) Invasive mould infections of the naso-orbital region of cats: a case involving *Aspergillus fumigatus* and an aetiological review. *Journal of Feline Medicine and Surgery* **12**, 714–723

Grosso FV, ter Haar G and Boroffka SAEB (2015) Gender, weight, and age effects on prevalance of caudal aberrant nasal turbinates in clinically healthy English bulldogs: a computed tomographic study and classification. *Veterinary Radiology and Ultrasound* **56**, 486–493

Gunnarsson L, Zakrisson G, Christensson D and Uggla A (2004) Efficacy of selamectin in the treatment of nasal mite (*Pneumonyssoides caninum*) infection in dogs. *Journal of the American Animal Hospital Association* **40**, 400–404

Hedlund CS (1998) Rhinotomy techniques. In: *Current Techniques in Small Animal Surgery*, ed. MJ Bojrab, pp.346–354. Williams & Wilkins, Baltimore

Hedlund CS (2007) Surgery of the upper respiratory system. In: *Small Animal Surgery, 3rd edn*, ed. TW Fossum, CS Hedlund, DA Hulse *et al.*, pp. 817–866. Mosby, St. Louis

Hedlund CS, Tangner CH, Elkins AD and Hobson HP (1983) Temporary bilateral carotid artery occlusion during surgical exploration of the nasal cavity of the dog. *Veterinary Surgery* **12**, 83–85

Henderson SM, Bradley K, Day MJ *et al.* (2004) Investigation of nasal disease in the cat – a retrospective study of 77 cases. *Journal of Feline Medicine and Surgery* **6**, 245–257

Holmberg DL, Fries C, Cockshutt J and Van Pelt D (1989) Ventral rhinotomy in the dog and cat. *Veterinary Surgery* **18**, 446–449

Holt D, Prymak C and Evans S (1990) Excision of tumors in the nasal vestibule of two dogs. *Veterinary Surgery* **19**, 418–423

Hunt GB, Perkins MC, Foster SF *et al.* (2002) Nasopharyngeal disorders of dogs and cats: A review and retrospective study. *Compendium on Continuing Education for the Practicing Veterinarian* **24**, 184–200

Johnson EG and Wisner ER (2007) Advances in respiratory imaging. *Veterinary Clinics of North America: Small Animal Practice* **37**, 879–900

Johnson LR, Drazenovich TL, Herrera MA and Wisner ER (2006) Results of rhinoscopy alone or in conjunction with sinuscopy in dogs with aspergillosis: 46 cases (2001–2004). *Journal of the American Veterinary Medical Association* **228**, 738–742

Kano R, Itamoto K, Okuda M *et al.* (2008) Isolation of *Aspergillus udagawae* from a fatal case of feline orbital aspergillosis. *Mycoses* **51**, 360–361

Kano R, Shibahashi A, Fujino Y and Sakai H (2013) Two cases of feline orbital aspergillosis due to *Aspergillus udagawae* and *A. viridinutans*. *Journal of Veterinary Medical Science* **75**, 7–10

Karnik K, Reichle JK, Fischetti AJ and Goggin JM (2009) Computed tomographic findings of fungal rhinitis and sinusitis in cats. *Veterinary Radiology and Ultrasound* **50**, 65–68

Kirpensteijn J, Withrow SJ and Straw RC (1994) Combined resection of the nasal planum and premaxilla in three dogs. *Veterinary Surgery* **23**, 341–346

Kuehn NF (2014) Diagnostic imaging for chronic nasal disease in dogs. *Journal of Small Animal Practice* **55**, 341–342

LaDue TA, Dodge R, Page RL *et al.* (1999) Factors influencing survival after radiotherapy of nasal tumors in 130 dogs. *Veterinary Radiology and Ultrasound* **40**, 312–317

Lawrence JA, Forrest LJ, Turek MM *et al.* (2010) Proof of principle of ocular sparing in dogs with sinonasal tumors treated with intensity-modulated radiation therapy. *Veterinary Radiology and Ultrasound* **51**, 561–570

Lefebvre J, Kuehn NF and Wortinger A (2005) Computed tomography as an aid in the diagnosis of chronic nasal disease in dogs. *Journal of Small Animal Practice* **46**, 280–285

MacEwen EG, Withrow SJ and Patnaik AK (1977) Nasal tumors in the dog: retrospective evaluation of diagnosis, prognosis, and treatment. *Journal of the American Veterinary Medical Association* **170**, 45–48

Mathews KG, Davidson AP, Koblik PD *et al.* (1988) Comparison of topical administration of clotrimazole through surgically placed *versus* nonsurgically placed catheters for treatment of nasal aspergillosis in dogs: 60 cases (1990–1996). *Journal of the American Veterinary Medical Association* **213**, 501–506

Mathews KG, Koblik PD, Richardson EF, Davidson AP and Pappagianis D (1996) Computed tomographic assessment of noninvasive intranasal infusions in dogs with fungal rhinitis. *Veterinary Surgery* **25**, 309–319

McCarthy TC (2005) Rhinoscopy: the diagnostic approach to chronic nasal disease. In: *Veterinary Endoscopy for the Small Animal Practitioner*, ed. TC McCarthy, pp. 137–200. Elsevier, St. Louis

McEntee MC (2006) Veterinary radiation therapy: review and current state of the art. *Journal of the American Animal Hospital Association* **42**, 94–109

Merveille AC, Battaille G, Billen F *et al.* (2014) Clinical findings and prevalence of the mutation associated with primary ciliary dyskinesia in old English sheepdogs. *Journal of Veterinary Internal Medicine* **28**, 771–778

Miles MS, Dhaliwal RS, Moore MP and Reed AL (2008) Association of magnetic resonance imaging findings and histologic diagnosis in dogs with nasal disease: 78 cases (2001–2004). *Journal of the American Veterinary Medical Association* **232**, 1844–1849

Mitten RW (1988) Nasopharyngeal stenosis in four cats. *Journal of Small Animal Practice* **29**, 341–345

Moore AH (2003) Use of topical povidone-iodine dressings in the management of mycotic rhinitis in three dogs. *Journal of Small Animal Practice* **44**, 326–329

Movassaghi AR and Mohri M (1988) Nasal mite of dogs *Pneumonyssus* (*Pneumonyssoides*) *caninum* in Iran. *Veterinary Record* **142**, 551–552

Mukaratirwa S, van der Linde-Sipman JS and Gruys E (2001) Feline nasal and paranasal sinus tumours: clinicopathological study, histomorphological description and diagnostic immunohistochemistry of 123 cases. *Journal of Feline Medicine and Surgery* **3**, 235–245

Novo RE and Kramek B (1999) Surgical repair of nasopharyngeal stenosis in a cat using a stent. *Journal of the American Animal Hospital Association* **35**, 251–256

Oechtering GU (2010) Brachycephalic syndrome – new information on an old congenital disease. *Veterinary Focus* **20**, 2–9

Oechtering GU, Hueber J, Kiefer I and Noeller C (2007a) Laser assisted turbinectomy (LATE) – a novel approach to brachycephalic airway syndrome. *Veterinary Surgery* **36**, E11

Oechtering GU, Hueber J, Oechtering TH and Noeller C (2007b) Laser assisted turbinectomy (LATE) – treating brachycephalic airway distress at its intranasal origin. *Veterinary Surgery* **36**, E18

Pavletic MM (2010) Facial reconstruction. In: *Atlas of Small Animal Wound Management and Reconstructive Surgery, 3rd edn*, ed. MM Pavletic, pp. 433–480. Wiley-Blackwell, Ames

Peeters D, Day MJ and Clercx C (2005) An immunohistochemical study of canine nasal aspergillosis. *Journal of Comparative Pathology* **132**, 283–288

Pownder S, Rose M and Crawford J (2006) Radiographic techniques of the nasal cavity and sinuses. *Clinical Techniques in Small Animal Practice* **21**, 46–54

Pratschke KM (2003) Inflammatory polyps of the middle ear in five dogs. *Veterinary Surgery* **32**, 292–296

Priddy NH, Pope ER, Cohn LA and Constantinescu GM (2001) Alveolar mucosal approach to the canine nasal cavity. *Journal of the American Animal Hospital Association* **37**, 179–182

Reiter AM and Holt DE (2012) Palate. In: *Veterinary Surgery: Small Animal*, ed. KM Tobias and SA Johnston, pp. 1707–1717. Elsevier Saunders, St Louis

Richardson EF and Mathews KG (1995) Distribution of topical agents in the frontal sinuses and nasal cavity of dogs: comparison between current protocols for the treatment of nasal aspergillosis and a new non-invasive technique. *Veterinary Surgery* **24**, 476–483

Russo M, Lamb CR and Jakovljevic S (2000) Distinguishing rhinitis and nasal neoplasia by radiography. *Veterinary Radiology and Ultrasound* **41**, 118–124

Saunders J, Clercx C and Snaps FR (2004) Radiographic, magnetic resonance imaging, computed tomographic, and rhinoscopic features of nasal aspergillosis in dogs. *Journal of the American Veterinary Medical Association* **225**, 1703–1712

Saunders J and Van Bree H (2003) Comparison of radiography and computed tomography for the diagnosis of canine nasal aspergillosis. *Veterinary Radiology and Ultrasound* **44**, 414–419

Schmiedt CW and Creevy KE (2012) Nasal planum, nasal cavity, and sinuses. In: *Veterinary Surgery: Small Animal*, ed. KM Tobias and SA Johnston, pp. 1691–1706. Elsevier Saunders, St Louis

Schuenemann RM and Oechtering G (2012) Cholesteatoma after lateral bulla osteotomy in two brachycephalic dogs. *Journal of the American Animal Hospital Association* **48**, 261–268

Schuenemann RM and Oechtering GU (2014a) Inside the brachycephalic nose: intranasal mucosal contact points. *Journal of the American Animal Hospital Association* **50**, 149–158

Schuenemann RM and Oechtering G (2014b) Inside the brachycephalic nose: conchal regrowth and mucosal contact points after laser-assisted turbinectomy. *Journal of the American Animal Hospital Association* **50**, 237–246

Sharman M, Paul A, Davies D *et al.* (2010) Multi-centre assessment of mycotic rhinosinusitis in dogs: a retrospective study of initial treatment success (1998 to 2008). *Journal of Small Animal Practice* **51**, 423–427

Sharp NJH, Harvey CE and O'Brien JA (1991a) Treatment of canine nasal aspergillosis/penicilliosis with fluconazole. *Journal of Small Animal Practice* **32**, 513–516

Sharp NJH, Harvey CE and Sullivan M (1991b) Canine nasal aspergillosis and penicilliosis. *Compendium on Continuing Education for the Practicing Veterinarian* **13**, 41–46

Sharp NJH, Sullivan M, Harvey CE and Webb T (1993) Treatment of canine nasal aspergillosis with enilconazole. *Journal of Veterinary Internal Medicine* **7**, 40–43

Sissener TR, Bacon NJ, Friend E, Anderson DM and White RA (2006) Combined clotrimazole irrigation and depot therapy for canine nasal aspergillosis. *Journal of Small Animal Practice* **47**, 312–315

Smith LN and Hoffman SB (2010) A case series of unilateral orbital aspergillosis in three cats and treatment with voriconazole. *Veterinary Ophthalmology* **13**, 190–203

Tasker S, Knottenbelt CM, Munro EA *et al.* (1999) Aetiology and diagnosis of persistent nasal disease in the dog: a retrospective study of 42 cases. *Journal of Small Animal Practice* **40**, 473–478

ter Haar G, Buiks SC and Kirpensteijn J (2013) Cosmetic reconstruction of a nasal plane and rostral nasal skin defect using a modified nasal rotation flap in a dog. *Veterinary Surgery* **42**, 176–179

ter Haar G and Hampel R (2015) Combined rostrolateral rhinotomy for removal of rostral nasal septum squamous cell carcinoma: long-term outcome in 10 dogs. *Veterinary Surgery* **44**, 843–851

Theon AP, Madewell BR, Harb MF and Dungworth DL (1993) Megavoltage irradiation of neoplasms of the nasal and paranasal cavities in 77 dogs. *Journal of the American Veterinary Medical Association* **202**, 1469–1475

Tomlinson MJ and Schenck NL (1975) Autogenous fat implantation as a treatment for chronic frontal sinusitis in a cat. *Journal of the American Veterinary Medical Association* **167**, 927–930

Tomsa K, Glaus TM, Zimmer C and Greene CE (2003) Fungal rhinitis and sinusitis in three cats. *Journal of the American Veterinary Medical Association* **222**, 1380–1384

Turek MM and Lana SE (2013) Nasosinal tumors. In: *Small Animal Clinical Oncology, 5th edn*, ed. SJ Withrow, DM Vail and RL Page, pp. 435–451. Elsevier Saunders, St Louis

Venker-van Haagen AJ (2005) The nose and nasal sinuses. In: *Ear, Nose, Throat, and Tracheobronchial Diseases in Dogs and Cat*, ed. AJ Venker-van Haagen, pp. 51–81. Schlütersche, Hannover

White D (2006) Canine nasal mycosis – light at the end of a long diagnostic and therapeutic tunnel. *Journal of Small Animal Practice* **47**, 307

Whitney J, Beatty JA, Martin P *et al.* (2013) Evaluation of serum galactomannan detection for diagnosis of feline upper respiratory tract aspergillosis. *Veterinary Microbiology* **162**, 180–185

Wiestner TS, Koch DA, Nad N *et al.* (2007) Evaluation of the repeatability of rhinomanometry and its use in assessing transnasal resistance and pressure in dogs. *American Journal of Veterinary Research* **68**, 178–184

Wilkinson GT, Sutton RH and Grono LR (1982) *Aspergillus* spp. infection associated with orbital cellulitis and sinusitis in a cat. *Journal of Small Animal Practice* **23**, 127–131

Willard MD and Radlinsky MA (1999) Endoscopic examination of the choanae in dogs and cats: 118 cases (1988–1998). *Journal of the American Veterinary Medical Association* **215**, 1301–1305

Windsor RC, Johnson LR, Herrgesell EJ and De Cock HEV (2004) Idiopathic lymphoplasmacytic rhinitis in dogs: 37 cases (1997–2002). *Journal of the American Veterinary Medical Association* **224**, 1952–1957

Withrow SJ (2013) Cancer of the nasal planum. In: *Small Animal Clinical Oncology, 5th edn*, ed. SJ Withrow, DM Vail and RL Page, pp. 432–435. Elsevier Saunders, St Louis

Withrow SJ and Straw RC (1990) Resection of the nasal planum in nine cats and five dogs. *Journal of the American Animal Hospital Association* **26**, 219–222

Wolf AM and Troy GC (1995) Deep mycotic diseases. In: *Textbook of Veterinary Internal Medicine, 4th edn*, ed. SJ Ettinger and EC Feldman, pp. 455–458. WB Saunders, Philadelphia

Zonderland J-L, Störk CK, Saunders JH *et al.* (2002) Intranasal infusion of enilconazole for treatment of sinonasal aspergillosis in dogs. *Journal of the American Veterinary Medical Association* **221**, 1421–1425

OPERATIVE TECHNIQUE 4.1

Dorsal rhinotomy

PATIENT POSITIONING

The patient is positioned in sternal recumbency, with the dorsum of the head clipped and prepared aseptically for surgery. The tip of the nose should be pointing down slightly to facilitate blood exiting the nose, and a roll of bandage material is positioned between the upper and lower jaws to prevent injury to the soft tissues of the oral cavity caused by pressure from the teeth while performing the rhinotomy.

ASSISTANT

Optional.

SURGICAL TECHNIQUE

Approach

A dorsal midline skin incision is made from the caudal aspect of the nasal planum to the medial canthus of the eye for both unilateral and bilateral rhinotomy. For sinusotomy, the incision is extended caudal to the zygomatic crests of the frontal bone.

Surgical manipulations

1 The subcutaneous tissue and periosteum are sharply incised on the midline and elevated and reflected laterally on either or both sides of the nasal cavity with small periosteal elevators to expose the entire nasal bone.

2 Stay sutures can be placed through the skin and subcutis to aid in retraction. A rectangular window of bone should be exposed to allow for removal of the nasal bone and part of the frontal bone. The bone flap should be as narrow as possible, yet allow for the introduction of large curettes and rapid turbinectomy. In small dogs, part of the maxillary bone adjacent to the nasal bone can be removed if needed. →

→ OPERATIVE TECHNIQUE 4.1 CONTINUED

3 With an osteotome and mallet the bone flap is outlined first, by not cutting completely full thickness. Once this has been done, the incisions can be quickly deepened and the nasal cavity opened to immediately address any bleeding associated with the osteotomy itself. Alternatively, a sagittal saw can be used.

4 The nasal cavity is then systematically explored gently for foreign body removal or if biopsy specimens of specific areas are to be taken. Material is also harvested for culture and sensitivity testing.

5 Complete turbinectomy or nasal exenteration is then performed using a large bone or uterine curette that should follow the inside of the maxillary bone ventrally and scoop back a large amount of turbinate material. As haemorrhage will occur at this stage, curettage should be as swift and targeted as possible.

6 Once haemorrhage has reduced to minimal oozing, the rhinotomy site can be closed.

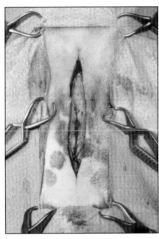

A midline incision is created over the nose through the skin and subcutis.

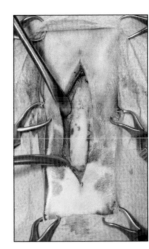

The incision is deepened to the level of the bone in the midline and the periosteum is elevated over the nasal bone of the side that requires exploration and turbinectomy.

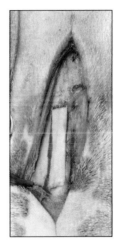

A rectangular flap of bone is outlined with rongeurs prior to full-thickness resection.

PRACTICAL TIP

Care should be taken to avoid damaging the cribriform plate caudomedially. Specific attention needs to be paid to removal of the rostral parts of the dorsal and maxillary turbinates within the nasal vestibule and in ensuring a patent nasopharyngeal meatus

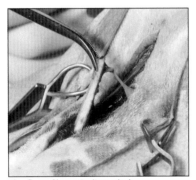

The flap of bone is discarded.

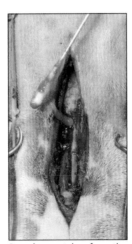

Samples are taken from the nasal cavity for cytology, culture and sensitivity testing.

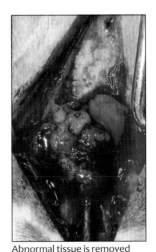

Abnormal tissue is removed with the associated turbinates using a large curette.

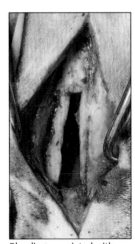

Bleeding associated with turbinectomy stops once all abnormal tissue and turbinates have been removed.

PRACTICAL TIP

Bleeding usually stops once turbinectomy is complete, but any ongoing haemorrhage is best controlled by direct pressure from gauze packing. After removal of the gauzes, active bleeding can usually be controlled with direct electrocautery, using metal Frazier or Adson suction cannulae as the conductor whilst 'fixating' the end of the vessel with the tip of the suction tube and clearing the surgical area of blood at the same time

→ **OPERATIVE TECHNIQUE 4.1 CONTINUED**

Closure

The periosteum is closed with 2–3 metric (2/0–3/0 USP) absorbable monofilament suture material in an interrupted pattern, followed by the subcutaneous tissues and skin in a routine fashion.

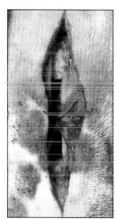

The periosteum is closed over the bony defect with simple interrupted sutures.

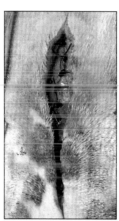

Complete closure of the periosteum and partial closure of the subcutaneous tissue.

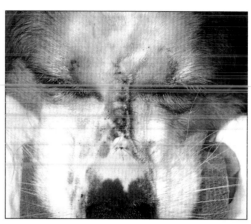

The skin is closed with simple interrupted sutures.

POSTOPERATIVE CARE

Routine analgesia and antibiotics based on culture and sensitivity results are required. Monitor for early postoperative complications including pneumocephalus and septic meningoencephalitis, subcutaneous emphysema, failure to mouth breathe, aspiration pneumonia, persistent anorexia and pain.

Chapter 5

Surgery of the ear

Karen M. Tobias and Christine Cain

Anatomy

The pinna of the ear gives dogs their distinctive look. Despite massive phenotypic variation among different breeds, the basic structure is the same for all. The auricular cartilage that forms the pinna is divided into two portions: a flat scapha and a tubular concha. A transverse fold on the concave base of the auricular cartilage, the antihelix, separates the two portions of the pinna. The cartilage of the pinna contains many small perforations that allow blood vessels and nerves to penetrate from the outer concave surface to the inner convex surface of the ear.

Trauma to the ear results in rupture of these blood vessels and significant haemorrhage or haematoma formation.

The external ear canal is formed by three overlapping tubes. The auricular cartilage, which is funnel-shaped at its base, twists and bends to form the majority of the vertical ear canal and the proximal portion of the horizontal ear canal. Its base surrounds and overlaps the annular cartilage, a ring of cartilage that forms the majority of the horizontal ear canal (Figure 5.1). The annular cartilage, in turn, overlaps the external acoustic meatus, a short bony extension of the skull that connects the cartilaginous ear canal to the tympanic cavity. These three tubes are

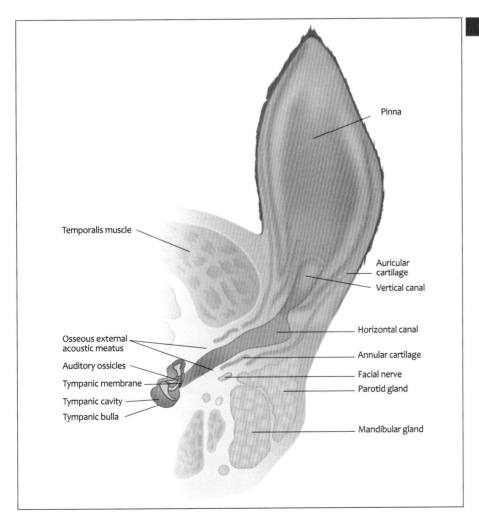

5.1 Anatomy of the canine external ear.

connected by fibrous tissue, permitting more movement and flexibility of the ear. The junctions of these tubes may be the sites of canal rupture and drainage when para-auricular abscesses and fistulae form.

The air-filled middle ear is separated from the external ear canal by the tympanic membrane; the middle ear is connected to the nasopharynx by the auditory, or Eustachian, tube. Within a small dorsal recess are the tiny auditory bones (ossicles) – the malleus, incus and stapes – that transmit sound vibrations. In the cat, a bony septum separates the dorsolateral portion of the tympanic bulla and the ossicles from the larger ventromedial tympanic cavity. A partial septum may also be seen in canine bullae (Figure 5.2). Across from the opening of the external ear canal are the cochlear (round) and vestibular (oval) windows, the openings to the inner ear, where the organs of hearing (cochlea) and balance (utriculus, sacculus and semicircular canals) reside. In the cat, the cochlear window is found in a gap within the septum between the two bulla compartments.

Innervation

The facial nerve exits the skull through the stylomastoid foramen, an opening just caudal to the external acoustic meatus. It splits into several branches after exiting the skull, but the major portion of the nerve continues rostrally to the face, travelling under and around the horizontal ear canal. Midway up the rostral surface of the ear canal, it splits into branches to the lower and upper lips, eyelids and front half of the pinna. From a lateral view the ear canal is almost completely surrounded by the nerve and its branches, making dissection without nerve damage very challenging.

Vasculature

The external carotid artery lies just ventral to the horizontal ear canal. Its caudal auricular branch travels up the caudal surface of the canal to the pinna. Damage to this vessel can result in necrosis and sloughing of the caudal half of the ear flap. The external carotid artery continues rostrally before splitting into superficial temporal and maxillary branches. The superficial temporal artery provides blood supply to the front half of the pinna. It is helpful to palpate for the external carotid artery and its branches during total ear canal ablation, since damage to this artery during dissection causes significant blood loss.

Surgery of the pinna

Because of its exposed position, the pinna is easily traumatized by animals and objects in the environment. Additionally, many dogs have the habit of vigorously shaking their heads and whipping their ears about, which can cause pinnal damage. Blood supply to the pinna is quite extensive, and blood loss can be dramatic and frightening to owners, although it is usually easily controlled with pressure. To prevent excessive bleeding and to improve visualization of the pinna, some veterinary surgeons (veterinarians) use lasers or cautery during dissection or resection.

Lacerations and defects

Treatment depends on the extent of the laceration and whether it is partial or full thickness.

- Linear lacerations of the skin usually heal by second intention, as long as the skin is still firmly attached to the underlying cartilage. If the skin becomes elevated from the cartilage, as in an L-shaped tear, it should be closed with simple interrupted skin sutures. Dead space, if present, can be closed with a continuous suction drain or mattress sutures placed through the

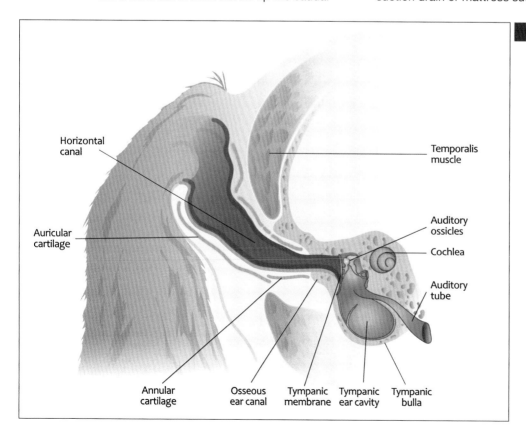

5.2 Anatomy of the canine bulla.

Horizontal canal

Temporalis muscle

Auricular cartilage

Auditory ossicles

Cochlea

Auditory tube

Annular cartilage

Osseous ear canal

Tympanic membrane

Tympanic ear cavity

Tympanic bulla

skin and underlying cartilage, as with treatment of aural haematomas (see below).

- Lacerations that extend through the underlying cartilage can be closed with simple interrupted sutures if the cartilage is not displaced, or can be pulled together with vertical mattress sutures, with the deeper bites of each stitch apposing the cartilage layer.
- Full-thickness lacerations require closure of both skin surfaces, using either a simple interrupted pattern on each side of the pinna or a simple interrupted pattern on one side and a vertical mattress pattern to realign the cartilage and skin on the other side.

Marginal defects

Defects of the pinna margins can be corrected by amputation of the affected part. For large defects, a pedicle flap can be used to replace the edge.

Partial amputation: A curved incision is made with a scalpel, cautery or laser along the margin, to excise as little tissue as possible. The medial and lateral skin edges are pulled together with 1.5 metric (4/0 USP) non-absorbable suture material in a continuous pattern. The ear is bandaged against the head or neck to prevent further trauma until the sutures can be removed.

Pedicle flap procedure: The pinna is brought to the side of the neck or face to determine which site will provide the most acceptable cosmetic appearance, based on hair length, the colour and direction of hair growth, and the least tension.

After aseptic preparation of the pinna, a small portion of the defect margin is removed to freshen and straighten the edges. If the pinna is thin, the defect can be left unsutured, covered with antibiotic ointment, and bandaged for 7 days to allow the skin of the pinna to thicken and become more vascular. Bandages are changed as needed to allow inspection of the margin.

Once the pinna is ready for closure, the pinna and donor site are aseptically prepared, and the margins of the pinna are debrided sparingly. The pinna is placed next to the donor site, and the outline of the defect is incised at the site. The outer skin of the defect is sutured to the elevated flap, and the pinna and site are gently bandaged. After 2 weeks, the flap is excised to free the pinna.

Medial defects

The medial portion of the pinna can be treated in several ways:

- Small defects can be allowed to heal by second intention
- For larger defects that cover the medial and lateral surfaces, a pedicle flap (described above) can be used. Once the flap has healed to the lateral margin, it is transected from its base such that the excess can be folded over and sutured to the pinna medially to cover any raw surfaces. This technique may cause obstruction of the blood vessels in the flap at the folded edge, leading to necrosis
- Alternatively, the original pedicle flap can be severed at 2 weeks and a second pedicle flap from the top of the head applied to its raw medial surface. The ear is bandaged in place for an additional 10–14 days until the second flap is cut down.

Aural haematomas

Pathophysiology

Aural haematomas are thought to be secondary to trauma. Vigorous head shaking in dogs with external ear canal irritation causes separation of the skin of the inner pinna from the cartilage, or separation between the cartilage layers or between the perichondrium and cartilage. The tiny vessels that perforate the cartilage rupture and bleed until pressure builds up sufficiently to stop the haemorrhage. If the dog continues to shake its head, further separation of the pinna layers allows continued or progressive accumulation of blood and clots.

Not all dogs and cats with aural haematomas have otitis externa (OE), and 15–45% of affected animals may have no evidence of external ear canal disease. Because head shaking is thought to be the underlying traumatic event that leads to haemorrhage, otoscopic and dermatological examinations and ear and skin cytology should be performed on all affected animals to rule out or diagnose predisposing conditions.

In animals with aural haematomas, the pinna is often infiltrated with eosinophils and mast cells. This suggests that many of the affected animals have underlying hypersensitivity. Fluid within the haematoma usually contains a low percentage of red blood cells, a few inflammatory cells and a moderate amount of protein. Fibrin, blood clots and other debris may also be present. Cartilage around the haematoma degenerates, and fibrovascular granulation tissue fills the defects, thickening the pinna and encouraging distortion of its shape during healing.

Conservative treatment

Conservative treatment involves drainage and flushing of the haematoma, either through a small incision or with a large needle, and administration of corticosteroids systemically or into the haematoma cavity. This may work best for small, acute haematomas. Two different protocols for steroid instillation have been used. It is important to keep in mind that recurrence of aural haematomas following drainage, with or without local infusion of corticosteroids, is common, and surgical intervention may be necessary for successful management of recurrent cases (Hall *et al.*, 2016).

After aseptic preparation of the pinna, the haematoma cavity can be aspirated with a 16 G needle and then flushed with physiological saline and reaspirated gently multiple times until the fluid becomes clear. The cavity is then injected once daily with dexamethasone (0.25 mg/kg diluted in sterile saline to 0.5–1 ml), or weekly with methylprednisolone acetate (0.5–1 ml) until the haematoma resolves. Injections must be performed using sterile technique to prevent infection. Bandaging of the ear is not necessary except to seal the drain hole or to prevent vigorous shaking (Kuwahara, 1986). Similar results are seen when steroids are administered systemically to animals after needle or incisional drainage of the ear. Haematomas treated with daily intralesional or systemic injections of dexamethasone usually heal within 3–6 days. Animals that receive intralesional methylprednisolone acetate may require a second or third injection, but most cases resolve with a single treatment (Kuwahara, 1986).

Surgical drainage

A variety of techniques have been proposed.

The haematoma can be drained and flushed through a long, S-shaped incision on the concave surface of the pinna. The pinna layers are then apposed with full-thickness mattress sutures placed parallel to the long axis of the pinna and avoiding blood vessels. Overtightening must be avoided because postoperative swelling is likely. A gap is left at the incision to allow continued drainage of the haematoma, and the ear is bandaged down across the neck or up over the head to prevent self-trauma and absorb additional fluid.

Other options for treatment include: fenestration of the medial pinna over the haematoma, using a carbon dioxide laser to make multiple drainage holes; passive drainage with a teat cannula placed through a stab incision at the apex of the haematoma, or a through-and-through Penrose drain; and continuous suction drainage with a closed system (Figure 5.3). Fenestrated silicone drains have been placed with a two-incision technique, first to introduce the drain into the haematoma cavity from the convex surface of the pinna and then to exit it at the base of the pinna through the cervical skin (Pavletic, 2015). The drain is sutured in place, attached to a commercial suction bulb (e.g. Jackson Pratt) and left for 18–21 days; during this time the dog wears an Elizabethan collar but does not require bandaging of the pinna.

- To make a small continuous suction drain, the syringe adaptor end of a 19 G butterfly catheter is removed and the remaining tube is fenestrated to a length slightly shorter than the haematoma cavity. Fenestrations are made by folding the tube over and cutting off a corner of the fold to make a hole less than 50% of the tube's diameter.
- The fenestrated portion of the tube is then inserted into the haematoma cavity through a stab incision on the concave surface of the ear.
- The stab incision is closed around the tube with a purse-string or mattress suture, and the tube is secured to the pinna with a fingertrap pattern or butterfly tape and mattress sutures.
- The needle end of the tube is inserted into a vacuum blood tube. If the vacuum blood tube loses its suction because of air introduction, it can be 'recharged' by using a needle and syringe to suction the air out of the blood tube.
- The ear is bandaged against the dog's head or neck, and the vacuum tube is changed as needed to maintain continuous suction and compression of the haematoma cavity.
- The tube is usually removed no sooner than 1 week after placement, and then the bandage is left in place for another week.

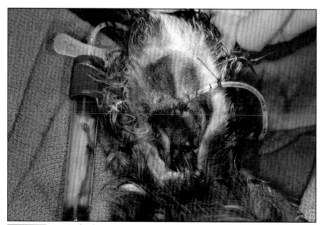

5.3 Auricular haematoma treated with oral steroids and a continuous suction drain made from a fenestrated butterfly catheter and vacuum tube. After the drain was placed, the dog's ear was affixed to its head with tape and a bandage to prevent head shaking.

Prognosis: Resolution occurs in 60–83% of dogs and cats after surgical drainage. Owners should be warned that cosmetic results can be variable, with some animals suffering thickening, longitudinal contraction or abnormal carriage of the pinna. Success for the surgical incision technique is best when drainage is maintained for more than 7–10 days and when the OE or underlying cause of aural pruritus is treated. Some surgeons recommend concurrent use of systemic corticosteroids (prednisolone: 1 mg/kg q12h for 2 weeks, then q24h for 2 weeks, then tapered) to help reduce inflammation and predisposing causes of pruritus and otitis.

Other pinnal conditions
Pinnal neoplasia
Various tumour types may occur on the pinna of dogs or cats, including histiocytomas, plasmacytomas, mast cell tumours, melanocytomas/melanomas, papilloma, haemangioma and squamous cell carcinoma. Squamous cell carcinoma of the pinna is most often encountered in white cats as a sequela to chronic actinic damage of the skin. Although round cell tumours of the pinna most often present as discrete nodules, squamous cell carcinoma (and its precursors, actinic keratosis and carcinoma *in situ*) may present as erythema, swelling, crusts and erosions or ulcers. Presurgical evaluation of tumours of the pinna may include fine-needle aspirates for cytological assessment, incisional biopsy for histopathology and staging procedures such as aspirates of local lymph nodes and thoracic radiographs.

The type of surgical procedure planned (e.g. marginal excision, partial pinnectomy or radical pinnectomy) will depend on the tumour type. Surgical resection is not typically recommended for canine histiocytomas because the vast majority will regress within 3 months (Clifford *et al.*, 2013). The outcome of surgical resection of pinnal neoplasms depends on tumour type and behaviour. For example, dogs with low-grade (grade 1 or grade 2) pinnal mast cell tumours have been shown to have a prolonged survival time following excision, whilst dogs with high-grade (grade 3) mast cell tumours had a more guarded prognosis and a median survival time of 10 months following surgical excision (Schwab *et al.*, 2014). A recent study of cats with pinnal squamous cell carcinoma reported a better response to surgical excision (radical pinnectomy with or without total ear canal ablation) in cats with actinic keratosis or squamous cell carcinoma restricted to the distal portion of the pinna than in cats with tumour extension to the proximal portion of the pinna and ear canal (Demirutku *et al.*, 2012). In that study, three of the eight cats had relapse of the tumour at the surgical site.

Pinnectomy for squamous cell carcinoma: For subtotal pinnectomy, the pinna is amputated with curved Mayo scissors at least 1–2 cm from the visible margin of the mass, ulceration or crusting. Haemostasis is achieved with cautery. The skin of the convex and concave surfaces is then sutured together. For complete pinnectomy, the skin is incised near the base along the convex surface of the ear and allowed to retract away from the pinna cartilage. The cartilage and the skin of the concave surface of the ear are transected with scissors. If skin apposition results in tension, the caudomedial edge of the wound can be elevated and advanced, or a single pedicle advancement flap is developed, to allow suture closure of the wound.

Pinnal necrosis

Necrosis of the pinna may be secondary to a number of underlying conditions, including ischaemic damage (vasculitis, proliferative thrombovascular necrosis of the pinna, cryoglobulinaemia) or frostbite (Halliwell, 2013). Clinical features of pinnal necrosis include cyanotic skin that is cool to the touch, sloughing skin, wedge-shaped ulcers of the pinnal tip or margin, bleeding and a deformed notched appearance to the pinnal margin. Management of pinnal necrosis relies upon identification and control of the underlying cause. Medical management of conditions such as pinnal margin vasculitis typically includes use of immunomodulatory medications and the rheological agent pentoxifylline. If necrosis is extensive or if bleeding of the pinnal tips or margins cannot be controlled with medical therapy alone, resection of the affected portions of the pinna via partial or complete pinnectomy may be indicated.

Otitis externa and media

Otitis is a very common extension of cutaneous inflammatory disease in dogs, though less so in cats. For descriptive purposes, it is often categorized as acute OE, chronic/recurrent OE and otitis media (OM). Clinically, the term otitis most often implies the presence of a bacterial or fungal infection, although sterile otitis can result from mass lesions (tumours, inflammatory polyps, foreign bodies), parasites, allergic diseases and irritating chemical or mechanical cleansing regimens. Primary secretory otitis media (PSOM) or otitis media with effusion (OME) is a breed-related condition resulting in sterile middle ear effusion and is recognized primarily in the Cavalier King Charles Spaniel (Cole, 2012). A similar condition has been reported in brachycephalic animals and is presumed to be the result of auditory tube dysfunction caused by anatomical differences in the position and shape of the tympanic bulla and auditory tube, and respiratory tract mucosal swelling (Hayes *et al.*, 2010). Bacterial and fungal (yeast) infections of the ear canals are thought to be secondary problems in the overwhelming majority of cases, and it is of utmost importance to control the primary otic disease in order to curtail repeated infections.

Aetiology

In cases of recurrent infection, all potential predisposing factors and direct/indirect causes of otic inflammation and immunosuppression must be considered. Infection may result when inflammation is persistent within the external auditory canal, regardless of the inciting cause. However, chronic/recurrent infectious otitis is most commonly associated with an uncontrolled primary allergic disease (e.g. atopy, adverse food reaction), endocrinopathy or iatrogenic immunosuppression. Chronic OE may lead to progressive pathological changes – such as glandular hyperplasia, fibrosis and osseous metaplasia – that necessitate surgical intervention. In such cases (referred to as 'end-stage otitis'), surgery may be the only option for correction of stenosis and the intractable secondary infections that result from a disrupted auditory canal microclimate.

OM, defined as inflammation of the tympanic bulla, is a common sequel to severe or chronic OE. Primary OM is thought to be rare in dogs but is implicated in cats with inflammatory polypoid disease (see below). Middle ear effusion in dogs and cats may also occur secondary to sinonasal or nasopharyngeal disease, presumably due to secondary dysfunction of the auditory tube (Detweiler *et al.*, 2006; Shanaman *et al.*, 2012; Foster *et al.*, 2015). In most instances, OM in dogs is thought to result from the extension of inflammatory disease from the external auditory canal into the bulla via a perforated tympanic membrane.

Diagnosis

The status of the tympanic membranes should be confirmed in all cases of chronic/recurrent otitis. If oedema or proliferative changes preclude visualization of the entire external canal to the level of the tympanum, topical antimicrobial therapy for the infection should be initiated, based upon cytological findings, and the patient should be discharged on an anti-inflammatory regimen of oral glucocorticoids. The potential for ototoxicity with topical antimicrobials (such as aminoglycosides) should be considered, particularly if the tympanic membrane cannot be visualized prior to initiating therapy (Oishi *et al.*, 2012). The patient should then be returned for otoscopic evaluation in 2–4 weeks.

It is not uncommon for a tympanic membrane to appear to be intact upon otoscopic examination, due to spontaneous repair, a subtle tear or poor visibility during otoscopy. The newer fibreoptic otoscopes, when compared with conventional otoscopes, allow superior visualization of deep structures. They provide magnification and a bright light source at the level of the tympanum, which may reveal tympanic defects that would have otherwise been missed with conventional otoscopes (Figure 5.4).

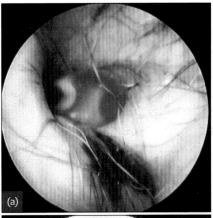
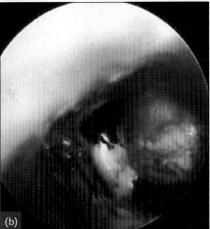

5.4 Otoscopic examination. (a) Normal tympanic membrane. (b) Ruptured membrane. As is often the case, the diseased tympanum is tearing away from its rostral attachment to the manubrium. This may be interpreted as an intact tympanum if the otoscopic visual field is obscured or the light source is poor.

Even with improved visual access, the diagnosis of OM can be quite challenging in the face of an intact tympanum. Collection of a culture sample from the bulla (via myringotomy when necessary) has been shown to be the most reliable method for diagnosis of bacterial or fungal otitis media, and superior to imaging techniques (Cole *et al.*, 2002). Sampling via myringotomy may be safely achieved by passing a sterile spinal needle through a sterilized otoscopic speculum to puncture the tympanic membrane.

Samples for cytology and culture/sensitivity testing are then collected from the tympanic bulla in a similar manner, using a micro-tip culturette. The external canal should be lavaged with sterile saline to clear exudates prior to passage of the speculum, to maintain as much asepsis of its internal surface as possible.

Indications for advanced imaging

Imaging studies can be helpful in any patient with chronic OE, particularly those with chronic pathological changes of the ear canals (e.g. glandular and epidermal hyperplasia, stenosis, suspected mineralization of the soft tissues of the ear canal) to evaluate for evidence of OM or osteomyelitis of the tympanic bulla: fluid within the tympanic bulla, sclerosis, or lysis/erosion of the wall of the tympanic bulla (Doust *et al.*, 2007). Advanced imaging studies are also useful to determine the presence or extent of suspected or known obstructive masses (i.e. neoplastic masses or inflammatory polyps), extension of middle ear disease to the petrous temporal bone or temporomandibular joint (particularly in patients presenting with reluctance to chew or open the mouth) or communication between abscesses or fistulous tracts and the ear canal (Bischoff and Kneller, 2004; Doust *et al.*, 2007). Other indications for advanced imaging include neurological signs consistent with OM/otitis interna (OI) (vestibular dysfunction, facial nerve paresis or paralysis, Horner's syndrome) or suspicion of brainstem abscessation or meningoencephalitis secondary to OM/OI (altered mentation, multiple cranial nerve deficits, seizures, gait abnormalities) (Sturges *et al.*, 2006; Martin-Vaquero *et al.*, 2011). Advanced imaging is also indicated to confirm middle ear effusion in Cavalier King Charles Spaniels with suspected PSOM. Clinical signs suspicious for PSOM may include head shaking or ear scratching, hearing loss, peripheral vestibular signs, facial nerve paresis or paralysis, frequent yawning, or bulging of the pars flaccida on otoscopic examination (Cole, 2012); affected dogs may present with only some of these clinical signs.

Available imaging modalities include bulla radiographs, computed tomography (CT), magnetic resonance imaging (MRI) or ultrasonography. CT is typically considered to be the ideal imaging modality to assess the tympanic bulla (Bischoff and Kneller, 2004). Radiography of the tympanic bulla is widely available, even to clinicians in primary care practice, but its utility may be limited to evaluation for mineralization of the ear canal or changes to the bone of the tympanic bulla. Interpretation of radiographs may be difficult owing to the need for precise positioning and the potential for superimposition of soft tissue structures (King *et al.*, 2007). Ultrasonography is also a readily available tool, and can potentially be performed without the need for sedation or general anaesthesia. The repeatability of ultrasound examination for detection of fluid within the tympanic bulla or changes to the bulla wall may be poor, however, and in cats visualization of the dorsal compartment of the tympanic bulla via ultrasonography may be limited (Dickie *et al.*, 2003; Doust *et al.*, 2007; King *et al.*,

2007). MRI is the modality of choice for differentiation of central vestibular disease and peripheral vestibular disease, and is also indicated when intracranial abscessation or meningoencephalitis as a sequela to OM/OI is suspected (Bischoff and Kneller, 2004; Sturges *et al.*, 2006; Martin-Vaquero *et al.*, 2011).

Medical treatment

Medical regimens for the successful treatment of infectious otitis may vary widely, depending upon the degree of pathological changes of the external ear canals, the status of the tympanic membranes and the specific microorganisms involved. Chronic OM is especially problematic, as impaction of the bulla can be difficult to resolve, and these cases often involve antibiotic-resistant bacteria. The continuing emergence of resistant *Pseudomonas aeruginosa* and *Staphylococcus* spp. is one of the most threatening factors to the successful practice of otology, and the spectrum of antimicrobial drugs capable of eliminating these organisms has been decreasing.

In addition to specific antimicrobial therapy, lavage of the middle ear cavity via a polypropylene or red rubber catheter inserted through the external auditory canal is considered by most veterinary dermatologists to be an important adjunct in the management of OM. In the case of bulla impaction with inflammatory exudates and debris, medical failure is virtually guaranteed without a thorough lavage. Prior to the advent of fibreoptic otoscopes, many cases of chronic OM with impaction or resistant bacterial infection were subjected to bulla osteotomy for curettage and lavage. However, fibreoptic otoscopes allow more efficient high-flow lavage through a working channel in the speculum. Additionally, an arthroscopic attachment will allow direct visualization of the bulla interior. Aggressive bulla lavage, when followed by long-term high-volume topical therapy, generally together with systemic antimicrobials based on middle ear culture and susceptibility, has been associated with an 82% rate of resolution for chronic OM, with a median time to resolution of 117 days (Palmeiro *et al.*, 2004). In some cases of OM associated with multi drug-resistant bacteria (particularly *P. aeruginosa*), oral antimicrobial options can be limited. In these cases, bulla lavage coupled with long-term high-volume topical therapy alone can be effective for resolution of chronic OM (Palmeiro *et al.*, 2004).

Indications for surgery

Despite the best efforts of the veterinary surgeon and owner, some cases will progress to end-stage otitis (Figure 5.5) due to progressive pathological changes that result in irreversible stenosis of the external auditory canals, and tissue ablation will then be necessary. Medically intractable OM due to impaction or resistant infection is also an indication for surgical intervention. For example, the American Cocker Spaniel is especially problematic. This breed is not only predisposed to allergic skin disease and idiopathic seborrhoea (both of which often contribute to intractable inflammation), but also responds to the inflammation differently from other breeds. These spaniels rapidly develop marked glandular hyperplasia of the external canals and may progress to end-stage otitis in as little as 2–3 months.

For any dog with end-stage OE, a total ear canal ablation (TECA) is the preferred method of treatment. Concurrent bulla osteotomy is mandatory, as persistent OM will continue to produce inflammatory exudates that no

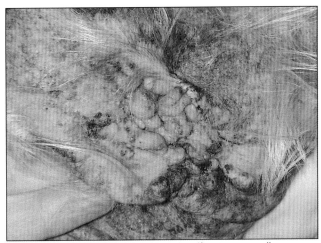

5.5 End-stage otitis in a Cocker Spaniel/Miniature Poodle crossbreed that had undergone lateral wall resection, with complete blockade of the ear canal opening. The obstructive tissue was a combination of hyperplastic glandular tissue with associated osseous metaplasia.

longer have a drainage pathway, and abscessation with fistulous tracts through soft tissues of the head is inevitable. In a minority of chronic otitis cases, the horizontal portion of the external canal will be deemed salvageable, and the surgeon may elect to ablate only the vertical canal. Conversely, a lateral wall resection may be chosen in cases where both the vertical and horizontal portions are fairly healthy, but continued episodes of otitis are expected. Lateral wall resections allow for improved air circulation and moisture evaporation and may also improve the owner's ability to medicate the ear. It must be stressed, however, that any procedure short of TECA is subject to failure if the veterinary surgeon is unable to prevent or successfully manage continuing episodes of otitis and secondary infection. Therefore, the early identification of candidates that might benefit from subtotal ablative procedures is recommended.

A more sound indication for lateral wall resection is the prophylactic surgical treatment of congenital anatomical abnormalities, such as infantile stenosis of the external canals (most commonly seen in the Shar-Pei) and excessively hirsute canals (most common in the Standard Poodle and some terrier breeds). In either situation, poor aeration and water trapping may result in recurrent OE without any underlying inflammatory disease. Improving the local microclimate of the canals by excising the lateral walls may be the only treatment necessary.

Surgical procedures

Lateral ear canal resection

Lateral ear canal resection, also known as lateral wall resection or Zepp's procedure, involves removal of most of the lateral wall of the vertical ear canal and the formation of a ventral cartilaginous and epithelial 'drainage board'. Lateral resections will improve the environment and drainage of the canal and facilitate application of topical medications. They may also be useful for removal of small benign tumours involving the lateral surface of the vertical ear canal.

Preoperative assessment: Appropriate patient selection is critical to success; many dogs with severe proliferative OE will progress despite improvements made to the canal

by lateral resection. Owners of pets with otitis secondary to other causes, particularly uncontrolled allergic dermatitis, should be warned that lateral ear canal resection is not curative and that continued local and systemic treatment will be necessary to control the disease. Lateral ear canal resection is usually unsuccessful in Cocker Spaniels with OE, even if surgery is performed before hyperplastic changes occur, because of disease progression despite medical treatment.

A thorough physical and dermatological examination should be performed to evaluate the animal's health and to look for evidence of underlying skin disease. The ear canals should be palpated and examined to verify that they are not mineralized or proliferative. If OM is suspected, radiography or CT of the bulla should be performed. OM can be present without radiographic changes, so a careful examination of the tympanic membrane under anaesthesia is warranted. Cytological assessment of the ear canal should be performed in all cases to guide topical antimicrobial therapy; culture of the deep external ear canal may also be considered, particularly if the animal has a history of recurrent or unresolved bacterial infections.

Surgical technique: Details of this procedure are given in Operative Technique 5.1. If OM is present, a myringotomy or ventral bulla osteotomy can be performed so that the tympanic bulla can be cultured and gently flushed.

Postoperative complications: The most common complications include dehiscence of the surgery site and progression of disease, particularly in patients with an uncontrolled or poorly controlled primary cause of otic inflammation. Dehiscence occurs in about 25% of patients because of self-trauma, tension, infection or poor technique. Extensive flap dehiscence that is not repaired may result in stenosis of the new opening. Stenosis can also occur with inadequate ventral reflection of the cartilage flap; this will require revision to prevent canal obstruction and subsequent otitis and fistulation. It may be necessary occasionally to clip the hair around the opening to improve ventilation and drainage.

Prognosis: Excellent results are seen in 41–50% of animals treated with lateral ear canal resection, but many of these patients will still require continued treatment to prevent recurrence of otitis. Animals that have congenital stenosis of the ear canal without hyperplastic changes usually have excellent outcomes. Ear disease will inevitably progress in Cocker Spaniels and in cases where the underlying cause of otitis has not been controlled, and many of these animals will require TECA within a few years.

Vertical ear canal resection

As with lateral resection, vertical ear canal resection alters the temperature and humidity of the ear canal environment, improves drainage and provides access to the horizontal ear canal to facilitate application of topical medications. Vertical resection is usually performed to remove tumours or polyps of the vertical ear canal that cannot be completely excised with a lateral resection. Vertical resection has also been used in animals with persistent or recurrent OE, as long as the horizontal ear canal is patent. Vertical resection removes more inflamed tissue, and is associated with less postoperative discharge and pain, fewer complications, and better healing and cosmetic appearance than lateral resection, although it can cause drooping of erect ears.

Preoperative assessment: Patient evaluation and prep-aration should be performed as for a lateral ear canal resection. Because the horizontal ear canal is often obstructed by hyperplastic tissue, it may be difficult to assess whether a vertical resection will be sufficient or whether TECA is needed.

Surgical technique: Details of this procedure are given in Operative Technique 5.2.

Postoperative complications: The most common compli-cations include dehiscence and stenosis. Primary repair of dehiscence is essential to prevent secondary stenosis and subsequent OM and fistulation. Facial nerve palsy and infection are uncommon, and most owners are satisfied with the cosmetic results.

Prognosis: Excellent results have been reported in 72–95% of dogs and cats. In one series, 95% of animals with end-stage OE were reported to be improved by the procedure, even when the horizontal canal, whilst still patent, was hyperplastic (McCarthy and Caywood, 1992). Operated patients still require continued therapy for otitis or its underlying causes, but they may require less fre-quent treatments. Animals that develop occlusion of the horizontal ear canal will need TECA and bulla osteotomy to resolve clinical signs.

Total ear canal ablation with lateral bulla osteotomy

TECA with lateral bulla osteotomy is an extremely chal-lenging procedure; supervised training and practice should be obtained by the veterinary surgeon before offer-ing this procedure to clients. Many practitioners will refer patients with end-stage otitis because of the difficulty of this surgery and high potential for complications. Referral may also be necessary to evaluate the animal for primary causes of otic inflammation, particularly uncontrolled or poorly controlled allergic dermatitis. Whilst removal of the ear canals provides relief to many animals, underlying skin conditions can still cause pruritus and proliferation of the remainder of the pinna; if these are not controlled, the owners will be dissatisfied with the results of surgery. TECA should be combined with bulla osteotomy to prevent recurrent fistulation and infection.

Preoperative assessment: Patients with end-stage otitis should have already undergone systemic and dermato-logical evaluations, as well as culture and cytology of the ear canals. Neurological function should be examined preoperatively. If the dog has a diminished blink reflex or drooping lip, then the facial nerve may be embedded in hyperplastic tissue or damaged by extensive inflammation, conditions that can make the surgery more challenging. Animals with head tilt and nystagmus may also be slightly worse after surgery.

Because TECA is almost always combined with bulla osteotomy, many veterinary surgeons forgo radiographic imaging of the skull in animals with obvious end-stage otitis. In brachycephalic breeds, however, CT is very useful for determining the location of the osseous bullae, because they may be difficult to reach from a lateral approach in some dogs. If unilateral OE is present or neo-plasia is suspected, skull radiography or CT is recom-mended to determine the extent of the disease. If a tumour has invaded the tympanic bulla, owners should be warned that surgical cure is unlikely and that other treatment modalities will be required, after surgical cytoreduction and histopathological confirmation of tumour type, to control the growth and spread of neoplasia. Patients sus-pected of having neoplasia should have thoracic radio-graphy or CT to determine whether gross metastatic disease is present. Metastasis of ceruminous gland adenocarcinomas may occur in half of affected cats.

Preoperative and perioperative medication: TECA with lateral bulla osteotomy is a very painful procedure, and pre-emptive analgesic administration should be used to ease the animal's recovery. The day before surgery, a fentanyl patch can be placed and non-steroidal anti-inflammatory drugs (NSAIDs) administered (if the patient has not been treated recently with steroids). Alternatively, pre-anaesthetic medication should include an opioid and an NSAID administered perioperatively. These drugs should be continued for several days after surgery once the animal has recovered enough to take oral medica-tions. Another option in dogs is placement of a wound soaker catheter to allow continuous delivery of lidocaine to the site for 38 hours after surgery. When compared with intravenous morphine, continuous local lidocaine infusion provided equipotent analgesia and produced less sedation in dogs undergoing TECA and bulla oste-otomy (Wolfe *et al.*, 2006).

Because thorough preparation of the ear canal is diffi-cult, this procedure is classified as 'dirty', justifying the use of perioperative antibiotics. Ideally, the choice of anti-biotics is based on results of prior cytology and culture and sensitivity testing. Intraoperative cultures of the bulla should be taken to confirm the bacterial species and anti-microbial susceptibility. Timing of intraoperative cultures is controversial, because isolates obtained before and after flushing differ in 70% of operated ears; if the primary concern is residual bacteria, then culture after flushing would make the most sense.

Surgical technique: Details of this procedure are given in Operative Technique 5.3.

Postoperative complications: Complications are seen in 29–68% of animals that undergo TECA with bulla osteot-omy and are reported in 82% of animals if bulla osteotomy is not performed, probably because of incomplete removal of affected epithelium within the osseous canal and bulla. Facial nerve paralysis occurs in 25–50% of dogs after the procedure and is permanent in 10–15% of all dogs. Temporary facial nerve palsy usually resolves in 1–4 weeks; administration of eye lubricants three times per day is recommended until eyelid function improves. Dogs with permanent facial nerve paralysis should undergo Schirmer tear tests to determine whether artificial tears are neces-sary to prevent keratoconjunctivitis sicca. Postoperative cellulitus and infection are also common complications, particularly if infected bulla lining or epithelial remnants lining the external acoustic meatus or cartilaginous attach-ments are not removed. Draining fistulas will appear 1–12 months after the surgery in 5–10% of animals; residual tissue must be removed through a lateral approach or a ventral bulla osteotomy.

Other complications include dehiscence, neurological abnormalities from inner ear damage (nystagmus, circling, head tilt, ataxia), hypoglossal nerve damage, Horner's syn-drome (particularly in cats) and avascular necrosis of the pinna. In patients with allergic dermatitis, persistent changes to the skin of the concave pinnae (e.g. erythema, pruritus, lichenification, glandular hyperplasia) may continue to be noted even after TECA. Additionally, animals that undergo bilateral TECAs may have postoperative pharyngeal swelling or hyoid apparatus damage from extensive dissection and may develop respiratory distress, requiring temporary tracheostomy. When faced with this daunting list of potential complications, many practitioners will opt to refer patients to a specialist veterinary surgeon for this procedure.

Prognosis: Long-term results are excellent in 58%, good in 34% and poor in 8% of animals undergoing the procedure. Surgery is successful in alleviating signs in 92–95%, and auditory function is usually not decreased because patients have been, and will be, reliant on bone and tissue vibration for conduction of sounds.

Ventral bulla osteotomy

The clinical features of OM may include hearing loss and pain when opening the mouth or on palpation of the bulla. However, in many patients with OM secondary to extension of infection through a compromised tympanic membrane, chronic OE is the only clinical sign of concurrent OM. With progression or chronicity, the vestibular portion of the inner ear may be damaged, causing signs of peripheral vestibular disease (ataxia, head tilt and nystagmus). Cats may develop Horner's syndrome because of damage to sympathetic fibres within the bulla. Septic OM often occurs as a result of OE, and patients that have both conditions usually require TECA and lateral bulla osteotomy. The decision on which procedure is appropriate depends on the condition of the horizontal ear canal and whether it is necessary to preserve air-conducted hearing. Bacterial OM can, however, occur with minimal or no external ear canal changes or secondary to sinonasal or nasopharyngeal disease (most commonly seen in cats), and ventral bulla osteotomy may be required to relieve clinical signs. Bacterial OM without concurrent OE is most commonly encountered in cats. Other conditions that can lead to signs of OM include congenital clefts of the hard and soft palate, *Cryptococcus neoformans* infection, polyps and neoplasia. Radiography of the tympanic bulla (Figure 5.6) is useful to evaluate for evidence of OM, as is CT.

Ventral bulla osteotomy provides drainage and removal of fluids and inflamed tissues, and allows access to the middle ear for cultures, biopsy and mass removal. It is most frequently performed in animals that have middle or inner ear disease and no significant changes in the external ear canal, and is particularly indicated in cats with

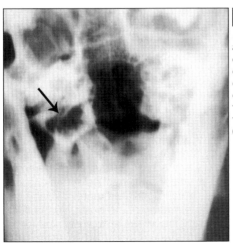

5.6
Radiographic appearance of otitis media in a dog. In this open-mouth view of the skull, soft tissue density fills the left bulla (arrowed).

inflammatory polyps (see section below) that are too extensive for removal by traction avulsion or have recurred following traction avulsion. Many dermatologists also consider ventral bulla osteotomy to be the treatment of choice for effusive OM in cats because thorough lavage of inflammatory exudates from both the dorsolateral and ventromedial compartments of the tympanic bulla can be difficult owing to the presence of the bony septum separating the compartments. Ventral bulla osteotomy may also be necessary in animals that develop recurrent infections and fistulas after TECA and (lateral or ventral) bulla osteotomy, particularly if the ear canal epithelium was completely removed at a prior surgery but the bulla was not opened or adequately cleared of infected contents.

Patient positioning: The animal is placed in dorsal recumbency with the legs pulled caudally, neck extended and head cradled by towels, a sandbag or suction cushion. The rostral mandible can be taped to the table to improve stability.

Surgical approach in dogs: The approach is through a ventral paramedian incision, starting medial to the ramus of the mandible and ending about 1 cm caudal to the level of the ear canal. In dogs the bulla is not palpable. Once the skin and subcutaneous tissues have been incised, the spiky paracondylar process, the caudal attachment site for the digastricus muscle, is located. The bulla is about 0.5 cm rostral and 0.5 cm medial to this bony process, dorsal to the digastricus muscle. The incision is centred at a point midway between the ramus and the wing of the atlas vertebra. The linguofacial vein is retracted if necessary.

Surgical technique in dogs: Blunt dissection is performed between the digastricus muscle laterally and the myelohyoideus and hyoglossus muscles and the hyoglossal nerve medially, keeping the scissors parallel to the long axis of the head to avoid damaging nerves and vessels. Self-retaining retractors, such as Gelpis, are used to keep the wound open. The digastricus muscle is retracted laterally and any remaining muscle tissues are bluntly dissected from the bulla. The stylohyoid bone can be palpated in the lateral part of the surgical field and can be followed dorsally to its insertion on the lateral aspect of the bulla.

The bulla is opened with an intramedullary pin or burr and the opening is enlarged with the burr or with rongeurs. If preservation of hearing is important, mechanical burrs should be used sparingly because the vibration caused by these instruments can have detrimental effects on the cochlear apparatus. Samples of the bulla contents are taken for culture and histological evaluation.

The ventral, medial and lateral portions of the bulla are curetted and all contents aspirated. Curettage of the epitympanic recess should be avoided because this will almost certainly damage the auditory ossicles. After it has been inspected for residual epithelial tissue, the bulla is flushed gently with warm saline. Closure is routine. Drains are usually not needed but may be placed into the area and exited through a new skin incision if severe infection is present.

Postoperative care: Antibiotics are given if infection is present, and treatment for OE is continued as needed.

Postoperative complications: Complications of ventral bulla osteotomy are usually from inner ear damage and include nystagmus, circling, head tilt and ataxia.

Otic and nasopharyngeal polyps

Cats

Otic and nasopharyngeal polyps are benign masses that probably originate from the lining of the middle ear in cats – they have also been presumed to originate from the lining of the auditory (Eustachian) tube, but it is not clear whether this is a site of origin or whether some polyps simply extend through the auditory tube from the middle ear to the nasopharynx. Their aetiology is unknown, although they are thought to be a response to inflammation, since their histological structure is that of inflammatory tissue.

- Ear polyps are red, smooth, round to oblong masses that may fill the horizontal ear cavity but do not adhere to its surface (Figure 5.7).
- Nasopharyngeal polyps are usually oblong and pinkish white; they can become inflamed or ulcerated with trauma. Although not readily visible on oral examination, they tend to displace the soft palate ventrally as they grow.

Histologically, inflammatory polyps are composed of well vascularized fibrous connective tissue covered by stratified squamous or columnar epithelium. Inflammatory cells – primarily lymphocytes, plasma cells and macrophages – are present within the stroma and are especially dense in the submucosal areas of the tissue.

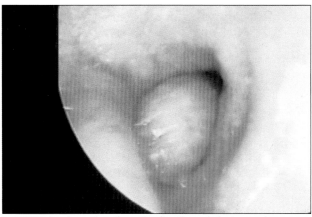

5.7 Aural, or otic, polyp extending through the tympanic membrane into the horizontal canal of a cat.

Clinical signs

Most cats with clinical signs of polyps present as young adults, although polyps have also been reported in older cats. Cats with inflammatory polyps extending to the ear canal exhibit signs of OE (head shaking, pawing at the ear) or otic discharge. Signs of OM or OI (e.g. Horner's syndrome, head tilt, ataxia or nystagmus) are occasionally seen.

Cats with nasopharyngeal polyps may present with nasal discharge, sneezing, stertorous or laboured breathing, dysphagia, gagging or voice change; occasionally they will also have OE or Horner's syndrome.

Diagnosis

The diagnosis of inflammatory polyps is made through otoscopic or nasopharyngeal evaluation and biopsy.

Histological or cytological evaluation of the mass should be performed to rule out malignant neoplastic conditions such as squamous cell carcinoma and lymphoma. Bulla radiography or CT may be recommended in cats with suspected inflammatory polyps that cannot be visualized or palpated via otoscopy or nasopharyngeal evaluation, to evaluate the size and extent of polyps prior to attempted removal by traction avulsion or ventral bulla osteotomy, or in older cats to evaluate for changes more consistent with neoplasia (e.g. invasion or lysis of the tympanic bulla).

The ear canal may need to be gently cleansed of exudates under heavy sedation or anaesthesia before a polyp is evident. Otic polyps usually do not extend externally beyond the horizontal canal. In some cases the tympanic membrane appears reddened or bulges outward if the disease is limited to the middle ear. In these cases, bulla radiographs, or ideally CT, are typically necessary to confirm the presence of the inflammatory polyp behind the tympanic membrane.

Nasopharyngeal polyps can be seen in anaesthetized cats by retracting the soft palate rostrally with a spay hook or stay sutures. On survey radiographs they are visible as a soft tissue density within the nasopharynx. CT findings of nasopharyngeal polyps may include a soft tissue density mass extending from the nasopharynx through the auditory tube to the tympanic bulla with an associated stalk-like structure, complete or partial filling of the dorsal or ventral portions of the tympanic bulla by soft tissue, and expansion of the tympanic bulla with sclerosis of the bulla wall (Oliviera *et al.*, 2012).

Dogs

Polypoid hyperplasia of the ear canal occurs commonly in dogs with chronic OE and represents focal areas of epidermal hyperplasia, inflammatory cell infiltration and glandular hyperplasia. Inflammatory polyps extending through the auditory tube to the nasopharynx have been rarely described in dogs. Similarly, inflammatory polyps originating within the tympanic bulla and extending into the external ear canal have also been rarely reported in dogs (Pratschke, 2003). In one report of five dogs, middle ear inflammatory polyps were composed of a fibrovascular stroma, multifocally infiltrated by inflammatory cells, and an overlying stratified squamous epithelium (Pratschke, 2003).

Surgical treatment

Otic polyps

Otic polyps may be removed from the ear canal by traction, and removal by traction avulsion is frequently the initial treatment of choice in cases in which the polyp may be accessed via the ear canal. Bulla radiographs or CT can be helpful to evaluate the size and extent of otic polyps prior to removal by traction avulsion. Removal by traction may be performed using tissue forceps, mosquito haemostats or a polypectomy snare. Polypectomy snares that insert through the working port of a fibreoptic otoscope are particularly helpful as they allow direct visualization of the polyp as the snare is placed. A perendoscopic transtympanic membrane traction technique has also been described, which combines removal of the otic polyp via traction with curetting of the dorsolateral and/or ventromedial compartments of the tympanic bulla (Greci *et al.*, 2014).

Administration of anti-inflammatory doses of gluco-corticoids, such as prednisolone at an initial starting dose of 1–2 mg/kg/day with tapering over 3–4 weeks, may be associated with a reduced risk of polyp recurrence following removal by traction (Anderson *et al.*, 2000; Greci *et al.*, 2014). In cases with radiographic evidence of severe changes to the tympanic bulla (e.g. pathological expansion, sclerosis or lysis of the bulla wall), those in which the polyp cannot be adequately removed by traction avulsion, or where there has been polyp recurrence following traction avulsion, ventral bulla osteotomy is the treatment of choice (see above for description of the technique in dogs). Ventral bulla osteotomy to loosen and remove the stalk of the polyp is usually performed before removal of the protruding part of the polyp in the horizontal ear canal. The remainder of the ear polyp can be removed from the canal with alligator forceps and gentle traction by a non-sterile assistant.

Ventral bulla osteotomy in cats: The cat is placed in dorsal recumbency, with the head and neck extended and stabilized and the forelegs pulled caudally. The large round bullae are readily palpable caudomedial to the mandible in this position. The approach and bulla entry are initially the same as for the dog (see above), but with the incision centred over the palpable bulla. The bulla is palpated frequently for orientation during dissection.

The initial osteotomy exposes the larger ventromedial compartment, which contains the cochlear (round) window on the dorsocaudal wall of the bulla near the septum, and the promontory, a bony process on the dorsomedial aspect of the bulla. The sympathetic nerve fibres course along the surface of the promontory, passing through a narrow fissure in the dorsal aspect of the septum into the dorsolateral compartment. The sympathetic nerve fibres continue along the dorsomedial wall of that compartment before entering the petrous temporal bone just medial to the opening of the auditory tube at the rostral apex of the bulla.

Once the outer bulla has been opened, the inner septum in the lateral half of the outer bulla is perforated with a Steinmann pin or burr; the perforation is enlarged gently with the burr, rongeurs or a curved haemostat. The bone in the septum is more fragile than that of the outer bulla and should be removed carefully to avoid trauma to the promontory.

The polyp's attachments to the bulla wall are removed gently, often by traction with a haemostat, and the extracted tissue is saved for culture and histological evaluation. Curettage to remove epithelial remnants is usually unnecessary; when this is performed, the surgeon must avoid curetting the caudomedial and dorsal portions of the bulla in cats to prevent damage to the round and oval windows, ossicles and sympathetic fibres.

The bulla is flushed gently with warm, sterile saline. As in dogs, a drain is usually unnecessary but should be placed if the bulla contains infected material that cannot be completely removed.

> **PRACTICAL TIP**
>
> In cats, once the ventral bulla wall has been removed, the inner septum will cross the rostrolateral third of the bulla. The septum can usually be removed in pieces with a small haemostat after it has been perforated with a Steinmann pin or haemostat tip

> **WARNING**
>
> In cats, the sympathetic fibres run along the surface of a bony prominence – the 'promontory' – on the dorsal surface of the bulla at the level of the septum and are easily damaged, particularly if the inner compartment of the bulla is curetted. The round window and oval window are also located on the dorsal surface of the bulla near the septum; curetting the rostrodorsal surface of the bulla could result in Horner's syndrome or signs of OI (ataxia, nystagmus, head tilt). Bulla lavage should be performed gently and with warm, sterile saline to prevent barotrauma

Prognosis: Regrowth of polyps has been reported in 17–50% of cats treated with traction removal alone. In a more recent study describing a technique of polyp removal via perendoscopic transtympanic traction, polyp recurrence was reported in only five of 37 cats (13.5%). Twenty-one of 37 cats in this study were also treated with glucocorticoids after polyp traction (Greci *et al.*, 2014). In one study, cats with normal bullae on radiographs had no recurrence of polyps after traction removal, whilst cats with radiographic evidence of OM had a 56% recurrence rate with traction removal (Veir *et al.*, 2002). In another study, recurrence was reported in nine of 14 cats that received traction alone and in none of the eight cats that received glucocorticoids after polyp traction (Anderson *et al.*, 2000).

Neurological damage often occurs during ventral bulla osteotomy and polyp removal. Horner's syndrome (Figure 5.8) from sympathetic nerve damage has been reported in >80% of cats after bulla osteotomy and can also occur with traction alone. Clinical signs (miosis, ptosis and third eyelid prolapse) usually resolve within a month. Intraoperative trauma to the sympathetic nerve fibres is most common with curettage of the ventromedial compartment, where the nerves are less protected by surrounding fibrous tissue. Persistent Horner's syndrome does not seem to affect a cat's behaviour. About 40% of cats may have signs of peripheral vestibular disease after bulla osteotomy for polyp removal (Faulkner and Budsberg, 1990; Trevor and Martin, 1993). The signs are transient in most cats.

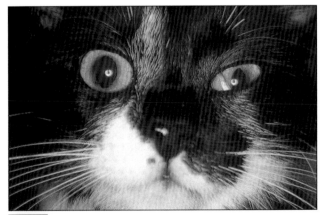

5.8 Horner's syndrome in a cat after ventral bulla osteotomy.

Nasopharyngeal polyps

These are removed under anaesthesia. The soft palate is retracted rostrally with stay sutures or a spay hook, and the polyp is digitally displaced ventrally into the oropharynx. Incision of the soft palate is usually not necessary for exposure. The stalk of the polyp, located dorsolaterally on digital or instrument palpation, is grasped blindly and gently with right-angled forceps or Allis tissue forceps. Alternatively, a portion of the polyp can be excised to expose the base. It is important not to crush the base of the polyp with the forceps as it may break off at that site, leaving tissue remnants attached to the auditory tube or bulla lining. Removal of the polyp is accomplished with gentle, continuous traction. If the entire polyp is removed, the stalk of the polyp should appear long and tapered; on otoscopic evaluation, blood may appear under the tympanic membrane of the affected side. The cat is then placed on an anti-inflammatory dose of glucocorticoids (e.g. 1–2 mg/kg q24h) for 2 weeks, after which the drug is tapered over 14–17 days.

Middle ear cholesteatomas in dogs

A cholesteatoma is an epidermoid cyst composed of a keratin core surrounded by a keratinizing stratified squamous epithelial lining and located within the middle ear cavity. In humans, cholesteatomas can be congenital or acquired. In dogs, middle ear cholesteatomas are thought to be acquired secondary to chronic OE and OM. The aetiology of middle ear cholesteatomas is not fully known, but they are thought to form secondary to invagination of the tympanic membrane into the middle ear cavity with subsequent cyst formation, or to migration of stratified squamous epithelium from the ear canal to the middle ear cavity through a compromised tympanic membrane. The progressive accumulation of keratin within the cyst can lead to cholesteatoma expansion and destruction of surrounding structures, particularly bone (Hardie *et al.*, 2008; Greci *et al.*, 2011). Middle ear cholesteatoma has been reported following TECA and lateral bulla osteotomy in two brachycephalic dogs; this may have been due to the relative difficulty in performing these procedures in brachycephalic breeds and the potential transfer of stratified squamous epithelium from the ear canal to the middle ear cavity during surgery (Schuenemann and Oechtering, 2012).

Clinical signs

Clinical signs of middle ear cholesteatomas depend on the severity and size of the cystic mass. Longstanding lesions may fill and expand the tympanic bulla, with associated bony lysis and clinical signs such as facial nerve paresis or paralysis, vestibular dysfunction, and pain on opening the mouth or on palpation of the tympanic bulla and/or temporomandibular joint (Hardie *et al.*, 2008; Greci *et al.*, 2011).

Diagnosis

Middle ear cholesteatoma may be suspected in dogs presenting with inability or discomfort on opening the mouth, as well as neurological signs consistent with vestibular and facial nerve dysfunction. CT findings consistent with cholesteatoma include filling and expansion of the middle ear cavity by non-contrast-enhancing soft tissue opacity material with sclerosis or lysis of the bone of the tympanic bulla (Travetti *et al.*, 2010; Greci *et al.*, 2011). Otoscopic examination may reveal a white or yellow mass or 'flakes' of keratin protruding from the middle ear cavity

into the horizontal ear canal (Greci *et al.*, 2011). Histopathology of material removed from the middle ear cavity via ventral or lateral bulla osteotomy is necessary for definitive diagnosis of cholesteatoma.

Surgical treatment

Middle ear cholesteatoma should be surgically addressed by ventral bulla osteotomy or TECA with lateral bulla osteotomy. As most affected dogs have a chronic history of OE, TECA with lateral bulla osteotomy is likely to be the more appropriate surgical approach. Cholesteatoma recurrence has been reported following ventral or lateral bulla osteotomy; the risk of recurrence is greater in dogs with evidence of more advanced disease on initial presentation (e.g. inability to open the mouth, neurological deficits or evidence of bony lysis on CT) (Hardie *et al.*, 2008).

Considerations for surgical success in patients with ear disease

Surgery of the ear is most often indicated in patients with a history of inflammatory skin disease. In these patients, control of the underlying inflammatory skin disease is key to improving comfort and preventing failure of surgical procedures such as aural haematoma repair. Consultation with a veterinary dermatologist may be necessary to address underlying dermatological disease, particularly chronic allergic dermatitis. Appropriate patient selection for surgical procedures should also be emphasized. For example, failure of lateral ear canal resection is often inevitable in dogs with end-stage otitis or poorly controlled inflammatory skin disease. Patients with chronic OE and OM have frequently been exposed to multiple topical and systemic antimicrobials, and antimicrobial-resistant infections, particularly with *Staphylococcus* spp. or *P. aeruginosa*, are common. Appropriate pre- and postsurgical antimicrobial therapy based on culture and susceptibility results is also integral to improved surgical outcomes.

References and further reading

Anderson DM, Robinson RK and White RAS (2000) Management of inflammatory polyps in cats. *Veterinary Record* **147**, 684–687

Bacon NAS (2012) Pinna and external ear canal. In: *Veterinary Surgery: Small Animal*, ed. KM Tobias and SA Johnston, pp. 2059–2078. Elsevier, St Louis

Bischoff MG and Kneller SK (2004) Diagnostic imaging of the canine and feline ear. *Veterinary Clinics of North America: Small Animal Practice* **34**, 437–458

Buback JL, Boothe HW, Carroll GL and Green RW (1996) Comparison of three methods for relief of pain after ear canal ablation in dogs. *Veterinary Surgery* **25**, 380–385

Clifford CA, De Lorimier LP, Fan TM and Garrett LD (2013) Neoplastic and non-neoplastic tumors. In: *Muller & Kirk's Small Animal Dermatology, 7th edn*, ed. WH Miller, CE Griffin and KL Campbell, pp. 774–843. Elsevier, St Louis

Cole LK (2012) Primary secretory otitis media in Cavalier King Charles Spaniels. *Veterinary Clinics of North America: Small Animal Practice* **42**, 1137–1142

Cole LK, Kwochka KW, Podell M, Hillier A and Smeak DD (2002) Evaluation of radiography, otoscopy, pneumotoscopy, impedance audiometry and endoscopy for the diagnosis of otitis media in the dog. In: *Advances in Veterinary Dermatology, 4th edn*, ed. KL Thoday, CS Foil and R Bond, pp. 49–54. Blackwell Science, Oxford

Demirutku A, Ozer K, Devecioglu Y *et al.* (2012) Pinnal squamous cell carcinoma in cats and the effectiveness of treatment with radical pinnectomy. *Veterinarni Medicina* **57**, 420–429

Detweiler DA, Johnson LR, Kass PH and Wisner ER (2006) Computed tomographic evidence of bulla effusion in cats with sinonasal disease: 2001–2004. *Journal of Veterinary Internal Medicine* **20**, 1080–1084

Dickie AM, Doust R, Cromarty L *et al.* (2003) Comparison of ultrasonography, radiography and a single computed tomography slice for identification of fluid within the canine tympanic bulla. *Research in Veterinary Science* **75**, 209–216

Doust R, King A, Hammond G *et al.* (2007) Assessment of middle ear disease in the dog: a comparison of diagnostic imaging modalities. *Journal of Small Animal Practice* **48**, 188–192

Dye TL, Teague HD, Ostwald DA Jr and Ferreira SD (2002) Evaluation of a technique using the carbon dioxide laser for treatment of aural hematomas. *Journal of the American Animal Hospital Association* **38**, 385–390

Faulkner JE and Budsberg SC (1990) Results of ventral bulla osteotomy for treatment of middle ear polyps. *Journal of the American Animal Hospital Association* **26**, 496–499

Foster A, Morandi F and May E (2015) Prevalence of ear disease in dogs undergoing multidetector thin-slice computed tomography of the head. *Journal of Veterinary Radiology and Ultrasound* **56**, 18–24

Greci V, Travetti O, Di Giancamillo M *et al.* (2011) Middle ear cholesteatoma in 11 dogs. *Canadian Veterinary Journal* **52**, 631–636

Greci V, Vernia E and Mortellaro CM (2014) Per-endoscopic trans-tympanic traction for the management of feline aural inflammatory polyps: a case review of 37 cats. *Journal of Feline Medicine and Surgery* **16**, 645–650

Halliwell REW (2013) Autoimmune and immune-mediated dermatoses. In: *Muller & Kirk's Small Animal Dermatology, 7th edn*, ed. WH Miller, CE Griffin and KL Campbell, pp. 432–500. Elsevier, St Louis

Hall J, Weir S and Ladlow J (2016) Treatment of canine aural haematoma by UK veterinarians. *Journal of Small Animal Practice* **57**, 360–364

Hardie EM, Linder KE and Pease AP (2008) Aural cholesteatoma in 20 dogs. *Veterinary Surgery* **37**, 763–770

Hayes GM, Friend EJ and Jeffrey ND (2010) Relationship between pharyngeal conformation and otitis media with effusion in Cavalier King Charles Spaniels. *Veterinary Record* **167**, 55–58

Hettlich BE, Boothe HW, Simpson RB *et al.* (2005) Effect of tympanic cavity evacuation and flushing on microbial isolates during total ear canal ablation and lateral bulla osteotomy in dogs. *Journal of the American Veterinary Medical Association* **227**, 748–755

Holt D, Brockman DJ, Sylvestre AM and Sadanaga K (1996) Lateral exploration of fistulas developing after total ear canal ablations: 10 cases (1989–1993). *Journal of the American Animal Hospital Association* **32**, 527–530

King AM, Weinrauch SA, Doust R *et al.* (2007) Comparison of ultrasonography, radiography and a single computed tomography slice for fluid identification within the feline tympanic bulla. *Veterinary Journal* **173**, 638–644

Kuwahara J (1986) Canine and feline aural hematomas: results of treatment with corticosteroids. *Journal of the American Animal Hospital Association* **22**, 641–647

Martin-Vaquero P, da Costa RC and Daniels JB (2011) Presumptive meningoencephalitis secondary to otitis media/interna caused by *Streptococcus equi* ssp. *zooepidemicus* in a cat. *Journal of Feline Medicine and Surgery* **13**, 606–609

McCarthy RJ and Caywood DD (1992) Vertical ear canal resection for end-stage otitis externa in dogs. *Journal of the American Animal Hospital Association* **28**, 545–552

Oishi N, Talaska AE and Schacht J (2012) Ototoxicity in dogs and cats. *Veterinary Clinics of North America: Small Animal Practice* **42**, 1259–1271

Oliviera CR, O'Brien RT, Matheson JS and Carrera I (2012) Computed tomographic features of feline nasopharyngeal polyps. *Veterinary Radiology and Ultrasound* **53**, 406–411

Palmeiro BS, Morris DO, Wiemelt SP and Shofer FS (2004) Evaluation of outcome of otitis media after lavage of the tympanic bulla and long-term antimicrobial drug treatment in dogs: 44 cases (1998–2002). *Journal of the American Veterinary Medical Association* **225**, 548–553

Pavletic MM (2015) Use of laterally placed vacuum drains for management of aural hematomas in five dogs. *Journal of the American Veterinary Medical Association* **246**, 112–117

Pratschke KM (2003) Inflammatory polyps in the middle ear of five dogs. *Veterinary Surgery* **32**, 292–296

Schwab TM, Popovitch C, DeBiasio J and Goldschmidt M (2014) Clinical outcome for MCTs of canine pinnae treated with surgical excision (2004–2008). *Journal of the American Animal Hospital Association* **50**, 187–191

Schuenemann RM and Oechtering G (2012) Cholesteatoma after lateral bulla osteotomy in two brachycephalic dogs. *Journal of the American Animal Hospital Association* **48**, 261–268

Shanaman M, Seiler G and Holt DE (2012) Prevalence of clinical and subclinical middle ear disease in cats undergoing computed tomographic scans of the head. *Veterinary Radiology and Ultrasound* **53**, 76–79

Spivak RE, Elkins AD, Moore GE and Lantz GC (2013) Postoperative complications following TECA-LBO in the dog and cat. *Journal of the American Animal Hospital Association* **49**, 160–168

Sturges BK, Dickinson PJ, Kortz GD *et al.* (2006) Clinical signs, magnetic resonance imaging features, and outcome after surgical and medical treatment of otogenic intracranial infection in 11 cats and four dogs. *Journal of Veterinary Internal Medicine* **20**, 648–656

Swaim SF and Bradley DM (1996) Evaluation of closed-suction drainage for treating auricular hematomas. *Journal of the American Animal Hospital Association* **32**, 36–43

Sylvestre AM (1998) Potential factors affecting the outcome of dogs with a resection of the lateral wall of the vertical ear canal. *Canadian Veterinary Journal* **39**, 157–160

Tobias KM (2000) Management of ear and nasopharyngeal polyps in cats. *Veterinary Forum* **17**, 46–53

Travetti O, Giudice C, Greci V *et al.* (2010) Computed tomography features of middle ear cholesteatoma in dogs. *Veterinary Radiology and Ultrasound* **51**, 374–379

Trevor PB and Martin RA (1993) Tympanic bulla osteotomy for treatment of middle-ear disease in cats: 19 cases (1984–1991). *Journal of the American Veterinary Medical Association* **202**, 123–128

Veir JK, Lappin MR, Foley JE and Getzy DM (2002) Feline inflammatory polyps: historical, clinical, and PCR findings for feline calici virus and feline herpes virus-1 in 28 cases. *Journal of Feline Medicine and Surgery* **4**, 195–199

White RAS (2012) Middle and inner ear. In: *Veterinary Surgery: Small Animal*, ed. KM Tobias and SA Johnston, pp. 2078–2089. Elsevier, St Louis

Wolfe TM, Bateman SW, Cole LK and Smeak DD (2006) Evaluation of a local anesthetic delivery system for the postoperative analgesic management of canine total ear canal ablation – a randomized, controlled, double-blinded study. *Veterinary Anaesthesia and Analgesia* **33**, 328–339

OPERATIVE TECHNIQUE 5.1

Lateral ear canal resection

- Clip the side of the face ventrally to the midline, rostrally to the lateral commissure of the eyelid, and for several centimetres caudal to the palpable ear canal.
- If the tympanic membrane is intact, the ear canal may be flushed with dilute chlorhexidine (0.05%). Because ototoxicity has been reported with antiseptics, some clinicians recommend using only sterile saline when flushing the horizontal ear canal, particularly if the tympanic membrane is perforated. Prepare the remainder of the surgical field with antiseptic solution and scrub.
- Some veterinary surgeons administer antibiotics prophylactically (e.g. cefazolin 22 mg/kg i.v. at induction and again within 2–6h) if the animal is not already on therapeutic perioperative antibiotics.

PATIENT POSITIONING

Lateral recumbency, with a folded towel under the side of the head. The pinna should be lying over the top of the head, away from the surgical site.

ASSISTANT

Optional.

ADDITIONAL INSTRUMENTS

Bipolar cautery is useful but not required.

SURGICAL TECHNIQUE

Approach

The skin overlying the vertical ear canal is cut in a U shape, starting at the tragohelicine notch and extending to a point 1–2 cm ventral to the junction between the vertical and horizontal ear canals, then returning to the intertragic incisure. The ear canal is exposed by dissection through the overlying subcutaneous tissue and retraction of the parotid salivary gland.

Surgical manipulations

1   Elevate the skin from the underlying ear canal and either remove it or leave it attached dorsally. Elevate the subcutaneous tissue from the lateral wall of the vertical canal using blunt and sharp dissection until the canal wall is exposed. The parotid gland may need to be retracted ventrally to expose the annular cartilage completely.

2   After the vertical canal is exposed, make two parallel incisions in the lateral wall to make a 'drainage board'. If the incisions are started at the canal opening, position yourself at the dorsum of the dog's head, looking down the ear canal. Make small cuts with Mayo scissors, starting at the tragohelicine and intertragic incisures, alternating sides until the flap extends to a level slightly below the midpoint of the horizontal canal circumference.

Alternatively, make two stab incisions with a No. 11 blade at the ventral-most extent of the proposed flap (at the junction between the conchal and annular cartilage). Insert a blade of the Mayo scissors into one of the perforations and extend the cut upwards to the incisure above. Repeat on the other side.

> **WARNING**
>
> Because the ear canal spirals slightly inward as it bends, it is easy to transect the flap accidentally. Therefore, make small cuts, alternating to either side, and recheck the flap position frequently

3   Grasp the skin flap or its attached cartilage with Allis tissue forceps and complete the lateral wall flap. The base of the flap should be located on each side of the horizontal canal, slightly below the midpoint of its circumference. The flap should lie flat, without obstructing the horizontal canal opening.

4   Remove the distal third to half of the lateral cartilage flap so that a 2–3 cm drainage board remains. Remove additional facial skin as needed so that the flap is pulled ventrally away from the opening.

→ **OPERATIVE TECHNIQUE 5.1 CONTINUED**

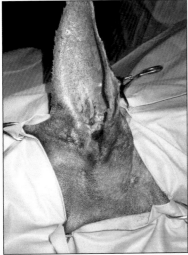

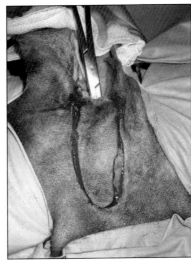

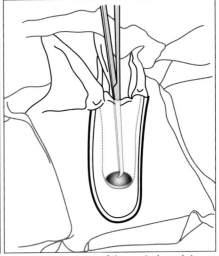

The patient is in lateral recumbency with the pinna lying over the head, away from the surgical site.

An instrument is inserted into the ear canal to identify the position of the vertical canal. A U-shaped incision is made over the lateral surface of the canal.

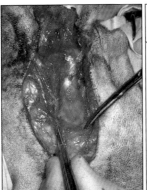

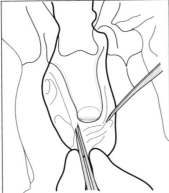

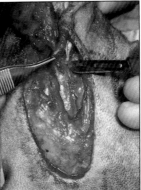

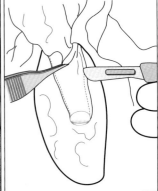

Subcutaneous tissues are dissected away from the lateral surface of the vertical canal.

To ensure the cuts in the vertical ear canal are in the correct site, it is helpful to score the cartilage with a scalpel tip. These marks can then be followed with the scissors (see next image).

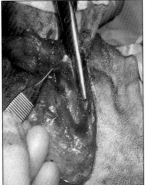

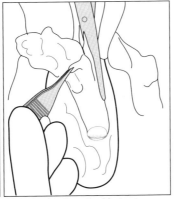

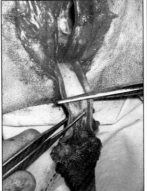

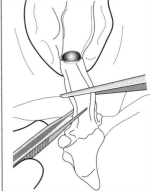

The lateral wall of the vertical canal is incised to form the 'drainage board'.

The distal third of the cartilage flap is transected to complete the 'drainage board'.

PRACTICAL TIP

The 'drainage board' must lie flat and should not obstruct the horizontal canal. Make sure the base of this flap originates slightly below the midpoint of the horizontal canal circumference. If the flap is calcified, dissect between the epithelium and cartilage and transect the cartilage to make a hinge. The final opening should be circular or slightly ovoid

→ **OPERATIVE TECHNIQUE 5.1 CONTINUED**

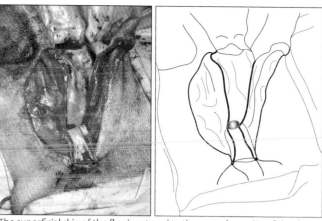

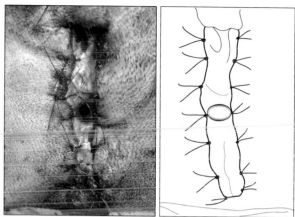

The superficial skin of the flap is sutured to the ventral margins of the skin incision. The horizontal canal opening should be checked before closure continues.

Closure is completed with figure-of-eight or simple interrupted skin sutures.

Closure

The cartilage of the drainage board can be secured to underlying subcutaneous tissue with absorbable sutures to reduce tension on the flap. Use nylon or polypropylene sutures (1.5 or 2 metric (3/0 or 4/0 USP)) to appose canal epithelium to skin.

Simple interrupted or figure-of-eight sutures can be preplaced along the new horizontal canal opening and at the corners of the drainage board to ensure that there is no excessive tension or redundant skin at those sites before completing the closure.

The margins of the remaining vertical canal can also be sutured to the skin above the new opening with a simple continuous pattern.

Closure is routine. It may be necessary to take partial-thickness bites of the facial skin to appose it to the epithelium of the vertical canal.

POSTOPERATIVE CARE

- Protect the ear from trauma after surgery with an Elizabethan collar or by securing the pinna to the head with tape.
- Place antibiotic ointment on the suture line to prevent blood and other materials from adhering to the sutures. The owners may need to gently clean the area daily until the sutures are removed.
- Continue treatment of any primary causes of otitis or dermatitis.

OPERATIVE TECHNIQUE 5.2

Vertical ear canal resection

PATIENT PREPARATION

- Clip the side of the face ventrally to the midline, rostrally to the lateral commissure of the eyelid, and for several centimetres caudal to the palpable ear canal. Clip the entire pinna and include it within the surgical field.
- If the tympanic membrane is intact, the ear canal may be flushed with dilute chlorhexidine (0.05%). Because ototoxicity has been reported with antiseptics, some clinicians recommend using only sterile saline when flushing the horizontal ear canal, particularly if the tympanic membrane is perforated. Prepare the remainder of the surgical field with antiseptic solution and scrub.
- Some veterinary surgeons administer antibiotics prophylactically (e.g. cefazolin 22 mg/kg i.v. at induction and again within 2–6h) if the animal is not already on therapeutic perioperative antibiotics.

PATIENT POSITIONING

Lateral recumbency, with a folded towel under the side of the head. The pinna should be lying over the top of the head, away from the surgical site.

ASSISTANT

Optional.

ADDITIONAL INSTRUMENTS

Bipolar cautery and Gelpi retractors are useful but not essential.

SURGICAL TECHNIQUE

Approach

Expose the affected ear canal through a lateral T-shaped incision that encircles the vertical canal opening and extends to a point ventral to the junction between vertical and horizontal ear canals (as for lateral wall resection). Make the initial skin incision around the opening of the vertical canal and just above the antihelix projection on the concave portion of the pinna. Use Mayo scissors to extend the skin incision through the cartilage of the medial wall of the vertical ear canal.

Surgical manipulations

1 Use blunt or sharp dissection with a sponge or scissors to free the vertical canal to the level of the annular cartilage. To dissect with a sponge, hold the proximal (dorsal) portion of the ear canal with Allis tissue forceps and, with a gauze sponge, wipe downwards along the canal (similar to stripping the spermatic cord in a castration). This will remove all the fat and expose the muscular attachments, which can be transected with scissors or cautery.

2 Once the canal is exposed to the junction of the annular and auricular (conchal) cartilage, transect the horizontal cartilage at least 1 cm beyond any tumour margin. It is advisable to leave a small portion of the vertical canal to make cartilage flap extensions dorsally and ventrally to reduce postoperative stenosis, although this is not necessary in all cases.

3 Incise the remaining vertical ear canal cranially and caudally to create both a ventral and a dorsal 'drainage board' to reduce postoperative stenosis.

PRACTICAL TIP

The ear canal can be dissected free of soft tissues by stripping it with a gauze sponge. This will expose muscular attachments that can be transected, with scissors, cautery or a laser, at their insertion sites on the ear canal

WARNING

The facial nerve can occasionally be damaged by vigorous dissection or retraction ventral or lateral to the horizontal canal

→ **OPERATIVE TECHNIQUE 5.2 CONTINUED**

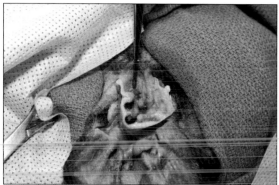

The skin and auricular cartilage are cut circumferentially around the external opening of the vertical canal.
(© Karen M. Tobias)

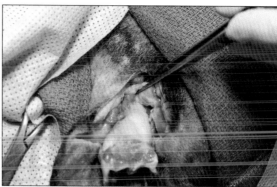

The vertical canal is dissected free of soft tissue attachments.
(© Karen M. Tobias)

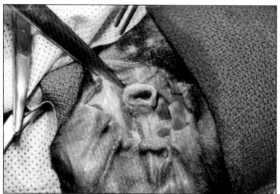

The vertical canal is transected, leaving a small amount of auricular cartilage.
(© Karen M. Tobias)

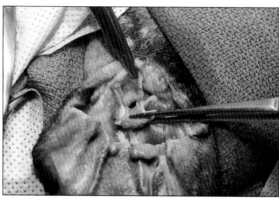

The auricular cartilage is transected midway along its rostral and caudal circumferences to make two cartilage flaps.
(© Karen M. Tobias)

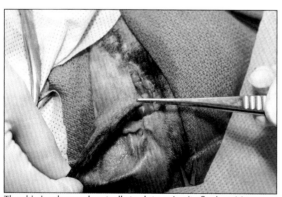

The skin is advanced rostrally to determine its final position.
(© Karen M. Tobias)

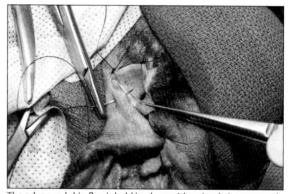

The advanced skin flap is held in place with a simple interrupted suture, and then the epithelium covering the cartilage flaps is sutured to the adjacent skin.
(© Karen M. Tobias)

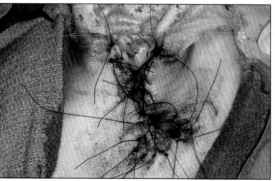

Final appearance of a vertical ear canal ablation in a dog with congenital stenosis of the vertical ear canal.
(© Karen M. Tobias)

→ **OPERATIVE TECHNIQUE 5.2 CONTINUED**

Closure

Before suturing the ear canal flaps to the skin, advance the skin edges towards one another to determine their final position and to see whether further skin elevation will be needed. Place one or two simple interrupted skin sutures between the advanced skin and the incision margin along the pinna to keep the skin in position.

Suture the ear canal epithelium from the drainage boards to the adjacent skin edges with non-absorbable monofilament sutures in a figure-of-eight or simple interrupted pattern. If the drainage boards are under tension, secure the cartilage of those flaps to the subcutaneous tissues before apposing the skin edges to the flap epithelium, making sure that the new opening is not obstructed by folds or sags in the flaps. Appose the remaining skin in a T-shape.

PRACTICAL TIP

Before placing any sutures, pull the skin flaps over the site to determine how best to close the skin. Often the skin incision must be extended ventrally or excess skin removed from around the proposed opening to prevent obstruction of the new ostium whilst reducing tension on the closure

POSTOPERATIVE CARE

Protect the surgical site from trauma with an Elizabethan collar. In dogs that shake their ears vigorously, the pinna should be taped to the head. Continue topical therapy and control of primary factors and clip the hair away from the opening as needed to maintain ventilation and drainage.

OPERATIVE TECHNIQUE 5.3

Total ear canal ablation and lateral bulla osteotomy

PATIENT PREPARATION

- Clip the side of the face ventrally and dorsally to the midline, rostrally to the lateral commissure of the eyelid, and for 5–7 cm caudal to the palpable ear canal. Additionally, clip the convex and concave surfaces of the pinna.
- Flush the ear canal with sterile saline or dilute betadine solution. Prepare the surgical field with antiseptic solution and scrub. During preparation and draping, the pinna can be suspended using a towel clamp and tape attached to an intravenous fluid pole.
- Some veterinary surgeons administer antibiotics prophylactically (e.g. cefazolin 22 mg/kg i.v. at induction and again within 2–6h) if the animal is not already on therapeutic perioperative antibiotics.

PATIENT POSITIONING

Lateral recumbency, with a folded towel under the side of the head. The pinna is usually draped into the sterile surgical field.

ASSISTANT

Extremely useful.

ADDITIONAL INSTRUMENTS

Bipolar cautery and Gelpi or ring retractors are useful.

SURGICAL TECHNIQUE

Approach

Expose the affected ear canal through a lateral T-shaped incision that encircles the vertical canal opening and extends to a point ventral to the level of the bulla. Make the initial skin incision around the opening of the vertical canal just above the antihelix projection on the concave portion of the pinna. Use Mayo scissors to extend the skin incision through the cartilage of the medial wall of the vertical ear canal.

➡️

→ **OPERATIVE TECHNIQUE 5.3 CONTINUED**

Surgical manipulations

1 Use blunt or sharp dissection with a sponge or scissors to free the vertical canal to the level of the annular cartilage. To dissect with a sponge, hold the proximal (dorsal) portion of the ear canal with Allis tissue forceps and, with a gauze sponge, wipe downward along the canal (similar to vertical ear canal ablation). This will remove all the fat and expose the muscular attachments, which can be transected with scissors or cautery.

2 Continue to dissect carefully immediately adjacent to the canal, to the level of the skull, pausing intermittently to palpate the area ventral to the canal to locate the facial nerve and identify the pulse of the external carotid artery. Retract the soft tissues gently to facilitate exposure and dissection of the horizontal canal.

3 With Mayo or cartilage scissors, carefully transect the horizontal canal adjacent to the skull and osseous external acoustic meatus, avoiding damage to the facial nerve, and remove the canal. Examine the margins of the osseous external acoustic meatus to verify that all cartilage attachments have been removed.

4 With a periosteal elevator, gently expose the lateral surface of the bulla, and resect the ventral rim of the osseous external acoustic meatus and the lateral wall of the bulla with a rongeur or burr.

5 Carefully curette the osseous tympanic bulla, remaining osseous canal, and rostral, caudal and medial aspects of the lateral half of the tympanic cavity proper to remove any epithelium.

6 Gently flush the bulla with warm sterile saline and take samples of the area for culture before closure.

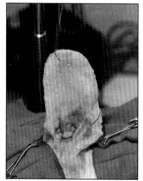

The pinna and lateral facial skin have been clipped and prepared. The ear is hung from a sterile towel clamp whilst drapes are placed.
(© Karen M. Tobias)

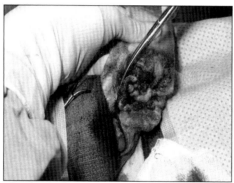

After the skin has been incised, the auricular cartilage is transected circumferentially around the vertical canal opening with curved Mayo or cartilage scissors.
(© Karen M. Tobias)

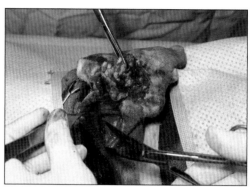

The soft tissues are carefully dissected away from the auricular cartilage.
(© Karen M. Tobias)

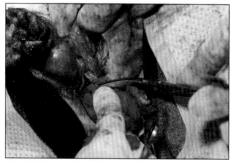

The facial nerve is visible along the ventrolateral surface of the annular cartilage.
(© Karen M. Tobias)

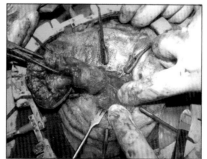

Ring retractors improve exposure during soft tissue dissection around the annular cartilage.
(© Karen M. Tobias)

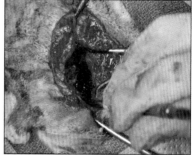

The bulla has been opened to expose debris and thickened lining, which will be removed with curettes, forceps or lavage.
(© Karen M. Tobias)

> **PRACTICAL TIP**
>
> Ring retractors may be helpful for improving exposure during deeper dissection

> **WARNING**
>
> The facial nerve can be damaged by vigorous dissection or retraction ventral or lateral to the horizontal canal. The external carotid artery may be torn during lateral bulla osteotomy if it is adherent to the bone or accidentally grasped with rongeurs

→ OPERATIVE TECHNIQUE 5.3 CONTINUED

Closure

If desired, place one or two sutures of 2 metric (3/0 USP) rapidly absorbable suture material to appose the deep tissues, being careful to avoid the facial nerve and external carotid artery. Position the skin to determine the best method for apposing skin to the incised pinna margin (usually a T- or L-shaped closure). Most surgeons use 2 metric (3/0 USP) nylon in an interrupted pattern to close the skin.

PRACTICAL TIP	**PRACTICAL TIP**
Subcutaneous sutures, when needed, should only be placed in the ventral portion of the incision	If the canal has ruptured and become abscessed, the surgical site can be managed as an open wound

POSTOPERATIVE CARE

A light bandage (e.g. stockinette) can be placed over the head to limit ear movement and protect the site. Thick or heavy bandages may result in compression of the airways and subsequent respiratory distress.

PRACTICAL TIP
In animals with bilateral disease, some surgeons stage the procedure to avoid long anaesthetic periods and the potential increased risk of severe swelling or infection. If bilateral procedures are performed, a change of instruments and gloves is recommended between sides

Chapter 6

Brachycephalic airway disease

Gert ter Haar and Gerhard U. Oechtering

Introduction

Brachycephalic dogs such as English and French Bulldogs, Pugs, Pekingese, Shih Tzus, Shar-Peis and Boston Terriers, and Persian and Himalayan cats, frequently present with signs of upper airway obstruction as a result of an anatomical distortion of their faces caused by selective breeding. Breeding for exaggerated, shortened skull features has deformed the heads of brachycephalic animals in such a way that health and welfare are compromised in an increasing number of individuals (Roedler *et al.*, 2013; Oechtering *et al.*, 2016b; ter Haar, 2016a). Termed brachycephalic airway disease (BAD), but also referred to as brachycephalic airway obstruction syndrome (BAOS), brachycephalic obstructive airway syndrome (BOAS) and brachycephalic airway syndrome (BAS), the condition develops as a result of an inherited defect in the development of the bones of the base of the skull (Harvey, 1989), whereby the head is of normal width but significantly reduced length. Because the soft tissues of the head are not reduced proportionally, redundant tissue increases the resistance to the flow of air through the upper airway. Problems go beyond the usually quoted triad of stenotic nares, overlong soft palate and everted laryngeal saccules. The syndrome entails narrowing of the entire nasal passageways as a result of relative conchal hypertrophy, with increased mucosal contact points and obstructive and protruding aberrant conchae (Roedler *et al.*, 2013; Oechtering, 2010; Schuenemann and Oechtering, 2014b; Oechtering *et al.*, 2016b). The nasopharyngeal passage is a narrow bony cage further compromised by excessive redundant tissue, and the aforementioned protrusion of nasal conchae and is prone to collapse (Rubin *et al.*, 2015). The pharyngeal and laryngeal airway passages are narrow as well, with dorsoventral flattening of the pharynx, a thickened base of the tongue, tonsillar hypertrophy and protrusion, and diffuse pharyngeal mucosal oedema all contributing to the obstruction caused by the relatively or absolutely overlong soft palate. Whereas, classically, laryngeal collapse has been described as the limiting factor in laryngeal airflow, narrowing of the larynx as a result of narrow and oval-shaped cricoid dimensions appears to be equally important (Rutherford *et al.*, 2017).

The set of airway signs characterized by stertor (excessive noise during breathing), reduced tolerance to exercise and stress, respiratory distress and, in severe cases, cyanosis and collapse, is frequently encountered in brachycephalic breeds. Nearly all brachycephalic dogs are affected by upper airway obstruction to some degree, but the clinical signs depend on the severity of functional stenosis of the airway. The upper airway obstruction is usually associated with some combination of abnormalities and the clinical signs vary from mild respiratory noise to severe signs of airway occlusion, including rough stertorous respiratory sounds, abducted forelimbs, slow forceful inspiratory effort and rapid forceful expiratory effort, and pale or cyanotic mucus membranes.

Besides these obvious effects on breathing, the small nasal cavity is no longer capable of performing other natural functions, all of which depend upon air being able to flow through the nose in well defined patterns over the turbinates. For a dog, drastic reduction of nasal breathing means that it loses its principal organ of thermoregulation and is no longer capable of evacuating body heat efficiently in the event of physical effort, excitement or even warm ambient temperatures (Oechtering, 2010, 2017). This causes the internal body temperature to rise and can lead to collapse and death. This is why brachycephalic animals are particularly heat-sensitive, why many pant to no avail even at room temperature and without physical effort, and why they may need several hours to recover even after brief exercise (Roedler *et al.*, 2013). To date, it is unclear how much the last function of the nose, olfaction, is affected by the nasal abnormalities seen.

Furthermore, the abnormal morphology of the tympanic bulla (Mielke *et al.*, 2017) seen in these breeds may predispose to auditory tube dysfunction and subsequent middle ear effusion, leading to conductive hearing loss and further decreasing the quality of life of these animals. As a result of the chronic high negative intrathoracic pressure generated upon inspiration, secondary gastrointestinal abnormalities such as hiatal hernia, oesophagitis, gastritis and pyloric mucosal hyperplasia, evidenced by gagging, vomiting and regurgitation, can develop (Poncet *et al.*, 2005), especially in the French Bulldog. Relative or absolute tracheal hypoplasia is commonly seen in the English Bulldog and is likely to be an important predisposing factor for development of aspiration pneumonia at an early age in this breed. Excessive facial and nasal skin folds make the animal prone to skin fold dermatitis. Corneal ulceration, as a result of large corneal exposure, reduced tear production, reduced sensitivity of the cornea and distichiasis or medial canthal entropion, is commonly seen, especially in the Pug.

Diagnosis

The diagnosis of BAD is very straightforward and based on the combination of a brachycephalic dog breed and obstructive upper airway signs alone. Taking a full history, performing a complete and multi-organ-system physical examination, and appropriate advanced imaging followed by endoscopic assessment are all mandatory to assess the severity of disease and thus inform the options for management.

A full history of clinical signs should be taken, preferably based on a structured standardized questionnaire (Roedler *et al.*, 2013; Pohl *et al.*, 2016) so that the clinician can assess the presence and severity of clinical signs associated not only with the airway obstruction but with other brachycephaly-related conditions as well. Nasal stertor indicates obstruction of airflow through the nasal passages, snoring is typically associated with (naso) pharyngeal disease, whereas laryngeal stridor ('g'-sound or sawing sound) is associated with laryngeal disease. Coughing, gagging, retching, regurgitation, vomiting and flatulence are frequently present as well, and may indicate significant aerophagia, or secondary or concurrent lower airway or gastrointestinal disease. Hearing loss often goes unrecognized by the owner, but scratching at the ears, head shaking, discharge and aural pain may be present. Epiphora, rubbing the face and ocular abnormalities may have been observed by the owner, as well as conformational orthopaedic and/or neurological abnormalities. A detailed description of all concurrent possible brachycephaly-related abnormalities is beyond the scope of this chapter, which will focus on the airways.

Physical examination findings are usually unremarkable except for the possible audible stridor and the obvious brachycephalic conformation of the animal. In addition, most patients demonstrate some degree of stenosis of the nares, and increased referred respiratory noises are frequently heard upon thoracic auscultation. These noises make cardiac auscultation difficult, which nonetheless needs to be performed meticulously to rule out concurrent cardiac disease such as pulmonic stenosis.

Diagnostic imaging of the head, neck and chest is useful for recognition of obstructing structures in the pharynx and larynx, tracheal hypoplasia (Figure 6.1), and to detect secondary aspiration pneumonia or pulmonary oedema. The tracheal diameter can be measured at the thoracic inlet and expressed as a percentage of the thoracic inlet diameter. In bulldogs, the tracheal diameter is a mean of 12.7% of the thoracic inlet, compared with 20% in non-brachycephalic breeds (Harvey, 1982c). In some patients, a hiatal hernia can be identified. Radiography is limited in its ability to provide information on the degree of narrowing of pharyngeal and laryngeal dimensions and associated pharyngitis and laryngitis, and it does not allow a proper evaluation of the nasal passages (aberrant conchae) and nasopharyngeal diameter. Pharyngeal fluoroscopy may be a useful diagnostic test for assessment of the degree of naso-pharyngeal collapse in brachycephalic patients (Rubin *et al.*, 2015). Computed tomography (CT) imaging is recommended in brachycephalic animals to allow assessment of all of the anatomical abnormalities using a single modality. This allows a much more accurate evaluation of the bony abnormalities and measurements of airway diameter, with assessment of the presence of nasopharyngeal turbinates and potential concurrent middle ear disease, also related to brachycephaly (Figure 6.2) (Grand and Bureau, 2011; Grosso *et al.*, 2015; Kaye *et al.*, 2015; Heidenreich *et al.*, 2016; Oechtering *et al.*, 2016a; Rutherford *et al.*, 2017; Mielke *et al.*, 2017).

Direct inspection of the pharynx and larynx with a laryngoscope is the most important diagnostic procedure for the subjective assessment of pharyngeal and laryngeal dimensions, the length of the soft palate and the degree of eversion of tonsils and mucosa of the lateral ventricles, and for evaluation of laryngeal collapse (Figures 6.3 and 6.4). With flexible or rigid endoscopes the nasal passages and nasopharyngeal area can be completely inspected, and evaluated for aberrant turbinates and increased mucosal contact points and protrusion of turbinates into the naso-pharynx (Figure 6.5). Endoscopic evaluation of the trachea helps in differentiating true tracheal hypoplasia from diffuse tracheal mucosal swelling and allows samples to be taken for cytological evaluation and culture in patients suspected of having aspiration pneumonia (Figure 6.6).

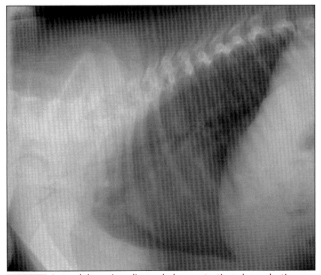

6.1 Lateral thoracic radiograph demonstrating a hypoplastic trachea in a 13-week-old Boston Terrier.

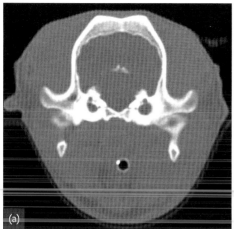
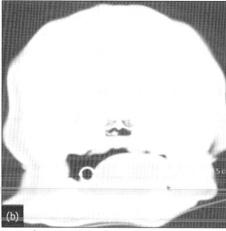
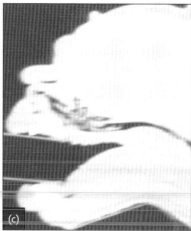

6.2 (a) Transverse computed tomographic (CT) image of a 4-year-old English Bulldog with non-aerated bullae and bilateral tympanic bulla wall thickening. (b) Transverse CT image of a 2-year-old Pug with severe nasopharyngeal turbinate protrusion. (c) Sagittal CT image of the same animal as in (b).

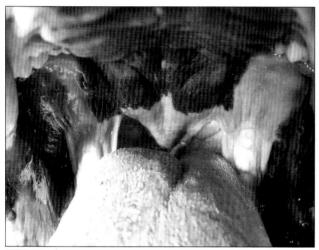

6.3 Throat examination in a 3-year-old French Bulldog demonstrating mild to moderate pharyngeal narrowing with mild dorsoventral flattening of the pharynx, mild protrusion of the tonsils, mild thickening of the base of the tongue, a moderate degree of pharyngeal oedema and a mildly elongated soft palate.

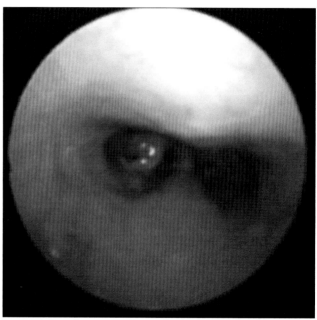

6.5 Nasopharyngoscopic examination in a French Bulldog demonstrating protrusion of the turbinates into the nasopharynx bilaterally.

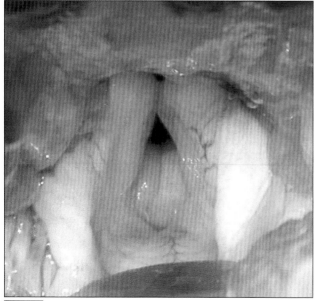

6.4 Everted laryngeal saccules in a French Bulldog.

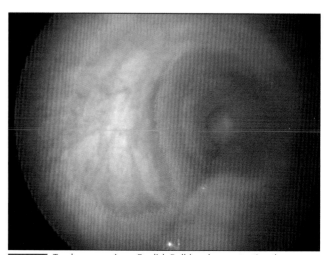

6.6 Tracheoscopy in an English Bulldog demonstrating the relatively narrow diameter of the trachea and mild tracheal hypoplasia.

Treatment

Animals in severe respiratory distress need to be evaluated quickly and intubated if respiratory arrest is imminent. Most animals respond to cold intravenous fluids, sedation with acepromazine (0.01 mg/kg i.v.), oxygen supplementation and dexamethasone (0.05–0.1 mg/kg i.v.) to decrease pharyngeal and laryngeal swelling. Intravenous access is mandatory in either case but should be obtained with as little restraint and stress to the animal as possible (Reiter and Holt, 2012). Long-term treatment of BAD is aimed at reducing airway resistance and alleviating obstruction, either medically and/or surgically (ter Haar, 2016b). Maintaining an appropriate bodyweight and condition, a clean, fresh and cool environment and regular controlled exercise are advised. Corticosteroids can be used to treat mucosal swelling, whereas broad-spectrum antibiotics, based on culture and sensitivity testing of tracheal aspirates/bronchoalveolar lavage samples, are indicated in cases with (aspiration) pneumonia. Any pre- or postoperative gastrointestinal signs are aggressively treated with a proton pump inhibitor (omeprazole 0.7 mg/kg orally q24h), a prokinetic (cisapride 0.2 mg/kg orally q8h or metoclopramide constant rate infusion at 1–2 mg/kg/day i.v.) and an antacid (Poncet et al., 2005; Reiter and Holt, 2012; Roedler et al., 2013; Oechtering et al., 2016b). Maropitant (1 mg/kg s.c. q24h) is a neurokinin (NK₁) receptor antagonist that may be useful in reducing the likelihood of regurgitation during anaesthesia. The components of the syndrome that are amenable to surgical correction are stenotic nares, aberrant turbinates, elongated soft palate, everted laryngeal saccules and laryngeal collapse.

Correction of stenotic nares and staphylectomy are techniques that, provided they are executed meticulously, improve patient welfare significantly and are associated with minimal complications. These two procedures form the first-stage surgical treatment for patients affected by BAD and can be performed in animals as young as 6 months of age (for instance, when presented for neutering).

Nasal airway resistance can be significantly reduced by resection of turbinates with laser under endoscopic guidance laser-assisted turbinectomy (LATE) (Oechtering et al., 2016b). The complication rate associated with the procedure in the hands of experienced surgeons appears to be low (Oechtering, 2010; Oechtering et al., 2016b). A recent report evaluating the LATE procedure in Pugs that had shown no or limited response to first-stage surgery has indicated that turbinectomy results in a good outcome, as assessed with barometric plethysmography (Liu et al., 2017).

Sacculectomy and laryngoplasty procedures (partial laryngectomy, arytenoid lateralization) are associated with higher perioperative risks (see section on surgical procedures), and therefore should only be employed if conservative treatment, in combination with the aforementioned surgical techniques, does not result in a significant improvement, or should be reserved for those cases where they are deemed absolutely necessary to improve outcome. In appropriately selected patients and when performed using magnifying loupes, or a surgical microscope and using meticulous technique, beneficial results can be obtained using sacculectomy, in selected patients with grade 1 laryngeal collapse, in particular, and occasionally in dogs with severe malformations.

Technique for correction of stenotic nares and resection of aberrant turbinates

Surgical correction of stenotic nares can be performed at a very early age (3–6 months). It significantly reduces upper airway resistance and decreases the rate of progression of other components of BAD (Harvey, 1982a; Lorinson et al., 1997; Huck et al., 2008). Several techniques have been described for correction of stenotic nares, using either scalpel blades, laser or electrosurgery. However, in the authors' experience, the use of excessive thermal energy, such as that generated by electrocautery and diode lasers, should be avoided because deep thermal damage, scarring and constrictive wound healing are commonly seen sequelae.

Patients are placed in sternal recumbency with the nose perpendicular to the table or slightly elevated. Adequate cosmetic and functional results of 'Trader's technique', which involves amputation of the ventral portion of the dorsal lateral nasal cartilage and healing by second intention, have been reported in immature Shih Tzu dogs with stenotic nares (Huck et al., 2008; Schmiedt and Creevy, 2012). In mature dogs, a lateral, vertical or horizontal wedge resection of the dorsal lateral cartilage can be performed (Venker-van Haagen, 2005; Schmiedt and Creevy, 2012). The authors recommend a modified horizontal wedge resection that includes a partial ala-vestibulectomy.

A wedge extending deep into the cartilage is resected, following the outer curvature of the ala from its medial dorsal-most aspect at the naris ventrally towards the lateral aspect and back over the body of the naris, connecting the start and end of the incision (see Operative Technique 6.1). A Beaver scalpel holder with a 6500 pointed blade allows accurate incision and determination of adequate depth. The initial suture is then placed from the middle of the remaining ventromedial part of the ala to the more dorsolateral aspect of the naris to open up the nasal vestibule adequately and create a maximal opening medially. Closure can be performed with 1–1.5 metric (4/0–5/0 USP) monofilament absorbable suture material in a single layer using a simple interrupted suture pattern.

Guided by preoperative cross-sectional imaging and rhinoscopy, LATE using a diode can be used to remove aberrant conchae and enlarge the ventral nasal meatus (Oechtering et al., 2016a,b). These recent reports indicate that this technique can reduce intranasal airway resistance by approximately 50% in brachycephalic dogs when performed by experienced surgeons. Grading of the degree of turbinate protrusion has recently been reported in English Bulldogs (Rooney, 2009; Rooney and Sargan, 2010; Palmer, 2012; Vilaplana Grosso et al., 2015). Pugs appear to have the most severe degree of turbinate protrusion amongst the brachycephalic breeds. Currently, the degree of protrusion that is clinically tolerated is unknown, but LATE has proven to be an effective treatment for intranasal obstruction, owing to a significant reduction in the number of contact points. Based on published results, morbidity and mortality rates associated with the procedure are low, and postoperative owner questionnaires (Pohl et al., 2016) and plethysmographic assessment (Liu et al., 2017) indicate substantial improvement. Whilst conchal regrowth after LATE is seen in most cases, it rarely leads to a need for revision surgery. A degree of regrowth may even be desirable as it allows for an increased capacity to fulfil important physiological functions (Schuenemann and Oechtering, 2014b).

Staphylectomy for elongated/overlong soft palate

The dog is positioned in sternal recumbency for soft palate resection (see Operative Technique 6.2). A bar is placed over the front of the surgery table from which the upper jaw is suspended by placing gauze, tape or bandage material around the maxillary canine teeth. The proposed lateral levels of palate resection, the caudal borders of the palatine tonsils when a minimal amount of rostral retraction is applied to the tongue, are tagged with two stay sutures. An Allis tissue forceps is placed on the caudal edge of the palate on the midline and used to pull the palate rostrally. The palate is then resected in an arch shape, making sure to remove more tissue medially than laterally. Resection can be performed with scalpel blades, scissors (Harvey, 1982b; Bright and Wheaton, 1983; Riecks et al., 2007), a carbon dioxide laser (Clark and Sinibaldi, 1994; Davidson et al., 2001; Riecks et al., 2007) or an electrothermal feedback-controlled bipolar sealing device (Brdecka et al., 2009). However, as for resection of the nares, the use of laser and electrothermal devices is not recommended for staphylectomy by the authors: 'cold' resection techniques are advised. After resection, the oropharyngeal and nasopharyngeal mucosa are apposed using 1.5–2 metric (3/0–4/0 USP) monofilament rapidly absorbable suture material.

Serious complications of staphylectomy include death as a result of aspiration pneumonia, dyspnoea and cyanosis requiring tracheostomy, or failure to recover from anaesthesia (Harvey, 1982b; Lorinson et al., 1997; Torrez and Hunt, 2006). Less severe complications include coughing, noisy respiration, and gagging and retching (Reiter and Holt, 2012). The prognosis of dogs after soft palate resection is good to excellent in 90% of cases, especially in dogs younger than 1 or 2 years of age (Harvey, 1982b; Poncet et al., 2005; Riecks et al., 2007; Reiter and Holt, 2012). A recent report (Liu et al, 2017), on the other hand, found that younger animals may actually have a worse prognosis. However, age was only one of several factors influencing outcome reported by this study and it also showed that dogs undergoing modern multilevel surgery have a better prognosis than those undergoing traditional surgery.

Everted laryngeal saccules and laryngeal collapse

Traditionally, three different stages of laryngeal collapse are clinically recognized (Leonard, 1960; Pink et al., 2006; Monnet and Tobias, 2012; Oechtering et al., 2016b; Liu et al., 2017). Stage I is relatively mild, consisting of laryngeal saccule eversion. In stage II, medial collapse of the cuneiform process of the arytenoid cartilage as a result of lack of rigidity is seen. In stage III, the corniculate processes of the arytenoid cartilages collapse, resulting in significant airway obstruction (Leonard, 1960; Harvey, 1982a; Lorinson et al., 1997; Pink et al., 2006; Huck et al., 2008; Monnet and Tobias, 2012). This classification does not do justice, however, to the wide range of laryngeal abnormalities seen in the brachycephalic breeds and the breed-specific laryngeal anatomy. Most animals have some degree of eversion of the saccules (i.e. the mucosa of the lateral ventricles), even in absence of obvious clinical signs (Kaye et al., 2015). In addition, pure stage II or III collapse is uncommon because most animals with more advanced laryngeal collapse demonstrate a varying degree of collapse of both the corniculate and cuneiform processes. It seems logical that primary developmental abnormalities of the larynx such as underdeveloped cartilages with chondromalacia and narrow glottic (cricoid) dimensions (Rutherford et al., 2017) play an important role in the aetiopathogenesis of the syndrome. More research into the specific primary and secondary laryngeal abnormalities is needed, however.

Whether or not all brachycephalic animals with respiratory problems benefit from sacculectomy is controversial, and the benefit of sacculectomy in the overall outcome has not been assessed.

Medical management, including weight loss, exercise restriction and drugs to reduce airway swelling (e.g. glucocorticoids) or oedema (e.g. furosemide), can be attempted in animals with signs secondary to persistent laryngeal collapse (Monnet and Tobias, 2012) and narrow laryngeal and tracheal dimensions. Patients that do not respond to the first-stage surgical and medical management may require sacculectomy, partial laser laryngectomy or laryngeal tie-back; however, the effectiveness of these procedures for resolution of airway obstruction has not been extensively evaluated (Pink et al., 2006; White, 2012; Monnet and Tobias, 2012). In the authors' opinion, temporary as well as permanent tracheotomy procedures in brachycephalic dogs should be avoided if possible because inherent tracheal hypoplasia, granulation tissue and scar formation, and increased loss of rigidity as a result of this procedure significantly complicate a successful outcome. In addition, breathing through a temporary as well as permanent tracheotomy site has been shown to lead to warming of cerebral arterial blood and the brain itself (Baker et al., 1974), adding to the disturbed thermoregulation in these breeds.

Postoperative care

In general, after rhinoplasty and staphylectomy, dogs should be observed and kept calm during recovery until at least 1 hour after extubation, which should take place only when they are almost fully awake and consciously aware of the tube (Brainard and Hofmeister, 2012; Monnet and Tobias, 2012). The dog's pulse, temperature, and respiratory rate and effort are monitored frequently. Food and water are withheld only until complete recovery. Dogs are monitored for any gagging, retching or vomiting, stridor and development of dyspnoea. After recovery, dogs are offered water and a small amount of soft food under supervision, and swallowing is carefully observed. After laryngeal procedures, dogs must be observed in an intensive care unit. If postoperative dyspnoea occurs, animals are best heavily sedated (for 8–12 hours, with an additional dose of corticosteroids administered) and re-intubated with a small tube. They can generally be successfully extubated and recovered uneventfully after this period.

References and further reading

Baker MA, Chapman LW and Nathanson M (1974) Control of brain temperature in dogs: effects of tracheostomy. Respiratory Physiology 22, 325–333

Brainard BM and Hofmeister EH (2012) Anesthesia principles and monitoring. In: Veterinary Surgery: Small Animal, ed. KM Tobias and SA Johnston, pp. 248–291. Elsevier Saunders, St Louis

Brdecka DJ, Rawlings CA, Perry AC and Anderson JR (2009) Use of an electrothermal, feedback-controlled, bipolar sealing device for resection of the elongated portion of the soft palate in dogs with obstructive upper airway disease. Journal of the American Veterinary Medical Association 233, 1265–1269

Bright RM and Wheaton LG (1983) A modified surgical technique for elongated soft palate in dogs. *Journal of the American Animal Hospital Association* **19**, 288–292

Clark GN and Sinibaldi KR (1994) Use of a carbon dioxide laser for treatment of elongated soft palate in dogs. *Journal of the American Veterinary Medical Association* **204**, 1779–1781

Davidson EB, Davis MS, Campbell GA *et al.* (2001) Evaluation of carbon dioxide laser and conventional incisional techniques for resection of soft palates in brachycephalic dogs. *Journal of the American Veterinary Medical Association* **219**, 776–781

Grand JG and Bureau S (2011) Structural characteristics of the soft palate and meatus nasopharyngeus in brachycephalic and non-brachycephalic dogs analysed by CT. *Journal of Small Animal Practice* **52**, 232–239

Grosso FV, ter Haar G and Boroffka SAEB (2015) Gender, weight, and age effects on prevalance of caudal aberrant nasal turbinates in clinically healthy English bulldogs: a computed tomographic study and classification. *Veterinary Radiology and Ultrasound* **56**, 486–493

Harvey CE (1982a) Upper airway obstruction surgery. 1. Stenotic nares surgery in brachycephalic dogs. *Journal of the American Animal Hospital Association* **18**, 535–537

Harvey CE (1982b) Upper airway obstruction surgery. 2. Soft palate resection in brachycephalic dogs. *Journal of the American Animal Hospital Association* **18**, 538–544

Harvey CE (1982c) Tracheal diameter: analysis of radiographic measurements in brachycephalic and nonbrachycephalic dogs. *Journal of the American Animal Hospital Association* **18**, 570–576

Harvey CE (1989) Inherited and congenital airway conditions. *Journal of Small Animal Practice* **30**, 184–187

Heidenreich D, Gradner G, Kneissl S and Dupré G (2016) Nasopharyngeal dimensions from computed tomography of pugs and French bulldogs with brachycephalic airway syndrome. *Veterinary Surgery* **45**, 83–90

Huck JL, Stanley BJ and Hauptman JG (2008) Technique and outcome of nares amputation (Trader's technique) in immature Shih Tzus. *Journal of the American Animal Hospital Association* **44**, 82–85

Kaye BM, Boroffka SAEB, Haagsman AN and ter Haar G (2015) Computed tomographic, radiographic and endoscopic tracheal dimensions in English Bulldogs with grade 1 clinical signs of brachycephalic airway syndrome. *Veterinary Radiology and Ultrasound* **56**, 609–616

Leonard HC (1960) Collapse of the larynx and adjacent structures in the dog. *Journal of the American Veterinary Medical Association* **137**, 360–363

Liu NC, Oechtering GU, Adams VJ *et al.* (2017) Outcomes and prognostic factors of surgical treatments for brachycephalic obstructive airway syndrome in three breeds. *Veterinary Surgery* **46**, 271–280

Lorinson D, Bright RM and White R (1997) Brachycephalic airway obstruction syndrome – a review of 118 cases. *Canine Practice* **22**, 18–21

Mehl ML, Kyles AE, Pypendop BH, Filipowicz DE and Gregory CR (2008) Outcome of laryngeal web resection with mucosal apposition for treatment of airway obstruction in dogs: 15 cases (1992–2006). *Journal of the American Veterinary Medical Association* **233**, 738–742

Mielke B, Lam R and ter Haar G (2017) Computed tomographic morphometry of tympanic bulla shape and position in brachycephalic and mesaticephalic dog breeds. *Veterinary Radiology and Ultrasound* **58**, 552–558

Monnet E and Tobias KM (2012) Larynx. In: *Veterinary Surgery: Small Animal*, ed. KM Tobias and SA Johnston, pp. 1718–1733. Elsevier Saunders, St. Louis

Oechtering GU (2010) Brachycephalic syndrome – new information on an old congenital disease. *Veterinary Focus* **20**, 2–9

Oechtering GU (2017) Diseases of the nose, nasopharynx and sinuses. In: *Textbook of Veterinary Internal Medicine, 8th edn*, ed. SJ Ettinger, EC Feldman and E Cote, pp. 1059–1077. Elsevier, Philadelphia

Oechtering GU, Pohl S, Schlueter C *et al.* (2016a) A novel approach to brachycephalic syndrome. 1. Evaluation of anatomical intranasal airway obstruction. *Veterinary Surgery* **45**, 165–172

Oechtering GU, Pohl S, Schlueter C and Schuenemann R (2016b) A novel approach to brachycephalic syndrome. 2. Laser-assisted turbinectomy (LATE). *Veterinary Surgery* **45**, 173–181

Palmer C (2012) Does breeding a bulldog harm it? Breeding, ethics and harm to animals. *Animal Welfare* **21**, 157–166

Pink JJ, Doyle RS, Hughes JM, Tobin E and Bellenger CR (2006) Laryngeal collapse in seven brachycephalic puppies. *Journal of Small Animal Practice* **47**, 131–135

Pohl S, Roedler FS and Oechtering GU (2016) How does multilevel upper airway surgery influence the lives of dogs with severe brachycephaly? Results of a structured pre- and postoperative owner questionnaire. *Veterinary Journal* **210**, 39–45

Poncet CM, Dupre GP, Freiche VG *et al.* (2005) Prevalence of gastrointestinal tract lesions in 73 brachycephalic dogs with upper respiratory syndrome. *Journal of Small Animal Practice* **46**, 273–279

Reiter AM and Holt DE (2012) Palate. In: *Veterinary Surgery: Small Animal*, ed. KM Tobias and SA Johnston, pp. 1707–1717. Elsevier Saunders, St. Louis

Riecks TW, Birchard SJ and Stephens JA (2007) Surgical correction of brachycephalic syndrome in dogs: 62 cases (1991–2004). *Journal of the American Veterinary Medical Association* **230**, 1324–1328

Roedler FS, Pohl S and Oechtering GU (2013) How does severe brachycephaly affect dog's lives? Results of a structured preoperative owner questionnaire. *Veterinary Journal* **198**, 606–610

Rooney NJ (2009) The welfare of pedigree dogs: cause for concern. *Journal of Veterinary Behaviour: Clinical Applications and Research* **4**, 180–186

Rooney NJ and Sargan DR (2010) Welfare concerns associated with pedigree dog breeding in the UK. *Animal Welfare* **19**, 133–140

Rubin JA, Holt DE, Reetz JA and Clarke DL (2015) Signalment, clinical presentation, concurrent diseases, and diagnostic findings in 28 dogs with dynamic pharyngeal collapse (2008–2013). *Journal of Veterinary Internal Medicine* **29**, 815–821

Rutherford L, Beever L, Bruce MM and ter Haar G (2017) Assessment of computed tomography derived cricoid cartilage and tracheal dimensions to evaluate degree of cricoid narrowing in brachycephalic dogs. *Veterinary Radiology and Ultrasound* **58**, 634–646

Schmiedt CW and Creevy KE (2012) Nasal planum, nasal cavity, and sinuses. In: *Veterinary Surgery: Small Animal*, ed. KM Tobias and SA Johnston, pp. 1691–1706. Elsevier Saunders, St Louis

Schuenemann R and Oechtering GU (2014a) Inside the brachycephalic nose: intranasal mucosal contact points. *Journal of the American Animal Hospital Association* **50**, 149–158

Schuenemann R and Oechtering G (2014b) Inside the brachycephalic nose: conchal regrowth and mucosal contact points after laser-assisted turbinectomy. *Journal of the American Animal Hospital Association* **50**, 237–246

ter Haar G (2016a) Diseases of the nasal cavity and sinuses. In: *Ear, Nose and Throat Diseases of the Dog and Cat, 1st edn*, ed. RG Harvey and G ter Haar G, pp. 287–334. CRC Press, London

ter Haar G (2016b) Surgery of the nose. In: *Ear, Nose and Throat Diseases of the Dog and Cat, 1st edn*, ed. RG Harvey and G ter Haar G, pp. 449–474. CRC Press, London

Torrez CV and Hunt GB (2006) Results of surgical correction of abnormalities associated with brachycephalic airway obstruction syndrome in dogs in Australia. *Journal of Small Animal Practice* **47**, 150–154

Venker-van Haagen AJ (2005) The nose and nasal sinuses. In: *Ear, Nose, Throat, and Tracheobronchial Diseases in Dogs and Cats*, ed. AJ Venker-van Haagen, pp. 51–81 Schlütersche, Hannover

Vilaplana Grosso F, ter Haar G and Boroffka SAEB (2015) Gender, weight, and age effects on prevalence of caudal aberrant nasal turbinates in clinically healthy English Bulldogs: a computed tomographic study and classification. *Veterinary Radiology and Ultrasound* **56**, 486–493

White RN (2012) Surgical management of laryngeal collapse associated with brachycephalic airway obstruction syndrome in dogs. *Journal of Small Animal Practice* **53**, 44–50

OPERATIVE TECHNIQUE 6.1

Modified horizontal wedge resection of the nares

PATIENT POSITIONING

The patient is positioned in sternal recumbency, with the nose pointed slightly upwards and at the end of the operating table. The nasal planum should be aseptically prepared for surgery.

ASSISTANT

Optional.

SURGICAL TECHNIQUE

Approach

The naris is slightly lifted by pushing on the base using the thumb of the non-dominant hand. A wedge extending deep into the cartilage is to be resected.

Surgical manipulations

1   The first incision is started at the medial dorsal-most aspect of the naris, whilst applying some pressure on it with a finger or thumb, ensuring that the Beaver scalpel blade is angled in a slight mediolateral direction. Care should be taken to incise deep into the underlying cartilage.

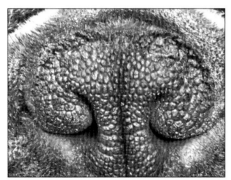 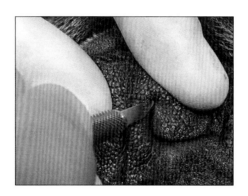

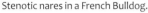
Stenotic nares in a French Bulldog.

2   The incision should be approximately 1 cm deep and should follow the outer curvature of the ala ventrally towards the lateral aspect of the naris, changing the angle of the blade to more horizontal for the most ventral part of the incision. The incision is continued laterally as far as deemed necessary.

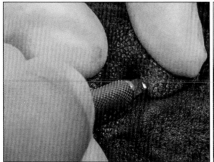 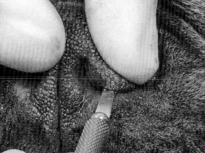 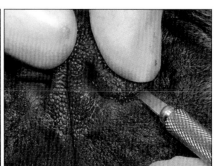

➡ **OPERATIVE TECHNIQUE 6.1 CONTINUED**

3 The part of the naris that is to be excised is grasped with tissue forceps and lifted.

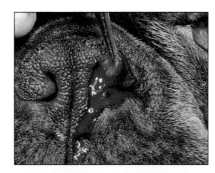

4 The incision is now continued over the body of the naris, connecting the start and end of the incision, and the excised part of the naris is removed.

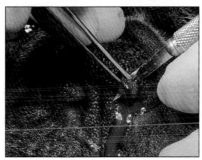

5 The initial suture is then placed from the middle of the remaining ventromedial part of the ala to the more dorsolateral aspect of the naris to open up the nasal vestibule adequately and create a maximal opening medially.

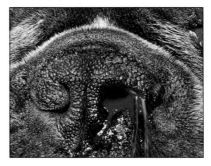

6 Two or three more interrupted sutures are placed to close the wound completely. A larger opening results, allowing airflow into the nasal vestibule.

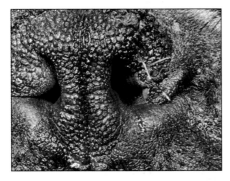 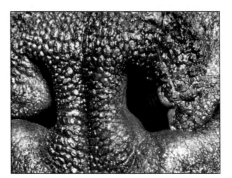

7 The procedure is repeated on the other side.

PRACTICAL TIP

The bleeding generally stops after placement of the first suture. Despite the bleeding associated with sharp excisional techniques, they are preferred over electrocautery or laser resection of the nares as these techniques cause more scar tissue formation

---

POSTOPERATIVE CARE

Postoperative care consists of removing the blood clots that will have formed in the nasal vestibules and close monitoring of the patient. Monitor for complications as described for staphylectomy (see Operative Technique 6.2).

OPERATIVE TECHNIQUE 6.2

Staphylectomy (soft palate resection)

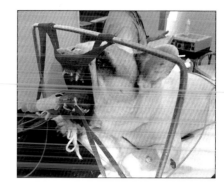

PATIENT POSITIONING

The dog is positioned in sternal recumbency for soft palate resection. A bar is placed over the front of the surgery table to which the upper jaw is suspended by placing gauze, tape or bandage material around the maxillary canine teeth. The lower jaw is attached to the surgery table as well, to achieve adequate exposure of the throat. A swab is placed deep in the laryngopharynx, just past the free edge of the soft palate, to aid in ventral deflection of the endotracheal tube.

ASSISTANT

Optional.

SURGICAL TECHNIQUE

Approach

An oral approach is used, which allows sufficient exposure of the soft palate in most dogs. In a dog with a very narrow pharynx or thick tongue, an assistant may be needed to deflect the tongue more ventrally as well as pulling the tongue out as needed to gain adequate exposure.

Surgical manipulations

1   An Allis tissue forceps is placed on the caudal edge of the soft palate on the midline and used to retract the palate rostrally.

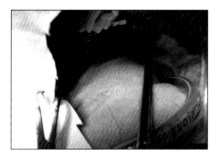

2   To mark the proposed lateral levels of soft palate resection, the free caudolateral edges of the palate are tagged with two stay sutures, applying only a minimal amount of rostral retraction to the tongue.

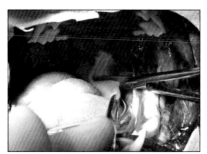 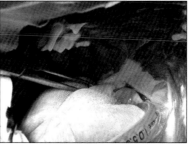

3   The soft palate is then resected in a wide arch shape, making sure that more tissue is removed medially than laterally. The highest point of the arch can be level with the mid- to rostral one-third of the tonsils. Resection is performed with scissors.

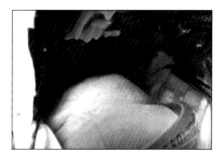 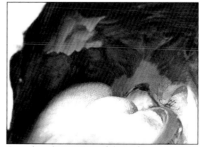

The incision is started laterally.   Half of the palate has been cut with scissors.   Completed resection of the soft palate; minimal blood loss is visible.

→ **OPERATIVE TECHNIQUE 6.2 CONTINUED**

4 The oropharyngeal and nasopharyngeal mucosa are then adapted using 1.5–2 metric (3/0–4/0 USP) monofilament or multifilament rapidly absorbable suture material in either an interrupted or a continuous pattern, starting in the middle of the incision, to complete the staphylectomy.

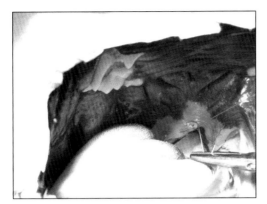 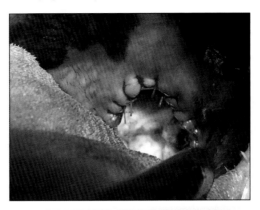

PRACTICAL TIP

The lateral stay sutures, when properly placed, will help to avoid cutting into the laterally located vessels and help minimize blood loss during the procedure. In addition, having an assistant pull on the stay sutures aids in stretching the soft palate, and helps subsequent excision and suturing

POSTOPERATIVE CARE

In general, after airway surgery, dogs should be observed and kept calm during recovery until at least 1 hour after extubation, which should take place only when they are almost fully awake and consciously aware of the tube. Food and water are withheld only until complete recovery. Dogs are monitored for any gagging, retching or vomiting, stridor and development of dyspnoea. If postoperative dyspnoea occurs, animals can either be heavily sedated (for 8–12 hours with an additional dose of corticosteroids administered) and re-intubated with a small tube, or a tracheostomy should be performed.

Chapter 7

Surgery of the larynx

Michael B. Mison and Gert ter Haar

Anatomy

The larynx is a fibroelastic membranous tube in which several stiff hyaline cartilages are embedded to maintain a patent airway. It separates the upper and lower airways and acts as a valve during swallowing. It maintains a patent airway whilst supporting two sets of valves, the passive, hinged epiglottis and the more refined, active glottis. There are five main cartilaginous structures (Figure 7.1):

- Cricoid cartilage
- Thyroid cartilage
- Paired arytenoid cartilages (with cuneiform, corniculate, muscular and vocal processes)
- Epiglottic cartilage
- Sesamoid cartilage/interarytenoid cartilage.

The larynx is anchored cranially to the thyrohyoid bone of the hyoid apparatus via a synovial joint with the cranial cornu of the thyroid cartilage. Its caudal attachment is from the cricoid to the trachea. The rima glottidis is the diamond-shaped airway formed dorsally by the arytenoid cartilages and ventrally by the vocal folds (Figure 7.2). This is the narrowest part of the larynx, thus its size (controlled by intrinsic laryngeal muscles) will determine the rate at which air can be passed into and out of the lungs. The glottis can be widened by contraction of the cricoarytenoid dorsalis muscles, causing abduction of the arytenoid cartilages as they rotate caudolaterally around the cricoarytenoid articulation. The glottis can also close very tightly when required (e.g. swallowing, laryngospasm) by the opposite rotation of the arytenoids caused by the cricoarytenoid lateralis, thyroarytenoid and transverse arytenoid muscles, which results in adduction of the arytenoids and closure of the vocal cords. The extrinsic muscles of the larynx suspend the larynx from the hyoid apparatus (Figure 7.3) and work to control the arytenoid cartilages.

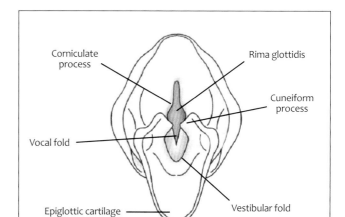

7.2 Anatomy of the larynx as viewed during laryngoscopy.

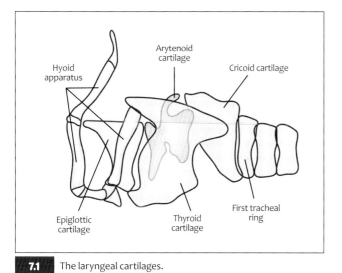

7.1 The laryngeal cartilages.

7.3 Muscles surrounding the larynx.

The laryngeal ventricles are located medial to the thyroid cartilage and lateral to the vestibular and vocal folds. The vocal folds and adjacent laryngeal ventricles control phonation. The slit-like opening is bordered cranially by the vestibular fold and caudally by the vocal fold (Basenji dogs have severely reduced or absent laryngeal ventricles, which fits with the speculation that they cannot or do not bark).

The recurrent laryngeal nerve is a branch of the vagus nerve that innervates all intrinsic muscles of the larynx except the cricothyroideus (tensor) muscle. The somatic fibres arise from the nucleus ambiguus before joining the vagus nerve. The recurrent laryngeal nerve branches from the vagus nerve at the level of the aortic arch, where the left recurrent laryngeal nerve courses around the ligamentum arteriosum before ascending cranially. On the right side, it arises from a similar level and wraps around the right subclavian artery before continuing on its course cranially. The nerve courses over the lateral aspects of the trachea to the level of the larynx and oesophagus, and terminates as the caudal laryngeal nerve bilaterally. The cricothyroideus muscle is innervated by branches of the cranial laryngeal nerve, in addition to pharyngeal branches of the vagus nerve. Less cited recurrent laryngeal nerve branches form the pararecurrent laryngeal nerves, which innervate the cervical and cranial thoracic oesophagus.

Functions of the larynx

The functions of the larynx include:

- Preventing inhalation of food or liquids during swallowing by adduction of the arytenoids and vocal folds and passive coverage by the epiglottis
- Regulating airflow and minimizing resistance to the passage of air when demand is increased:
  - At rest: abduction of arytenoids during inspiration, passive during expiration
  - With vigorous exercise: maximal abduction during inspiration and expiration
- Vocalization, mediated by the vocal folds and laryngeal ventricles. This can be important in working dogs. A change in bark may be the earliest sign of laryngeal paralysis. A loss of purring can be an early sign in the cat
- The larynx is also important in coughing, parturition, eructation and vomiting.

These functions are regulated by the intrinsic musculature and innervation of the larynx. The cricoarytenoideus dorsalis muscle is responsible for arytenoid cartilage abduction during inspiration. The recurrent laryngeal nerve innervates this muscle. An injury to the recurrent laryngeal nerve at any point along its length, or to the cricoarytenoideus dorsalis muscle, can lead to laryngeal paresis or paralysis. Laryngeal dysfunction can be unilateral or bilateral.

Laryngeal paralysis

Aetiology of paralysis

Interruption in the transmission of impulses through the recurrent laryngeal nerves and caudal laryngeal nerves can lead to denervation of adductor and abductor muscles of the larynx. Consequently, the vocal folds and arytenoid cartilages remain in a paramedian position. Upper airway obstruction occurs because of the greatly increased resistance to airflow at the level of the rima glottidis. Laryngeal oedema may develop as a consequence of turbulent airflow, causing further obstruction.

- **Congenital laryngeal paralysis** occurs at a young age (typically before 1 year of age) in Bouviers des Flandres, Bull Terriers, Dalmatians, Rottweilers and Huskies. Bouviers and Bull Terriers tend to be of European lineages, whilst affected Dalmatians and Huskies tend to be reported in the USA. Wallerian degeneration of the recurrent laryngeal nerves and abnormalities of the nucleus ambiguus are present.
- An **inherited laryngeal paralysis** has been documented in young Bouviers des Flandres. It can be uni- or bilateral and is autosomal dominant, involving a loss of motor neurons in the nucleus ambiguus. Similar findings have been reported in young Siberian Huskies and crosses, and in Bull Terriers.
- A suspected hereditary **laryngeal paralysis–polyneuropathy** complex has been reported in Dalmatians, Rottweilers and Leonbergers in which affected dogs manifest signs of a generalized neuropathy.
- There have been several reports of a **neurodegenerative disease** in Rottweilers, different from the above. These dogs demonstrate progressive ataxia, tetraparesis and laryngeal paralysis, and have widespread neuronal vacuolation and spongiform changes in their nervous systems.
- **Myasthenia gravis** has been reported with laryngeal paralysis, and laryngeal paralysis can occasionally be the presenting clinical sign.
- Four cases of **spontaneous laryngeal paralysis** in juvenile white-coated German Shepherd Dogs have been reported.
- **Traumatic laryngeal paralysis** occurs sporadically with injuries to the neck or cranial thorax (e.g. bite wounds).
- **Iatrogenic trauma** to the recurrent laryngeal nerve(s), during procedures such as tracheal surgery, patent ductus arteriosus surgery and pharyngostomy tube placement, could potentially result in temporary or permanent dysfunction.
- **Tumours** such as thyroid neoplasia and cranial mediastinal masses can disrupt recurrent laryngeal nerve function, resulting in the condition.
- Laryngeal paralysis can be a manifestation of any **generalized neuropathy or myopathy**, e.g. vagal neuropathy, and is seen associated with **hypothyroidism** (up to 17% of hypothyroid dogs have been reported to have laryngeal paralysis).
- By far the majority of dogs with laryngeal paralysis fall into the category **idiopathic laryngeal paralysis (ILP)**. ILP is seen mostly in middle-aged to older, medium to large breeds such as Labrador and Golden Retrievers, Irish Setters, pointers, Afghan Hounds, and some giant breeds. Male dogs seem to be more frequently affected than bitches, but not all studies support this observation.

History and examination findings

Presenting signs are similar for both congenital and acquired forms of laryngeal paralysis. Signs can be progressive over months to years. Early signs may include a change in 'voice' (dysphonia) and gagging or coughing associated with eating and drinking. Exercise tolerance decreases over time and inspiratory stridor becomes more apparent. The most severely affected animals may have episodes of severe dyspnoea, cyanosis and syncope. Various degrees of dysphagia may also accompany laryngeal paralysis, due to pararecurrent laryngeal nerve dysfunction, and this is correlated with an increased likelihood of aspiration pneumonia. The physical examination findings for an animal with laryngeal paralysis are typically unremarkable with the exception of the respiratory system. Inspiratory stridor that does not improve with open-mouth breathing is often present. Referred upper airway noise can be heard on thoracic auscultation. Animals with concurrent pneumonia or non-cardiogenic pulmonary oedema may have pulmonary crackles on auscultation.

Laboratory findings

Consistent bloodwork abnormalities are uncommon in patients with laryngeal paralysis. If concurrent pneumonia is present, leucocytosis with neutrophilia may be present. Animals with hypothyroidism can have hypercholesterolaemia, hyperlipidaemia and elevated liver enzymes. Thyroid testing is recommended in these cases. If myasthenia gravis is suspected, edrophonium chloride testing or acetylcholine receptor antibody titres can be performed.

Radiographic examination

Radiographic examination is typically utilized to evaluate the thoracic cavity for evidence of pneumonia, megaoesophagus or any mediastinal mass that could be the cause of laryngeal paralysis. Secondary cardiac changes (right ventricular hypertrophy) due to chronic upper airway obstruction can be seen. Hiatal hernia has been reported in association with laryngeal paralysis and is probably secondary to the extreme subatmospheric intrathoracic pressure generated in dogs during an upper airway obstructive crisis. Cervical radiographs tend to be unremarkable, although caudal retraction of the larynx can be seen in animals that are dyspnoeic.

Laryngeal examination

A sedated laryngeal examination is the most definitive diagnostic tool for laryngeal paralysis. Historically, sodium thiopentone was used to induce a light plane of anaesthesia for functional examination of the larynx; more recently, propofol or alfaxalone has been used. To evaluate the larynx, the patient must be at a deep enough plane of anaesthesia to allow the mouth to be opened, but not so deep that the pharyngeal and laryngeal reflexes are compromised. If the anaesthetic plane is thought to be too deep, the patient should be given time to recover from the anaesthetic event until the pharyngeal gag reflex or cough reflex returns.

With the animal in sternal recumbency and the mouth opened at the level of normal head carriage, the arytenoid cartilages and ventrally located vocal folds should retract laterally during each inhalation and return to a neutral position on exhalation. Subjectively decreased or absent movements and/or 'paradoxical motion' of the arytenoid cartilages or 'paradoxical flutter' signifies paresis or paralysis. For animals taking short shallow breaths, doxopram can be administered intravenously to increase the tidal volume and respiratory rate. It is also helpful for an assistant to mark each attempt at inhalation so that the laryngeal observer can focus on the corresponding laryngeal

motion. In patients with signs of chronic upper airway obstruction, or following a recent dyspnoeic event, the mucosa overlying the laryngeal cartilages may show a varying degree of oedema and erythema due to turbulent instead of laminar airflow.

Emergency treatment

Animals with laryngeal paralysis can be presented in either a stable or unstable condition, depending on the severity of the dysfunction (paresis *versus* complete paralysis) and prevailing environmental conditions. In an emergency presentation, patients are presented with severe breathing difficulty, cyanosis or collapse, as a result of their upper airway obstruction. Excitement, exercise or increased ambient temperature is usually the catalyst for such an event in an animal with laryngeal paralysis. With prompt medical therapy, most patients recover initially. Excitement and increased ambient temperature lead to an increased respiratory rate and laryngeal oedema. As the speed of air flowing over the arytenoid cartilages increases, the air pressure decreases. This tends to draw the arytenoids further towards each other. The upper airway obstruction causes distress to the animal and leads to greater inspiratory effort, which exacerbates the turbulent airflow through the rima glottidis, worsening the laryngeal oedema and paradoxical laryngeal motion.

Initial stabilization should include sedation with anxiolytics (acepromazine at a dose of 0.02–0.1 mg/kg i.v., maximum dose 3 mg). If the patient's stress level is increased by the restraint needed to facilitate intravenous injection, intramuscular injection is a reasonable second option. Intravenous corticosteroids may be used to reduce laryngeal oedema. Dexamethasone at a dose of 0.2–1 mg/kg i.v. q12h or prednisolone sodium succinate at a dose of 1 mg/kg i.v. q24h may be used initially. Supplemental oxygen therapy is indicated after the sedation has been administered. Patients in an acute crisis are often hyperthermic, and active cooling should be instituted using water baths, ice packs or alcohol applied to the foot pads. Finally, for animals with refractory upper airway obstruction, intubation or emergency tracheostomy can be considered.

Medical management

Medical management is considered conservative management and is reserved for patients with mild clinical signs. Laryngeal paralysis is a progressive disease and clinical signs will worsen with time. The hallmarks of medical management are lifestyle changes. This means avoiding strenuous exercise, maintaining a low ambient temperature, and sedation as needed. Clients need to be counselled on the fact that clinical signs will progress and that their pet could have an acute respiratory event at any time. Ultimately, surgery is recommended when medical management is not sufficient to control clinical signs.

Surgical management

The goal of surgery in the treatment of laryngeal paralysis is to palliate the clinical signs associated with inspiratory failure. This may be achieved by the permanent removal or repositioning of the laryngeal cartilages to widen the rima glottidis. According to Poiseuille's law, the resistance to fluid flow through a cylinder is proportional to the radius of the cylinder (at its narrowest point) to the fourth power, which means that even a modest change in glottic radius can make a profound difference in resistance to airflow.

Reported procedures include unilateral arytenoid lateralization (cricoarytenoid or thyroarytenoid), bilateral arytenoid lateralization, ventricular cordectomy and partial arytenoidectomy via an oral or ventral approach, modified castellated laryngofissure, reinnervation of the laryngeal musculature, nitinol stenting and permanent tracheostomy.

The technique with the best reported outcome is unilateral arytenoid lateralization, and this is the most common procedure performed. Patients do well with unilateral surgery and the risk of aspiration pneumonia is minimized. Both a cricoarytenoid technique and a thyroarytenoid technique have been described, with good clinical outcomes (see Operative Techniques 7.1 and 7.2). The increase in total rima glottidis size with cricoarytenoid lateralization is considerable, but this does not have long-term clinical significance when compared with thyroarytenoid lateralization. Regardless of the technique performed, one or two monofilament non-absorbable sutures are placed to retract the arytenoid cartilage. A swaged-on needle is preferred to reduce the possibility of fracturing the fragile cartilages. The suture is tightened to the point of abduction created by the indwelling endotracheal tube. Extubation and laryngeal examination should be performed at that time to confirm appropriate placement before closure of the surgical site.

A final salvage procedure is permanent tracheostomy, which effectively bypasses the upper airway altogether (see Chapter 8). This is a viable option for animals with significant risk of aspiration pneumonia (myasthenia gravis, diffuse myopathy or other compounding gastrointestinal disease) because the laryngeal anatomy is not altered. This technique is fraught with management complications such as stoma occlusion by mucous accumulation because animals are more prone to inhaling foreign material, require grooming around the tracheal stoma and must be prohibited from swimming throughout the rest of their lives.

Postoperative complications and care

The major benefit of the arytenoid lateralization technique is that no temporary tracheostomy is necessary. There is also no disruption of the laryngeal mucosa and therefore the risk of scar formation is removed. The risks associated with this procedure are cartilage fracture and suture failure if animals are anxious or bark excessively. Postoperative aspiration pneumonia is the most concerning risk, with reported rates of around 20–25% at some point during the patient's life postoperatively. However, use of a unilateral technique, instead of bilateral, diminishes the risk of aspiration pneumonia. In addition, certain strategies can be employed to minimize this risk in the perioperative period, which is the time of highest risk. With regard to anaesthesia, strict fasting for 8–12 hours prior to surgery to ensure complete gastric emptying is recommended. Premedication with high emetogenic properties (hydromorphone) should be avoided. Patients are premedicated with maropitant (1 mg/kg s.c. q24h) and famotidine (1 mg/kg i.v., s.c., i.m. q24h) at the time of induction to reduce the risk of vomiting and regurgitation in the perioperative period. Dexamethasone sodium phosphate (0.2 mg/kg i.v. once) is administered to reduce airway oedema during the perioperative period. Patients are intubated swiftly at the time of surgery to reduce the time during which their airway is not protected, and endotracheal cuff inflation is carefully checked.

Postoperatively, patients are extubated only when they have a strong swallowing/gag reflex. Patients should be monitored closely for respiratory distress and given appropriate analgesics. They are maintained on intravenous fluids until they are drinking. Soft food may be offered after full recovery but the patient should be observed for clinical signs consistent with aspiration. This is most critical for dogs that routinely eat vigorously and 'inhale' their food. Soft food is recommended because it does not particulate when chewed. Water should be offered in small shallow volumes to slow the rate of drinking. Initially, patients will often cough when eating and drinking, which is a normal response to their altered airway.

Prognosis

The overall prognosis for laryngeal paralysis is variable, based on the severity of signs and confounding factors. With certain lifestyle adjustments, animals can have a good quality of life without surgery, but ultimately the clinical signs will progress as the cricoarytenoideus muscles degenerate. Once clinical signs progress to the point of affecting quality of life, surgical intervention is strongly recommended. Animals have an immediate resolution of upper airway obstruction postoperatively. Reported owner perception of improvement in quality of life is around 90% with unilateral arytenoid lateralization. Whilst the reported incidence of aspiration pneumonia should not be dismissed, with the specific management strategies listed above, the risk can be minimized.

Recently, geriatric onset laryngeal paralysis and polyneuropathy (GOLPP) syndrome has been described and reported. GOLPP is a common problem of older large- and giant-breed dogs. It is a disease of the nervous system, characterized by the slow but progressive degeneration of some of the longer nerves in the body. It results in laryngeal paralysis, oesophageal dysfunction, and hind limb paresis. It is important for pet owners to understand that GOLPP is a progressive syndrome and that dogs vary widely in their presentation and progression of this neurological disease. Dogs with more severe oesophageal dysfunction are more likely to develop aspiration pneumonia with or without surgical treatment of the airway. In dogs with mild oesophageal and/or other peripheral nerve deficits, unilateral arytenoid lateralization surgery has a good prognosis for return to good, pet-quality function. However, other peripheral nerve deficits will continue to progress and may become severe enough over the remainder of the pet's life to affect their abilities to walk, urinate, and defecate.

Laryngeal trauma

Aetiology and clinical signs

Blunt laryngeal trauma can result from road traffic accidents, severe straining or harsh pulling on the leash. Penetrating laryngeal trauma can be caused by animal bites, sticks, knives or bullets. Traumatic or incautious insertion of an endotracheal tube can also cause blunt laryngeal injury, especially in cats. Acute injuries to the larynx can produce laryngeal contusion and obstruction as a result of haematoma and oedema formation. Respiratory obstruction may increase rapidly, and careful observation of breathing rate and pattern and the degree of stridor is mandatory for a successful outcome. Extrinsic penetrating injuries are usually more extensive than suggested by the skin wounds, especially when caused by dog bites to the neck. Subcutaneous emphysema and dyspnoea are the most important indicators of a penetrating laryngeal wound, but the perforation may include the trachea, pharynx and oesophagus, vessels and nerves, and neck muscles.

Diagnostic imaging and laryngoscopy

Laryngoscopy should always be performed to assess the presence of intralaryngeal perforations and lacerations, to estimate the degree of obstruction caused by haematoma and oedema, and to determine the need for tracheostomy tube placement. After thorough inspection, patients can be intubated with a small tube before diagnostic imaging commences. Diagnostic imaging is always recommended after acute injury as it will help detect fractures of the hyoid bones and laryngeal cartilages and will allow assessment of concurrent pulmonary contusions or pulmonary oedema. More detailed information can be obtained using computed tomography (CT) or magnetic resonance imaging (MRI).

Treatment

Affected dogs or cats should be hospitalized and monitored when there are no fractures of the larynx and the laryngeal mucosa is seen to cover the laryngeal cartilages. In cases of severe dyspnoea, if a significant increase in swelling in the post-imaging period is expected, or if non-dislocated laryngeal fractures are seen, a tracheotomy should be performed.

Fractures with discontinuity of the laryngeal cartilages should be repaired immediately or granulation tissue will cause contraction and narrowing of the laryngeal passageway. Associated soft tissue injuries of the skin, subcutaneous tissues and pharyngeal and laryngeal muscles necessitating repair can be attended to in the same surgical session. Surgery is always recommended for patients with penetrating injuries, such as after bite incidents or stick injury, to retrieve foreign material, debride necrotic tissue, repair fractures and soft tissue trauma and drain the area, as bacterial contamination inevitably will be present. For all injuries, a ventral midline approach is recommended for exploration of the neck. Any obviously devitalized tissue or heavily infected tissue should be removed if possible. Lacerations of the pharynx, larynx, trachea and oesophagus are closed after careful debridement. Thorough flushing of the area is performed to decrease bacterial contamination further. Continued post-operative drainage should be provided by placement of active or passive wound drains. Broad-spectrum antibiotics and analgesia are given and the patient is hospitalized for careful monitoring during the first few days.

Laryngeal tumours

Benign masses, cysts and neoplastic disease in the larynx are rare in dogs and cats. Cysts are very rare, but can be recognized by radiographic and ultrasonographic examination of the larynx and localized precisely by laryngoscopy, when they can also be incised and drained or surgically excised. In cats, obstructive laryngeal disease with granuloma formation can mimic neoplastic disease, and the conditions need to be differentiated by biopsy and histopathology (Figure 7.4).

Reported canine laryngeal tumours include rhabdomyoma (oncocytoma), lipoma, osteosarcoma, chondroma, myxochondroma and chondrosarcoma, extramedullary

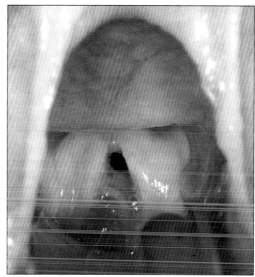

7.4 Laryngoscopic view of a large red granulomatous mass in a cat with chronic laryngitis, mimicking neoplastic disease.

plasmacytoma, melanoma, granular cell tumour, undifferentiated carcinoma, fibropapilloma and fibrosarcoma, mast cell tumour, adenocarcinoma and squamous cell carcinoma. Most laryngeal tumours are very locally invasive and have a significant metastatic potential. Feline laryngeal neoplasms are most commonly lymphomas, although squamous cell carcinoma and adenocarcinoma have been reported. Except for laryngeal oncocytomas, which appear to occur in younger mature dogs, most dogs and cats with laryngeal cancer are middle-aged to older. Neoplasms such as lymphoma (Figure 7.5) and thyroid adenocarcinoma may secondarily invade the larynx, although the latter usually invades the trachea.

Diagnosis

Dyspnoea and a progressive change in voice or bark (hoarseness and 'breaking voice') are usually the presenting clinical signs of animals with laryngeal cancer, although exercise intolerance and dysphagia are sometimes reported as well. The laryngeal stridor is usually only inspiratory at first; however, when the obstruction is large enough it will be both inspiratory and expiratory.

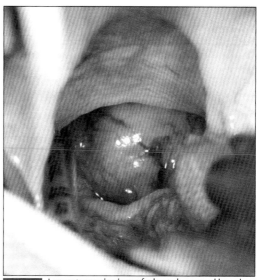

7.5 Laryngoscopic view of a large laryngeal lymphoma obstructing the entire rima glottidis in a cat.

On physical examination in dogs usually no abnormalities are detected, with the exception of the stridor; however, in cats, tumours can sometimes be palpated because feline tumours are more likely to involve multiple laryngeal structures and the larynx is softer and more flaccid than in the dog.

Diagnostic imaging

Ultrasonography, radiography, CT and MRI can be used to characterize and stage laryngeal cancer. Although ultrasonography and radiography can reveal the general location of the tumour and give some idea of its extension, both CT and MRI will show finer anatomical detail and provide more useful information about invasion of the cartilage, extralaryngeal extension and the status of the local lymph nodes. Laryngoscopy is essential for further assessment and facilitates biopsy for cytological or histological diagnosis.

Therapy

Benign laryngeal cancers can usually be removed successfully with preservation of function via either an endoscopy-assisted oral approach or ventral laryngotomy. Temporary tracheostomy is advised for the initial recovery period (2–3 days). Complete laryngectomy with a permanent tracheostomy is technically demanding but feasible in dogs and cats; however, the permanent tracheostoma created with this technique will need constant attention and protection. Radiation should be able to control lymphoma or granular cell tumour, mast cell tumour, adenocarcinoma and squamous cell carcinoma, but chemotherapeutic treatment of feline lymphoma yields excellent results as well.

Benign lesions of the trachea and larynx have a good prognosis if they can be completely resected; the prognosis for malignant lesions appears to be poor.

References and further reading

Demetriou JL and Kirby BM (2003) The effect of two modifications of unilateral arytenoid lateralization on rima glottidis area in dogs. *Veterinary Surgery* **32**, 62–68

Griffin JF and Krahwinkel DJ (2005) Laryngeal paralysis: pathophysiology, diagnosis, and surgical repair. *Compendium on Continuing Education for the Practicing Veterinarian* **27**, 857–869

Griffiths LG, Sullivan M and Reid SWJ (2001) A comparison of the effects of unilateral thyroarytenoid lateralization *versus* cricoarytenoid laryngoplasty on the area of the rima glottidis and clinical outcome in dogs with laryngeal paralysis. *Veterinary Surgery* **30**, 359–365

Hammel SP, Hottinger HA and Novo RE (2006) Postoperative results of unilateral arytenoid lateralization for treatment of idiopathic laryngeal paralysis in dogs: 39 cases (1996–2002). *Journal of the American Veterinary Medical Association* **228**, 1215–1220

Monnet E (2003) Laryngeal paralysis and devocalization. In: *Textbook of Small Animal Surgery, 3rd edn*, ed. D Slatter, pp. 837–845. Saunders Elsevier, Philadelphia

Stanley BJ, Hauptman JG, Fritz MC *et al.* (2010) Esophageal dysfunction in dogs with idiopathic laryngeal paralysis: a controlled cohort study. *Veterinary Surgery* **39**, 139–149

ter Haar G (2016) Surgical management of laryngeal paralysis. In: *Complications in Small Animal Surgery*, ed. DJ Griffon and A Hamaide, pp. 178–184. Wiley-Blackwell, Ames

Venker-van Haagen AJ (2005) The larynx. In: *Ear, Nose, Throat, and Tracheobronchial Diseases in Dogs and Cats*, ed. AJ Venker-van Haagen, pp. 121–165. Schlütersche, Hannover

OPERATIVE TECHNIQUE 7.1

Cricoarytenoid lateralization

PATIENT POSITIONING

The patient is placed in lateral recumbency (most surgeons prefer right lateral recumbency). The entire neck should be aseptically prepared for surgery.

ASSISTANT

Optional but preferred.

SURGICAL TECHNIQUE

Approach

The larynx is exposed through a left lateral cervical approach. A lateral skin incision is made just ventral to the jugular vein, starting from the caudal angle of the mandible and extending caudally approximately 2–3 cm from the larynx.

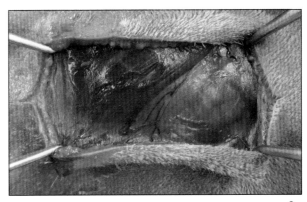

→ **OPERATIVE TECHNIQUE 7.1 CONTINUED**

Surgical manipulations

1   The subcutaneous tissues, platysma and parotidauricularis muscles are incised and blunt dissection is performed to expose the sternocephalicus and sternohyoideus muscles. Care must be taken to avoid damaging the jugular vein.

2   The sternocephalicus muscle and jugular vein are retracted dorsally and the sternohyoid ventrally to expose the laryngeal area.

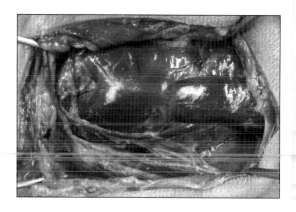

3   Palpate the dorsal edge of the thyroid cartilage and incise the thyropharyngeus muscle along the dorsolateral margin of the thyroid cartilage. Stay sutures (or Lone Star hooks) are placed to retract and rotate the thyroid cartilage laterally.

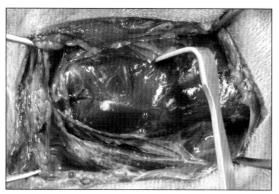 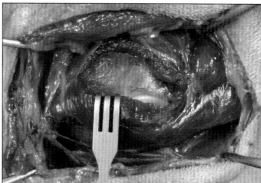

4   The cricothyroid articulation is disarticulated to expose the cricoarytenoideus dorsalis muscle and the muscular process of the arytenoid cartilage.

5   A stay suture is placed in the thyroid cartilage to aid in retraction. The cricoarytenoid articulation is disarticulated and the arytenoid is dissected free from its attachments without entering the laryngeal lumen. Transection of the sesamoid band (interarytenoid ligament) is optional.

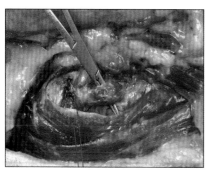

The cricothyroid articulation is disarticulated with scissors.

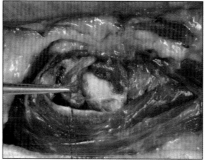

The cricoarytenoideus dorsalis muscle is incised and the muscular process is identified.

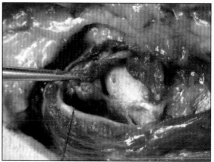

The cricoarytenoid articulation is disarticulated at the muscular process.

→ **OPERATIVE TECHNIQUE 7.1 CONTINUED**

6 Two monofilament synthetic non-absorbable sutures are placed through the muscular process of the arytenoid cartilage and the caudal one-third of the cricoid cartilage near the origin of the cricoarytenoideus muscle, to mimic the function/action of the muscle.

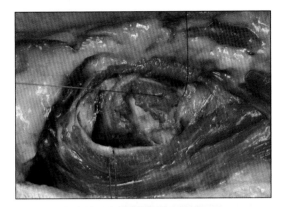
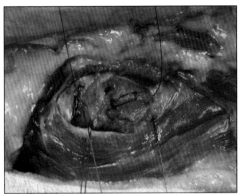

7 The abduction is verified via intraoral visualization.

PRACTICAL TIP

The use of Lone Star ring retractors is helpful in providing exposure. Inadvertent penetration into the laryngeal lumen and oesophageal laceration can be prevented by having a thorough knowledge of local anatomy and using careful surgical technique with appropriate instruments. Do not lavage the surgical site until the muscles are closed

---

PRACTICAL TIP

Fragmentation of the arytenoid is less likely to occur if the arytenoid is pulled into position towards the caudal cricoid, after dissection and preplacement of the sutures, using an Allis forceps on the remnants of the cricoarytenoideus dorsalis muscle instead of pulling on the sutures themselves. The arytenoid cartilage is already abducted by the endotracheal tube, so avoid excessive caudal traction

---

Closure

The thyropharyngeal muscle can be apposed with a simple continuous pattern with absorbable material. The subcutaneous tissues and the skin are closed routinely.

POSTOPERATIVE CARE

Postoperative care consists of close monitoring of the patient and providing broad-spectrum antibiotics and analgesics. Monitor for complications such as haematoma formation, suture avulsion, discomfort during swallowing, temporary glottic dysfunction and coughing after eating or drinking, sometimes resulting in aspiration pneumonia.

OPERATIVE TECHNIQUE 7.2

Thyroarytenoid lateralization

PATIENT POSITIONING

The patient is positioned in dorsal recumbency; the entire neck should be aseptically prepared for surgery. A lateral approach or a ventral paramedian approach can be used, depending on the surgeon's preference. The ventral paramedian approach allows for concurrent tracheotomy, if indicated, without repositioning the patient, and will be reviewed here.

ASSISTANT

Optional.

SURGICAL TECHNIQUE

Approach

A paramedian skin incision is made on the left side from 2 cm caudal to the larynx, extending to the caudal angle of the mandible.

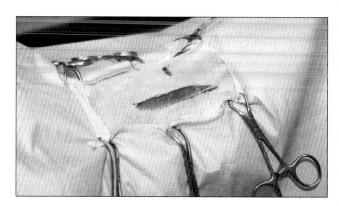

Surgical manipulations

1 The subcutaneous tissues and platysma are incised and blunt dissection is performed lateral to the sternohyoid and sternocephalic muscles until the dorsal edge of the thyroid can be palpated and lifted (pulled ventrally).

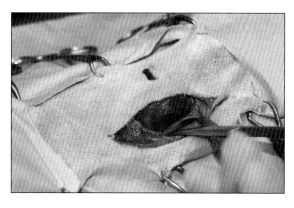
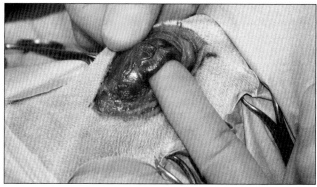

2 An incision is made in the thyropharyngeal muscle along the dorsolateral edge of the thyroid to expose the thyroid. Stay sutures are then placed, to retract and rotate the larynx laterally, after which the thyropharyngeal muscle is opened as far as needed.

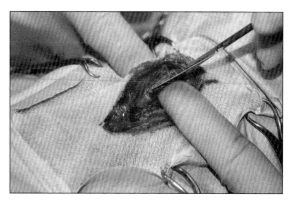
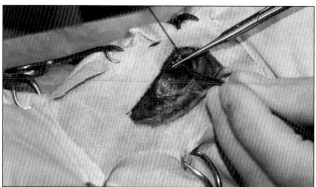

→ **OPERATIVE TECHNIQUE 7.2 CONTINUED**

3 The cricothyroid articulation can be disarticulated with scissors if more exposure is needed, after which the dorsal cricoarytenoideus muscle and muscular process of the arytenoid can be identified. The dorsal cricoarytenoideus muscle is grasped with an Allis forceps to aid disarticulation.

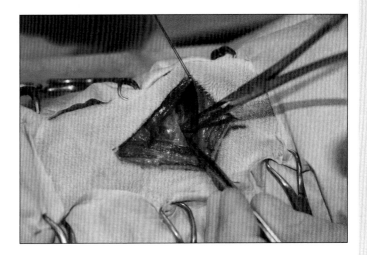

4 The cricoarytenoideus muscle is cut to allow cricoarytenoid disarticulation. The arytenoid is dissected free from its attachments without entering the laryngeal lumen and the interarytenoid ligament is dissected last.

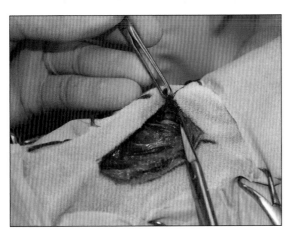
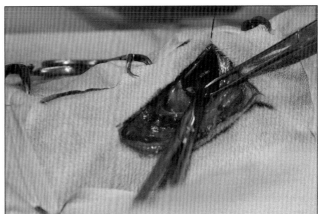

5 Two synthetic non-absorbable sutures are placed through the most caudodorsal part of the thyroid to the muscular process of the arytenoid to lateralize the arytenoid. The second suture is placed 5 mm cranial to the first in the caudal thyroid and 5 mm dorsal through the arytenoid cartilage.

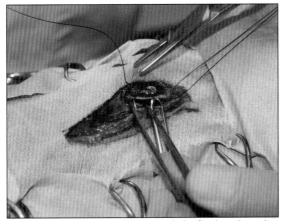
Placement of the first suture starts with the first bite through the most caudodorsal part of the thyroid.

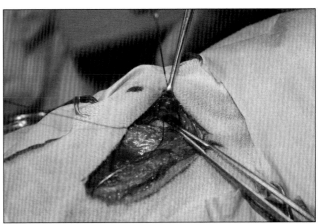
This suture then incorporates the muscular process of the arytenoid.

→ **OPERATIVE TECHNIQUE 7.2 CONTINUED**

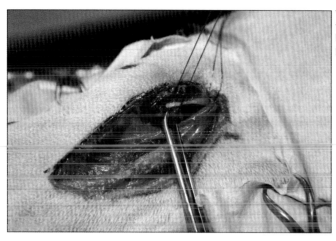

The caudal suture has been tied after the arytenoid has been brought into position by pulling on the Allis forceps.

6 The abduction is now verified with the help of the anaesthetist, using intraoral visualization.

> **PRACTICAL TIP**
>
> Care should be taken to avoid damaging the cranial laryngeal nerve. Inadvertent penetration into the laryngeal lumen and oesophageal laceration can be prevented by having a thorough knowledge of local anatomy and using careful surgical technique with appropriate instruments

> **PRACTICAL TIP**
>
> Fragmentation of the arytenoid is less likely to occur if the arytenoid is pulled into position towards the caudal thyroid, after dissection and preplacement of the sutures, using an Allis forceps on the remnants of the cricoarytenoideus dorsalis muscle instead of pulling on the sutures themselves

Closure

The thyropharyngeus muscle can be apposed with a simple continuous pattern with absorbable material. The subcutaneous tissues and the skin are closed routinely.

POSTOPERATIVE CARE

Postoperative care consists of close monitoring of the patient and providing broad-spectrum antibiotics and analgesics. Monitor for complications such as haematoma formation, suture avulsion, discomfort during swallowing, temporary glottic dysfunction and coughing after eating or drinking, sometimes resulting in aspiration pneumonia.

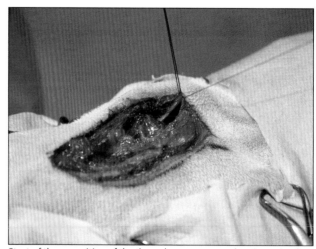

Start of the apposition of the thyropharyngeus muscle using a simple continuous pattern with absorbable material.

Chapter 8

Surgery of the extrathoracic trachea

Zoë J. Halfacree and Chick Weisse

Anatomy and physiology

The trachea extends from the cricoid cartilage of the larynx to the carina at the level of the heart base, where it divides to form the mainstem bronchi. It is composed of between 35 and 46 incomplete C-shaped cartilage rings that are united dorsally by the dorsal tracheal ligament and trachealis muscle and joined together by fibroelastic tissue, the annular ligaments, to form a circular tube in cross section (Figure 8.1). The trachea is lined by mucosa composed of a pseudostratified columnar epithelium, which contains ciliated epithelium and goblet cells. The cervical trachea has a delicate segmental blood supply, which arises as branches from the cranial and caudal thyroid arteries (Figure 8.2); venous drainage is via the internal jugular veins. The trachea is innervated by the vagus and recurrent laryngeal nerves.

The trachea serves as a conduit for passage of air to and from the lungs during ventilation, but also plays a role in warming and filtering the air following inhalation. The mucociliary escalator, provided by the ciliated epithelium, plays an essential role in clearing particulate matter from the lungs.

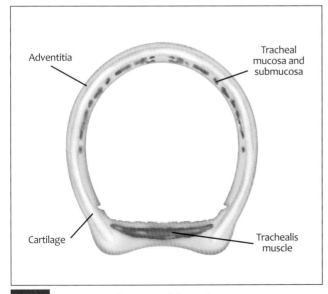

8.1 Cross-sectional anatomy of the trachea.

Adventitia

Tracheal mucosa and submucosa

Cartilage

Trachealis muscle

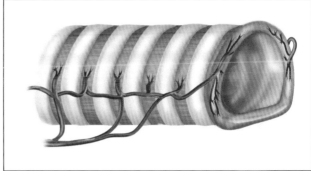

8.2 The segmental blood supply to the trachea is derived from the cranial and caudal thyroid arteries.

Indications for surgery of the extrathoracic trachea

- Tracheal trauma:
  - Perforation or avulsion of the trachea
  - Tracheal necrosis, e.g. secondary to endotracheal intubation injury.
- Management of segmental tracheal stenosis.
- Management of obstructive tracheal masses (mural or intramural).
- Management of tracheal collapse.
- Management of upper airway obstruction by temporary or permanent tracheostomy.

Tracheal trauma

Tracheal trauma may be caused by external or internal forces. External forces include bite wounds, cervical stick injury and choke chain injuries. Internal trauma to the trachea may be caused iatrogenically following inappropriate use of an endotracheal tube.

Owing to the complex nature of the forces exerted from a bite wound to the neck (penetrating, avulsion and crushing forces), a range of different injuries may be observed. Penetrating injuries may cause perforation of the trachea and the development of a 'sucking' cervical wound and extensive subcutaneous emphysema. Even in the absence of a full-thickness skin wound, tracheal avulsion or cricotracheal separation may occur, resulting in the development of subcutaneous emphysema alone. If a cervical bite wound is suspected, radiographs must be obtained of the neck and thoracic cavity. Radiography revealed subcutaneous or mediastinal emphysema in all animals with airway injury following cervical bite wounds in one study of 56 cases (Jordan *et al.*, 2013). Tracheoscopy may also be used to evaluate the presence, extent and location of tracheal injury. All animals with cervical bite wounds should undergo ventral midline neck exploration for appropriate wound management, particularly if emphysema has been detected indicating that airway repair may be required. Given the location of the trauma, injury to other important structures, such as neurovascular bundles, the spine, pharynx or oesophagus, may have occurred.

Following identification of an injury to the trachea, the tissue must be assessed for viability and debridement performed where necessary. Primary repair may be possible for a small defect (Figure 8.3); a fasciomuscular patch, such as sternohyoid muscle (Jordan *et al.*, 2013), can be used to augment the repair if necessary. Where a section of trachea is non-viable, a tracheal resection and anastomosis should be performed. In all cases, great care must be taken to preserve the segmental blood supply to the trachea and to avoid injury to the recurrent laryngeal nerves running in close approximation to the trachea. Airway examination should be conducted to assess laryngeal function both before and after the surgery. If the site of tracheal injury is evident, it is prudent to select a cuffed endotracheal tube that can be passed beyond the site of perforation and therefore allow controlled management of anaesthesia and ventilation if required. Significant airway swelling may be present in some patients and this, in addition to the absence of normal laryngeal function, may suggest that placement of a temporary tracheostomy tube is indicated, but this must be decided on an individual patient basis. The cervical wound must be thoroughly lavaged and can be closed over a drain once 'healthy'. The use of a Penrose drain may be most appropriate at this location as active suction drains could cause damage to important cervical neurovascular structures. If use of a closed suction drain is indicated then the most appropriate drain to select is a Jackson Pratt drain, which has a more consistent low level of suction than other drain types (Halfacree *et al.*, 2009).

Iatrogenic tracheal tears can occur acutely following endotracheal intubation, due to tube cuff overinflation, frequent changes in patient position without disconnecting the endotracheal tube (e.g. during anaesthesia for dental prophylaxis) or use of an overlong stylet. Pressure necrosis of the trachea following prolonged use of a low-volume high-pressure cuff can also cause gradual loss of tracheal integrity, therefore resulting in a delay in presentation of clinical signs. The clinical signs observed include coughing, dyspnoea and the development of subcutaneous emphysema. Radiography of the neck and thorax reveals subcutaneous emphysema and pneumomediastinum (Figure 8.4). The majority of cats can be treated conservatively with strict cage rest; however, surgery may be required (Mitchell *et al.*, 2000). The trachea is approached via a ventral midline cervical approach and the lesion in the dorsal tracheal ligament is debrided and repaired. The use of high-volume low-pressure cuffs, rather than low-volume high-pressure cuffs, is recommended to minimize the risk of this injury.

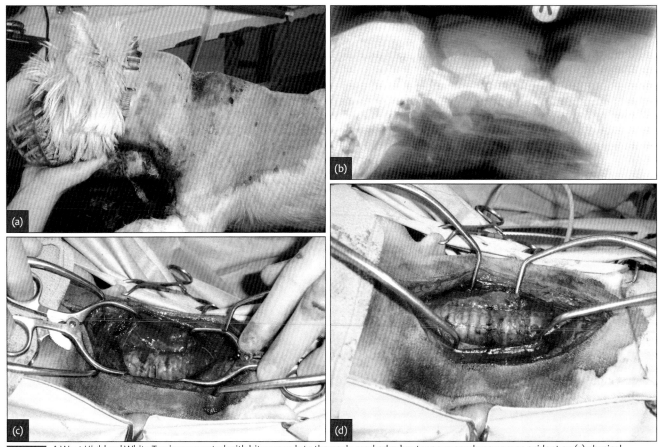

8.3 A West Highland White Terrier presented with bite wounds to the neck; marked subcutaneous emphysema was evident on (a) physical examination and (b) cervical radiography. (c) Ventral neck exploration revealed tracheal perforation through the annular ligament of the trachea. (d) Primary repair of the tracheal laceration was performed using simple interrupted sutures.

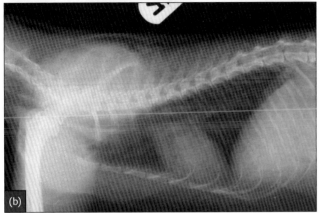

8.4 (a) Lateral cervical and (b) thoracic radiographs of a cat that developed extensive subcutaneous emphysema 10 days following general anaesthesia for routine ovariohysterectomy. The cat had a tear in the dorsal tracheal ligament at the level of the thoracic inlet consistent with an injury secondary to endotracheal tube cuff inflation.

Tracheostomy

Temporary tracheostomy

Placement of a temporary tracheostomy is indicated for emergency management of upper airway obstruction pending:

- Appropriate patient stabilization
- Definitive surgical correction of the upper airway (e.g. laryngeal paralysis requiring arytenoid lateralization when an experienced surgeon was not initially available)
- Response to medical therapy and bypass of the airway (e.g. severe airway swelling following anaphylaxis, management of the surgical complication of airway swelling following upper respiratory tract surgery)
- Receipt of biopsy results from a lesion in the upper respiratory tract.

Temporary tracheostomy is also indicated in a patient that requires a prolonged period of assisted ventilation, to avoid laryngeal trauma and reduce the depth of anaesthesia required by minimizing laryngeal stimulation. Patients with maxillary and mandibular fractures may benefit from temporary tracheostomy, rather than orotracheal intubation, to facilitate accurate assessment of dental occlusion during fracture reduction. Cuffed tracheostomy tubes would be required in these situations.

Temporary tracheostomy is performed by creating a transverse incision in the ventral tracheal wall, through one of the annular ligaments, at approximately the level of the third to fifth tracheal ring. The incision should ideally be no greater than 50% of the tracheal circumference (Figure 8.5). A step-by-step guide to the procedure is outlined in Operative Technique 2.1. Depending upon the size of the patient and/or the trachea, different tracheostomy tubes are

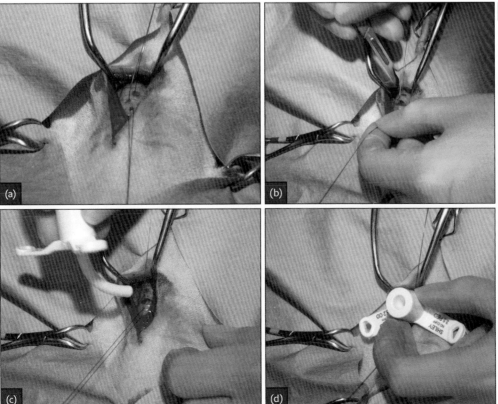

8.5 Temporary tracheostomy placement in a cat with upper respiratory tract obstruction secondary to laryngeal inflammation. (a) Stay sutures are placed through the trachea proximal and distal to the proposed site of annular ligament incision for the tracheotomy. (b) A tracheotomy is performed using a scalpel blade to incise through the annular ligament. (c) Manipulation of the stay sutures to open the tracheostomy can aid insertion of the tracheostomy tube. (d) The tracheostomy tube is inserted and will then be secured around the neck of the cat using umbilical tape.

available. For smaller patients, such as cats, small dogs and some brachycephalic dogs with hypoplastic tracheas, it is necessary to use paediatric tubes (Figure 8.6). Owing to their small size the tube is a simple design without a removable inner cannula. This means that cleaning and maintenance of the tube requires removal and reinsertion, therefore complicating management. Larger patients can accommodate a tube with a removable inner cannula (Figure 8.7); this facilitates regular cleaning to ensure that mucus plugs do not build up within the tube. The risks of tube occlusion, dyspnoea and fatal respiratory obstruction are accordingly lower in larger patients.

Following placement of a temporary tracheostomy, the patient requires constant monitoring and regular management of the tube. Complication rates are high, but with effective management the majority of patients survive until tube removal or definitive diagnosis (Guenther-Yenke and Rozanski, 2007; Nicholson and Baines, 2012). Dogs with tracheostomy tubes were found to be more likely to have an unsuccessful outcome if they were Bulldogs, younger dogs or if they experienced episodes of bradycardia (Nicholson and Baines, 2012). The main major complications are tube occlusion (Figure 8.8) and tube dislodgement. Equipment must be prepared to facilitate rapid replacement of a tracheostomy tube; spare tubes of a range of sizes should be close at hand. The conformation of certain dog breeds (e.g. abundant skin folds or short necks) can make it more challenging to secure the tube; Bulldogs were three times more likely to dislodge the tube than other breeds in one study (Nicholson and Baines, 2012).

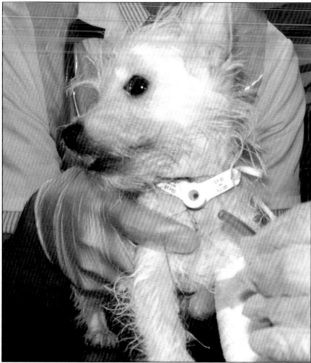

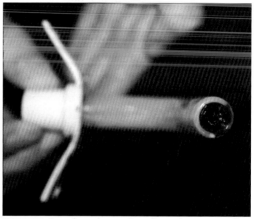

8.8 Complete obstruction of a tracheostomy tube with mucus secretions.

Bypass of the upper airways does not allow filtering, warming and humidification of air prior to entry into the trachea. The loss of these functions, in addition to disruption of the mucociliary escalator following tracheostomy, predisposes to the development of copious tenacious mucous, which can increase the risk of respiratory obstruction. The patient should receive intravenous fluid therapy to ensure they remain well hydrated, and regular saline nebulization should be performed. Minor complications include maceration of the skin around the tracheostomy site associated with drainage of respiratory secretions on to the skin. Regular cleaning should be performed followed by application of a barrier cream. Whilst careful management of these patients is essential, it should be noted that an increase in complications has been documented in patients under more frequent tube management regimens (Nicholson and Baines, 2012) and therefore excessive interference should be avoided. In particular, suction of the airway must be used only when absolutely required; suction can cause a drop in arterial oxygen saturation and will further irritate the airways, encouraging additional mucus production.

8.6 A paediatric tracheostomy tube used for management of upper respiratory tract obstruction in a puppy; owing to the small size of the tube there is no removable inner cannula.

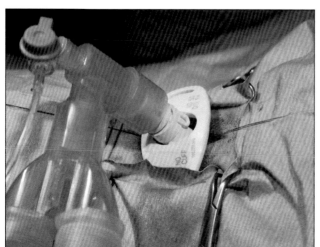

8.7 A tracheostomy tube with a removable inner cannula, which facilitates regular cleaning of the tube to prevent obstruction. The inner cannula can be interchanged between a cannula that can connect to an anaesthesia breathing circuit, for use during placement (as shown), and a shorter cannula for use in the conscious patient.

The tracheostomy tube is removed once it is no longer required and the stoma is left to heal via second intention. Brief temporary occlusion of the tracheostomy tube can be performed to assess upper airway patency in medium to large dogs; however, this should not be performed in cats, small dogs or brachycephalic breeds, because the tube can occupy up to 75% of the tracheal lumen and the test is not, therefore, representative of their functional airway and may compromise the patient. In some animals, airway examination under a light plane of general anaesthesia may be indicated to determine whether removal of the tracheostomy tube is appropriate.

Permanent tracheostomy

Permanent tracheostomy may be performed for management of end-stage upper respiratory tract obstruction, for example, advanced laryngeal collapse or palliation of upper respiratory tract neoplasia. Very careful client communication is required prior to this procedure, as there is a significant risk of postoperative complications and there must be a commitment to long-term aftercare. A permanent tracheostomy is achieved by removing the ventral portions of approximately four tracheal rings. The sternohyoid muscles are sutured together dorsal to the trachea and the tracheal wall is sutured to the surrounding cervical skin (Figure 8.9); the technique is described by Hedlund *et al.* (1982). A recent publication reporting the outcome following permanent tracheostomy in the dog indicated that a major complication occurred in around half of the patients; these complications were most commonly a need for stoma revision (due to skin fold occlusion or stenosis) or aspiration pneumonia. However, despite complications, 90% of dogs were discharged alive. Whilst some dogs achieved long-term survival at home without further problems (median survival time 328 days; 25% of patients survived 1321 days or longer), around a quarter of the dogs died acutely at some stage as a result of airway obstruction (Occhipinti and Hauptman, 2014).

Permanent tracheostomy in the cat is associated with particularly high rates of complications and mortality (Guenther-Yenke and Rozanski, 2007; Stepnik *et al.*, 2009). Dyspnoea is frequently encountered in the postoperative period and is most often due to respiratory obstruction

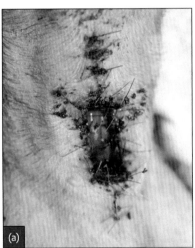

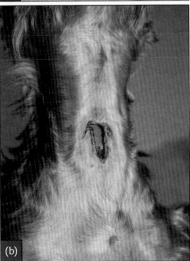

8.9 A permanent tracheostomy in a Yorkshire Terrier, which was performed for management of grade 3 laryngeal collapse and upper respiratory tract obstruction. (a) Three days postoperatively. (b) Two months postoperatively.

caused by a mucus plug at the stoma or elsewhere in the respiratory tract. Around 40% of cats in both studies died due to acute respiratory obstruction with a mucous plug. Stoma obstruction and death was 6.6 times more likely to occur in cats with inflammatory laryngeal disease (Stepnik *et al.*, 2009).

Patients that have undergone permanent tracheostomy require very intensive aftercare initially. The patient and the airway must be kept well hydrated by provision of intravenous fluids, and frequent nebulization and regular cleaning of the distal extent of the stoma is necessary. The irritation of the tracheal mucosa and secondary squamous metaplasia results in significantly increased mucous production following surgery, and dried mucous plugs may occlude the tracheal stoma. This change resolves over time, and around 16 weeks following surgery mucous production is reduced (Hedlund *et al.*, 1982) and management may become straightforward; however, regular stoma cleaning is still required. It is important that dusty environments are avoided and the animal must not be allowed to swim.

Tracheal collapse syndrome

The tracheal collapse syndrome comprises a variety of tracheal disorders, leading to a wide range of clinical signs associated with compromise of the tracheal lumen. The most commonly recognized 'traditional' form is a progressive degenerative condition of the tracheal rings (chondromalacia) and/or dorsal membrane (trachealis muscle) leading to dynamic respiratory difficulty, ranging from the classic 'honking' cough to severe respiratory distress (Figure 8.10ab). Another more recently recognized type (author's observation) is the tracheal 'malformation' variety in which the normally C-shaped cartilage rings are W-shaped, leading to a fixed luminal obstruction at the level of the thoracic inlet that can be associated with concurrent dynamic collapse elsewhere (Figure 8.10cd). Once the condition has been differentiated from other causes of respiratory difficulty, conservative medical management can be useful to palliate clinical signs. Unfortunately, medical management may often achieve only a temporary response (or may even be ineffective for cases involving malformation), and progressive respiratory difficulty requires more aggressive intervention. A number of surgical and interventional techniques have been described; each has its own indications, limitations and associated complications. No single technique has demonstrated clear superiority over others, or has delayed subsequent disease progression. Whilst the long-term prognosis remains guarded, the clinician can offer techniques to palliate these animals and, at least temporarily, improve the remaining quality of life.

Aetiology

Tracheal collapse is typically a disease of middle-aged small and toy breed dogs; Yorkshire Terriers, Poodles, Pomeranians, Chihuahuas and Maltese dogs are overrepresented. However, no genetic cause has yet been identified (Buback *et al.*, 1996). Whilst the underlying cause remains to be determined, a series of structural changes has been identified in tracheal collapse that helps explain the resulting syndrome. Trachealis muscle weakness suggests a possible centrally mediated neurological deficiency that results in atrophy, weakening and subsequent collapse of the trachealis muscle into the

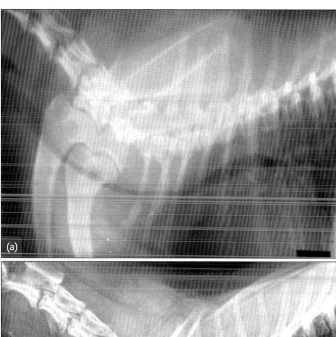

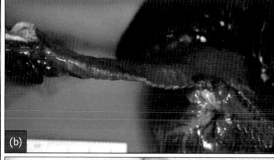

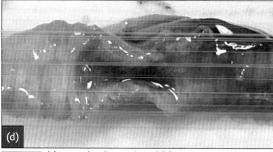

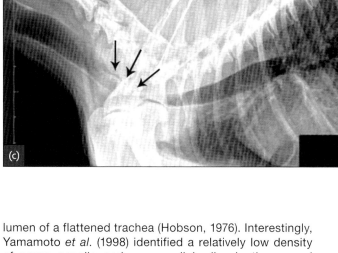

8.10 (a) Lateral radiograph and (b) post-mortem image of a dog with 'traditional' tracheal collapse characterized by flattened tracheal rings and weakened, stretched dorsal trachealis muscle. (c) Lateral radiograph and (d) post-mortem image of a dog with a tracheal 'malformation', characterized by W-shaped tracheal cartilage rings, located most commonly at the thoracic inlet. In (c), note the radiographic pathognomonic sign of a dorsally located tracheal lumen (arrowed) due to the deviated rings.

lumen of a flattened trachea (Hobson, 1976). Interestingly, Yamamoto *et al.* (1998) identified a relatively low density of nerve ganglia and nerve cell bodies in the normal canine trachea near the thoracic inlet, when compared with densities found in the same trachea at the level of the carina. An underlying structural abnormality of the tracheal ring hyaline cartilage has also been reported. Dallman *et al.* (1985, 1988) documented that the cartilage of collapsed tracheas contained fewer chondrocytes and reduced glycoprotein, calcium and chondroitin sulphate, and appeared less homogeneous than normal tracheal cartilage. The hyaline cartilage matrix in some collapsed tracheal rings was completely replaced by fibrocartilage (Dallman, 1981). Hamaide *et al.* (1998) confirmed a weak but significant correlation between proteoglycan content and biomechanical properties of normal canine tracheal ring cartilage. It remains unclear, however, whether these structural abnormalities are the result of a degenerative process occurring in normal hyaline cartilage, a failure of the normal development of tracheal hyaline cartilage, or the result of an underlying inflammatory process. More recently, one of the authors [CW] has encountered a tracheal 'malformation' which does not fall into either of the above classifications. In addition, over 50% of the cases treated at the author's practice fall within the 'malformation' classification in that there is a static, fixed luminal obstruction of the trachea located at the level of the thoracic inlet (see Figure 8.10cd).

Clinical signs

Middle-aged toy breed dogs are most frequently affected and present with a history of intermittent, progressively worsening cough and/or respiratory difficulty. Clinical signs range from a mild 'honking' cough to severe life-threatening dyspnoea, cyanosis and collapse.

Diagnosis

History and signalment, combined with an inducible cough during manual compression of the trachea, are sufficient criteria for a provisional diagnosis.

Physical examination

It is important for the clinician to remain mindful of the precarious respiratory status of such animals. Simple observation can often reveal the location of an airway obstruction:

- **Inspiratory stertor** suggests an *extrathoracic* airway obstruction, as the subatmospheric pressure generated during inspiration collapses the cervical trachea whilst the intrathoracic trachea expands with other structures within the thorax
- **Expiratory stertor** suggests an *intrathoracic* obstruction, as increased pressures generated within the thorax during expiration collapse the airways and vessels, and exhaled air expands the cervical trachea.

A general physical examination should proceed, with particular attention to the respiratory and cardiovascular systems. Careful thoracic auscultation for crackles, wheezes and murmurs may reveal underlying pulmonary or cardiac disease that may be amenable to medical therapy. The neck is gently palpated to search for compressive masses. Manual tracheal palpation often induces a cough and may reveal a flaccid, collapsible trachea.

Imaging

Survey lateral radiography of the entire trachea should include the cervical region and thorax (see Figure 8.10ac). Requesting three views is advised, with the forelimbs pulled caudally in one lateral radiograph and cranially in the contralateral radiograph to ensure that an unobstructed view of the entire trachea is obtained. Otherwise, the forelimbs will always be positioned over the thoracic inlet, obscuring this most commonly affected region. Whilst radiography is often diagnostic for collapse, fluoroscopy is preferred to standard radiography to evaluate the trachea throughout all phases of respiration. Whenever possible, fluoroscopy during a coughing episode is most useful to reveal dynamic collapse under more extreme physiological airway pressures; however, this is rarely performed if treatment is not imminent.

Tracheobronchoscopy is considered by some as the 'gold standard', particularly for evaluation of the mainstem bronchi and for the collection of samples for cytology and culture. Tracheoscopy also permits 'grading' of the tracheal collapse: grades 1, 2, 3 and 4 indicate a progressive decrease in tracheal lumen size from 25% reduction through 50% and 75% to almost 100%. Unfortunately, tracheobronchoscopy requires general anaesthesia, which is often dangerous for animals in respiratory distress.

General blood tests, including a complete blood count and biochemistry panel, should be performed, as should a cardiac evaluation when necessary and oral/laryngeal examination whenever possible. The latter is typically performed during an intervention to avoid an unnecessary anaesthetic episode.

Conservative management

Aggressive medical management with corticosteroids, antitussives, bronchodilators and/or sedatives/tranquillizers is always recommended prior to surgical treatment for tracheal collapse if there is no imminent threat of airway obstruction.

The role of antibiotics remains unclear. Johnson and Fales (2001) reported that 86% of cases of tracheal collapse in dogs had positive cultures obtained via tracheobronchoscopy. This finding, however, might be attributed to oropharyngeal contamination, as cytological evidence of inflammation was rare and mixed bacterial populations were common. Normal dogs often have positive cultures (Johnson and Fales, 2001). Antibiotics may be indicated if clinical signs suggest infection or a single bacterial population is cultured.

It is also imperative to manage obesity, to limit exposure to second-hand smoke and to replace neck leads with harnesses to help reduce clinical signs. Medical management for this disease has been described elsewhere, and readers are referred to these sources for a complete list of options (Fossum, 2002; Mason and Johnson, 2004).

Surgical treatment

The indication(s) for surgical management of tracheal collapse are still under debate. White and Williams (1994) reported a >70% long-term response (>12 months) with medical management alone. However, these authors agreed that surgery can play a role when conservative management fails and that animals could fail to continue to respond to medical management after some years of successful conservative therapy.

Surgical treatments, including dorsal membrane plication, chondrotomy, and tracheal resection and anastomosis, have been described. However, the most commonly performed procedure is the use of extraluminal polypropylene ring prostheses. Regardless of the technique used, serious complications are not uncommon, even in the hands of trained surgeons. For this reason, one cannot overemphasize the importance of identifying and treating concurrent causes of respiratory distress, and recommending surgery only for those animals that have failed to respond to aggressive conservative therapy and for whom tracheal collapse is the primary cause of their clinical signs.

Extraluminal polypropylene ring prostheses

Indications: Animals determined to be relatively good anaesthetic and surgical candidates, with cervical tracheal collapse extending no further caudally than the second intercostal space, are candidates for extraluminal prostheses. Buback et al. (1996) reported excessive morbidity rates when attempting to place prosthetic rings on the thoracic trachea; it is, therefore, not recommended at this time. More recently, Becker et al. (2012) have challenged this statement, demonstrating that some dogs with combined cervical and intrathoracic collapse may benefit from cervical rings, especially if the clinical signs are mostly inspiratory.

Prosthesis preparation: Prosthetic rings can be purchased commercially or manually crafted from a polypropylene syringe case or syringe. The size of the intended recipient will determine which of these is most appropriate. A saw, dental drill or pipe cutter can be used to cut the syringe or syringe case into sections that are 5–8 mm wide, with approximately five holes and one open end. Sandpaper or a dental drill burr is recommended to smooth any rough edges before use. These techniques are described in detail elsewhere (Hobson, 1976). The prostheses can be autoclaved and stored for future use. Commercially available tracheal ring prostheses are now recommended.

Technique: When possible, a brief oral/laryngeal examination and tracheoscopy are performed under sedation, followed by rapid induction of anaesthesia. Although uncommon in the authors' opinion, concurrent laryngeal paralysis would be important to address simultaneously and identify prior to surgical manipulation of the trachea. More commonly, long soft palates are identified that might require partial staphylectomy. Perioperative antibiotics are recommended, as the tracheal lumen is not a sterile environment, and full-thickness sutures and a prosthesis will be placed.

The patient is placed in dorsal recumbency with dorsoflexion of the neck as it is draped over a towel or sandbag with the forelimbs pulled caudally. This position increases exposure to the trachea as well as elevating it to a more superficial location.

A ventral midline cervical incision, from the caudal larynx to the thoracic inlet, exposes subcutaneous tissues and the paired sternohyoid muscles, which are carefully separated with sharp and blunt dissection. It is *imperative* for the surgeon to identify the delicate segmental tracheal blood supply located in the lateral pedicles (Figure 8.11a). In addition, care must be taken to avoid the recurrent laryngeal nerve, located in the lateral pedicle along the dorsolateral aspect of the trachea, tracking laterally and then ventro-laterally as it courses caudally towards the thoracic inlet (Figure 8.11b); the right recurrent laryngeal nerve may be located within the carotid sheath (Fossum, 2002). Damage to either of these important structures during the procedure can lead to tracheal necrosis or laryngeal paralysis, respectively. Excessive dissection around the trachea should be avoided by gentle blunt dissection and fenestration only where the ring is to be placed.

A pair of curved haemostats or right-angled Mixter forceps facilitates passage of the ring around the collapsed trachea, and 1.5 metric (4/0 USP) or 2 metric (3/0 USP) monofilament non-absorbable suture material is passed through the ring and trachea. It is imperative that at least one suture engages the dorsal tracheal membrane. Care is taken to avoid the endotracheal tube cuff during passage of the suture into the tracheal lumen. Temporarily leaving one of the ventral sutures long, for use as a stay suture, can facilitate cranial traction to increase exposure to part of the intrathoracic trachea without extension of the incision into a thoracotomy. Care must be taken to avoid penetration of the pleural cavity and subsequent pneumothorax. Rings are placed approximately 5 mm apart (Figure 8.11cd). The endotracheal tube is moved gently after each ring is placed

to ensure it has not been sutured; alternatively, the cuff is located prior to suture placement and avoided.

One report advocates concurrent left arytenoid lateralization to reduce catastrophic perioperative complications associated with iatrogenic laryngeal paralysis (White, 1995), but the authors of this chapter do not routinely perform this additional procedure. Repeat tracheoscopy is performed following the procedure to confirm appropriate luminal patency following placement of tracheal rings. During recovery and spontaneous breathing, one can attempt to evaluate for laryngeal paralysis although assessment can be difficult following general anesthesia. Monitoring would be recommended before surgical treatment would be indicated.

Results: The largest retrospective study evaluating the use of extraluminal polypropylene ring prostheses for tracheal collapse (Buback *et al.*, 1996) reported a 5% perioperative mortality rate, a 37% rate of immediate postoperative complications (24% coughing, 16% dyspnoea, and 11% incidence of laryngeal paralysis) and a 19% incidence of permanent tracheostomy (more than half of which were performed within 24 hours of surgery). Only 10% of the 90 dogs in this study had evidence of intrathoracic tracheal collapse for which the perioperative morbidity was excessive enough to recommend avoiding surgery. For those animals that recovered favourably, the median survival time was approximately 2 years; half of these animals died of causes unrelated to the respiratory system. Age at the time of surgery was the only prognostic factor identified: animals younger than 6 years had more severe tracheal collapse but a better prognosis.

Some smaller studies report more favourable results, such as a 4% complication rate and 75% success rate when concurrent left arytenoid lateralization is performed (White, 1995). More recently, two other studies have reported improved outcomes in terms of prolonged survival times (>2500 days for cervical collapse alone) and a reduced need for postoperative medications; however, rates of laryngeal paralysis and other respiratory complications were still high (Becker *et al.*, 2012; Chisnell and Pardo, 2015). Tinga *et al.* (2015) demonstrated similar major complications for dogs with stents or extraluminal rings, and no difference in median survival times when corrected for age.

In general, it appears that animals with concurrent cardiac or respiratory disease or mainstem bronchial collapse may have a worse prognosis. It is clear that careful patient selection and long discussions with the animal's owners are important to explain potential complications and expectations.

Intraluminal devices

Interventional radiology involves the use of imaging modalities, such as fluoroscopy, to gain access to structures to administer materials or devices for therapeutic reasons. Tracheal stenting, the minimally invasive, through-the-mouth placement of a stent (support) within the lumen of the trachea, has been investigated. Migration of balloon-expandable stents led researchers to evaluate various types of self-expanding stents made of stainless steel or nitinol (a nickel–titanium alloy) (Radlinsky *et al.*, 1997). Stenting provides a rapid, minimally invasive option that avoids dissection around the peritracheal neurovascular structures and other complications associated with upper airway surgery. Disadvantages include the need for fluoroscopy and complications associated with the presence of an intraluminal stent.

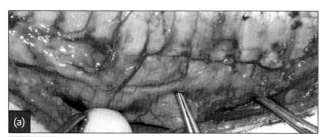

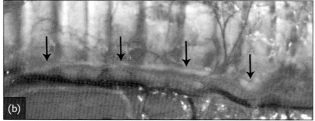

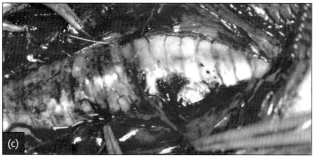

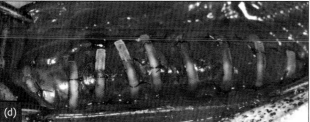

8.11 Serial images of canine tracheas. (a) Note the segmental blood supply originating from the dorsolateral tracheal margins. (b) The recurrent laryngeal nerve (arrowed) is often located on the lateral tracheal wall. (c) Initial placement of extraluminal tracheal ring prostheses in a patient with tracheal collapse. (d) Completed tracheal ring prostheses demonstrating closer but imperfectly re-established tracheal anatomy.

Indications: These have not yet been completely determined. Stenting may be indicated in animals that are refractory to aggressive medical management, have extensive intrathoracic tracheal collapse or are poor surgical candidates. The role for stenting in animals with cervical collapse alone is unclear and it is usually avoided unless surgery is contraindicated or denied.

Prostheses: A review of different stents and materials is beyond the scope of this chapter. The most commonly used devices include mesh nitinol self-expanding metallic stents (e.g. Vet Stent-Trachea™, Figure 8.12), or more uncommonly devices made of stainless steel (e.g. Wallstent™) or woven/braided nitinol (e.g. Ultraflex stents).

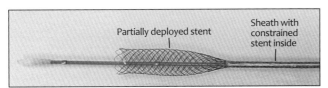

Partially deployed stent | Sheath with constrained stent inside

8.12 Partially deployed Vet Stent-Trachea™ within its delivery sheath, demonstrating the low-profile delivery system and stent foreshortening.

Technique: Briefly, an oral/laryngeal examination and tracheoscopy are performed under sedation, followed by rapid induction of anaesthesia. The patient is placed in lateral recumbency on the fluoroscopy table. Perioperative corticosteroids and antibiotics may be used. If available, a marker catheter is passed through the mouth into the oesophagus, to the level of the thoracic inlet, to account for magnification on the recorded images. The endotracheal tube is retracted until it is just caudal to the larynx. Positive pressure ventilation to 20 cmH$_2$O is generated whilst a radiograph including the cervical and thoracic trachea is obtained. The degree of magnification is calculated in order to determine the actual diameter of the trachea. A stent of appropriate diameter and length is chosen and the location of collapse previously determined via fluoroscopy in the awake animal is noted (in general most of the trachea is stented). The stent is deployed under fluoroscopic guidance (Figure 8.13). More complete discussions of tracheal stent placement can be found in Moritz *et al.* (2004) and Weisse (2015).

Results: Two studies report clinical improvement in 75–90% of animals treated with intraluminal self-expanding stainless steel stents (Moritz *et al.*, 2004). Most immediate complications were minor, including coughing, tracheal haemorrhage and pneumomediastinum. A perioperative mortality rate of approximately 10% has been reported, due to aspiration pneumonia, worsening clinical signs, incorrect stent placement and emphysema. Long-term complications included excessive granulation tissue, stent shortening, stent fracture and progressive tracheal collapse.

Masses causing tracheal obstruction

External compression is caused by an extramural mass lesion, such as a haematoma, abscess, cyst, granuloma, lymphadenopathy or neoplasia (e.g. thyroid carcinoma or oesophageal neoplasia). An intraluminal mass may be a haematoma, abscess, cyst, eosinophilic granuloma, inflammatory polyp, tracheal neoplasm, parasitic reaction (e.g. to *Oslerus* (formerly *Filaroides*) *osleri*), or a foreign body.

Obstructive diseases cause increased airway resistance at the point of the obstruction. Clinical signs depend on the degree of airway obstruction. Severe obstruction results in an obstructive breathing pattern, with a slow inspiratory phase followed by a more rapid expiratory phase. Many animals present with stridor and a rattling noise in the throat. Coughing may also occur. Respiratory distress is usually obvious.

Tracheal foreign bodies

Some tracheal foreign bodies can be removed endoscopically. Holding an anaesthetized patient head down and tapping the thorax gently may occasionally remove a foreign body or may move it into a more proximal position for easier tracheoscopic removal. Surgical removal, via tracheotomy, is indicated for foreign bodies that cannot be removed by tracheoscopy. Alternatively, graspers, or stone baskets or snares, can be used under fluoroscopic guidance in patients with airways too small to permit endoscopic removal, as described by Tivers and Hotston Moore (2006) (Figure 8.14).

Tracheal neoplasia

Tracheal neoplasia is rare in the dog and the cat. In both species, tracheal neoplasia includes lymphoma, osteosarcoma, chondrosarcoma, fibrosarcoma, adenocarcinoma, squamous cell carcinoma and mast cell tumour. In the cat, lymphosarcoma and squamous cell carcinoma predominate. Benign tracheal neoplasia includes plasmacytoma, ostechondroma and tracheal polyps. Osteochondral dysplasia of the trachea is a condition seen in young dogs; lesions stop growing at skeletal maturity and surgical resection of the lesion typically achieves cure.

Clinical signs of tracheal neoplasia include paroxysmal coughing of weeks' to months' duration, dyspnoea which progressively worsens and the presence of stridor. Retching with production of haemorrhagic discharge may occur occasionally. Large masses may be palpable on examination of the neck. Respiratory signs are usually only evident when 50% of the tracheal lumen is obliterated, so in general patients present with advanced disease.

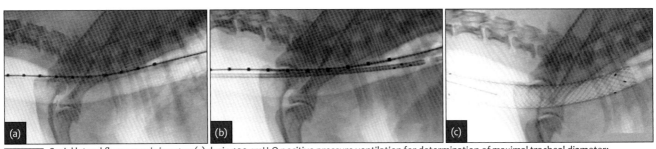

(a) (b) (c)

8.13 Serial lateral fluoroscopic images: (a) during 20 cmH$_2$O positive pressure ventilation for determination of maximal tracheal diameter; (b) during placement of a tracheal stent delivery system through the endotracheal tube and within the tracheal lumen; (c) immediately following stent deployment.

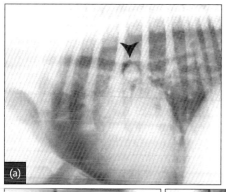

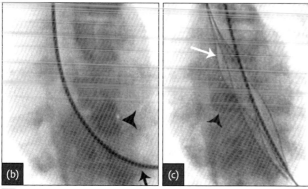

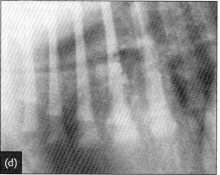

8.14 Series of radiographic images of an 8-week-old puppy with a tracheobronchial foreign body (a bead). (a) Bead (arrowhead) located at the carina, resulting in nearly complete airway obstruction. (b) Ventrodorsal radiograph with the bead (arrowhead) in the left mainstem bronchus and a 0.035-inch guidewire (arrowed) passed beyond the bead into the left bronchus. (c) Ventrodorsal radiograph with stone basket (arrowed) adjacent to the bead (arrowhead) bronchial foreign body. (d) Final lateral thoracic radiographic image demonstrating completed removal of the foreign body.

A diagnosis is achieved by diagnostic imaging of the neck and thoracic cavity. Radiography may reveal the location of a mass, due to deviation or narrowing of the air-filled trachea or due to mineralization of the mass. Computed tomography may provide further information regarding the mass and its association with adjacent structures. Tracheoscopy allows a definitive diagnosis to be achieved by visualization of the mass and obtaining brush cytology or grab biopsy samples. Additionally, laser ablation or instrument-assisted debulking can be performed under endoscopic guidance.

For lesions confined to the trachea and affecting a defined segment, surgical management is the treatment of choice. Benign neoplasms are readily cured if adequate margins are achieved, and the survival times for malignant neoplasms are also favourable following surgical resection. If surgical excision is not feasible and the mass is in the cranial cervical trachea, a permanent tracheostomy may give temporary relief. As these tumours are not uncommonly extensive, diffuse and/or closely associated

with important neighbouring neurovascular structures, complete excision may not be safely possible. Endoluminal tracheal stenting has been effective in re-establishing a patent airway in these patients in a palliative setting or to stabilize them prior to more definitive treatments such as radiation therapy (Figure 8.15).

Chemotherapy and/or radiation therapy are the most appropriate treatments for lymphoma. Squamous cell carcinoma, mast cell tumours and lymphoma are radio-sensitive, and radiotherapy can therefore be considered for management of these lesions.

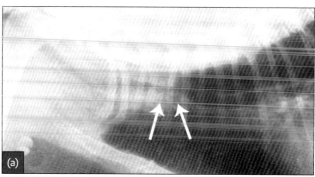

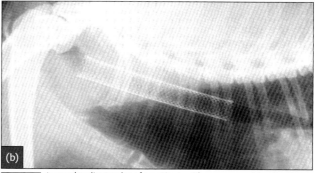

8.15 Lateral radiographs of a patient with a narrowed tracheal lumen due to malignant obstruction (arrowed). (a) Before and (b) following palliative tracheal stent placement.

Segmental tracheal stenosis

Segmental stenosis of the trachea is a rare congenital condition associated with congenital cartilage deformities (Mawby et al., 2006) and may also be acquired following trauma, including endotracheal tube injury associated with anaesthesia for dental prophylaxis or tracheostomy (Culp et al., 2007). Extensive tracheal narrowing has been treated using intraluminal self-expanding nitinol stents (Culp et al., 2007). Focal segmental tracheal stenosis may be managed by performing a tracheal resection and anastomosis (Figure 8.16).

Tracheal resection and anastomosis

Indications for tracheal resection and anastomosis

- Focal tracheal neoplasm.
- Congenital tracheal stenosis.
- Acquired tracheal stenosis following trauma.
- Resection of a traumatized section of trachea that is not amenable to primary repair.

Technique

Tracheal resection and anastomosis of the extrathoracic trachea should be performed in a controlled manner, with good surgical access and careful airway management. The procedure is technically demanding and requires careful planning and teamwork but does not require any specialized equipment, although the use of sterile endotracheal tubes is required. The aims of surgery are to achieve precise approximation and minimal tension at the anastomosis site, to allow rapid healing with minimal risk of complications. Tension at the anastomosis site has an important influence upon the nature of the healing: the degree of stenosis is increased when anastomosis tension is high, due to gap formation and consequent second intention healing (Demetriou et al., 2006).

The length of the segment of trachea to be resected is determined by findings on diagnostic imaging, tracheoscopy and assessment at surgery (Figure 8.16a). For mass lesions, cytological or histopathological samples will have ideally been obtained prior to surgery to allow thorough surgical planning. The maximum number of rings that can be resected is variably reported: up to 50% of the tracheal length (around 17–23 rings) has been documented in experimental dogs but this requires considerable use of dissection and tension-relieving techniques (Dallman and Bojrab, 1982). To minimize the risk of complications, removal of no greater than 25% of the tracheal length (8–10 tracheal rings) in the adult dog is recommended (Lau et al., 1980). Given the fragility of the trachea in the immature dog, no more than 20% of the tracheal length can be resected because the cartilage rings cannot withstand the necessary forces to support tension-relieving sutures with longer resections (Maeda and Grillo, 1973).

Prior to orotracheal intubation, an assessment of laryngeal function should be performed under a light plane of anaesthesia. The extrathoracic trachea is accessed via a ventral midline cervical approach; the paired sternocephalicus and sternohyoid muscles are separated on the midline. Dissection should avoid and preserve the recurrent laryngeal nerves; the use of monopolar cautery should be avoided. Once the limits of the resection are determined, the priority is to obtain access to the airway distally. This may be achieved by advancement of the orotracheal tube beyond the site of resection or by direct intubation of the distal tracheal segment, when passage of the tube is not possible (Figure 8.17). Sutures are placed as 'stay sutures' in the proximal and distal trachea to aid manipulation. When distal segment tracheal intubation is required, a tracheotomy incision is performed at the distal extent of the resection to allow insertion of a cuffed sterile endotracheal tube; a range of sizes should be available (see Figure 8.16b). The anaesthesia circuit is then detached from the orotracheal tube and connected to the sterile endotracheal tube inserted via the tracheostomy. Sterile drapes may be used to shroud the anaesthesia circuit, or sterile apparatus may be used. Following establishment of a reliable airway, the proximal portion of trachea can be carefully dissected, avoiding damage to the delicate vasculature and the recurrent laryngeal nerves. Once the section of trachea has been resected, the proximal and distal trachea can be brought into approximation; the sterile endotracheal tube is removed from the distal trachea and the orotracheal tube is advanced from the proximal to the distal trachea (see Figure 8.16c).

The precise site of tracheal transection should be selected carefully when the tracheal segment is resected, with tracheotomy performed either through ('split-ring') or between the tracheal cartilages. Tracheal anastomosis using the split-ring technique is reported to result in less stenosis than other techniques (Hedlund, 1984); however, this may be challenging to perform in small animals. The anastomosis is repaired using preplaced sutures of a monofilament absorbable material, such as polydioxanone (Fingland et al., 1995) (Figure 8.18). Sutures are placed dorsally in the dorsal tracheal ligament first and subsequently in the ventral tracheal rings; however, the dorsal

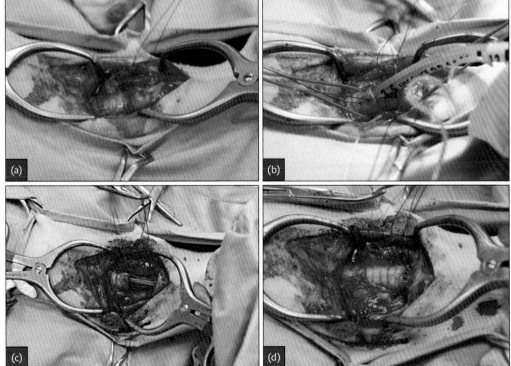

8.16 Resection and anastomosis of the cervical trachea in a Domestic Shorthaired cat for management of segmental tracheal stenosis at the site of a previous temporary tracheostomy (head to the right in all images). (a) A ventral midline exploration revealing the stenotic segment of trachea. (b) Following tracheotomy, a sterile endotracheal tube has been placed in the distal trachea to maintain anaesthesia and oxygenation. (c) Following resection of the stenotic segment, the orotracheal tube has been advanced from the proximal to the distal trachea and simple interrupted sutures have been preplaced ready to perform the anastomosis. (d) The distal and proximal sections of the trachea have been apposed and the sutures in the cartilage ring have been tied to achieve the anastomosis; the sutures in the dorsal tracheal ligament are tied last.

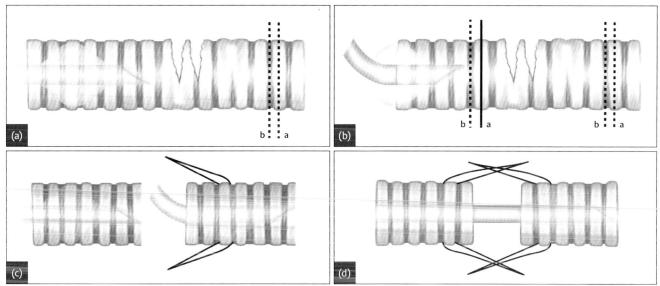

8.17 Tracheal resection. (a) The cartilage rings can be split (line a) in large dogs. In small dogs and cats, the cut in the trachea is most easily made between rings (line b). (b) Whenever possible, the endotracheal tube should be advanced beyond the site of tracheal excision. If this is not possible, the excision should be planned and the distal tracheal incision made first. (c) A sterile endotracheal tube should be available to secure the airway in the distal tracheal segment. Stay sutures will help to control the airway. The orotracheal tube should be left *in situ* and will be used once the anastomosis is complete. (d) Whenever possible, the endotracheal tube should be advanced beyond the site of tracheal excision. Stay sutures will help to maintain temporary tracheal alignment whilst sutures are preplaced.

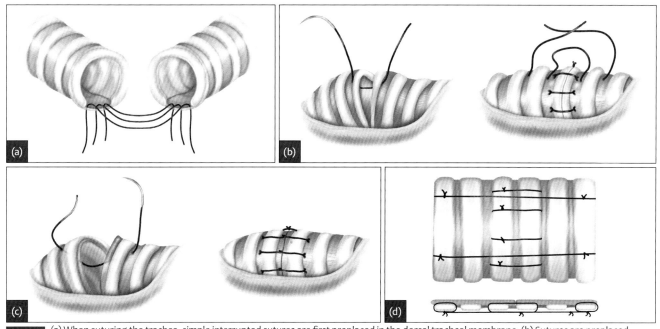

8.18 (a) When suturing the trachea, simple interrupted sutures are first preplaced in the dorsal tracheal membrane. (b) Sutures are preplaced around the tracheal rings. If the tracheal rings have been split, the sutures appose the cut cartilage edges. Tension-relieving sutures can be placed around the tracheal cartilages proximal and distal to the anastomosis site. (c) In small dogs and cats, sutures are placed around the tracheal rings, which, when tied, appose the tracheal membrane between rings. Care should be taken not to tighten these sutures such that cartilage rings overlap excessively. (d) Tension-relieving sutures can be placed around tracheal cartilages proximal and distal to the anastomosis site.

sutures are not tied first because the dorsal tracheal ligament is weaker and sutures may pull through (see Figure 8.16d). Various different suture patterns are described for performing the anastomosis: simple interrupted sutures, simple continuous and simple interrupted reinforced with horizontal mattress sutures. Sutures are placed to encircle each cartilage ring adjacent to the transection site. A biomechanical study in cadaveric canine tracheas suggests that a simple continuous technique should be selected when tension-relieving sutures are required for tracheal anastomosis. This offers the same advantages as simple interrupted reinforced with horizontal mattress sutures, but is superior to simple interrupted sutures alone (Demetriou *et al.*, 2006). However, a simple continuous suture pattern is reported to result in a less precise apposition of the tracheal segments (Fingland *et al.*, 1995) and should be avoided in growing animals owing to the potential to increase the risk of stenosis during growth (McKeown *et al.*, 1991).

Postoperative complications include subcutaneous emphysema due to air leakage, infection, decreased mucociliary clearance and stenosis. Strict rest is required for at least 2 weeks following surgery to allow satisfactory healing, and a harness should be used instead of a neck collar. Stenosis may be managed by bougienage; however, placement of an intraluminal stent (Culp *et al.*, 2007) or surgical revision of the anastomosis may be required.

References and further reading

Adamama-Moraitou K, Pardali D, Prassinos NN *et al.* (2010) Analysis of tidal breathing flow volume loop in dogs with tracheal masses. *Australian Veterinary Journal* **88**, 351–356

Becker WM, Beal M, Stanley BJ *et al.* (2012) Survival after surgery for tracheal collapse and the effect of intrathoracic collapse on survival. *Veterinary Surgery* **41**, 501–506

Bhandal J and Kuzma K (2008) Tracheal rupture in a cat: diagnosis by computed tomography. *Canadian Veterinary Journal* **49**, 595–597

Buback JL, Boothe HW and Hobson HP (1996) Surgical treatment of tracheal collapse in dogs: 90 cases (1983–1993). *Journal of the American Veterinary Medical Association* **208**, 380–384

Carb A and Halliwell WH (1981) Osteochondral dysplasia of the canine trachea. *Journal of the American Animal Hospital Association* **17**, 1040–1054

Chisnell HK and Pardo AD (2015) Long-term outcome, complications and disease progression in 23 dogs after placement of tracheal ring prostheses for treatment of extrathoracic tracheal collapse. *Veterinary Surgery* **44**, 103–113

Culp WTN, Weisse C, Cole SG *et al.* (2007) Intraluminal tracheal stenting for treatment of tracheal narrowing in three cats. *Veterinary Surgery* **36**, 107–113

Dallman MJ (1981) Normal and collapsed canine tracheas. A histochemical, scanning electron microscopic and statistical study. PhD thesis, University of Missouri–Columbia

Dallman MJ and Bojrab MJ (1982) Large segment tracheal resection and interannular anastomosis with a tension release technique in the dog. *American Journal of Veterinary Research* **42**, 217–223

Dallman MJ, McClure RC and Brown EM (1985) Normal and collapsed trachea in the dog: scanning electron microscopy study. *American Journal of Veterinary Research* **46**, 2110–2115

Dallman MJ, McClure RC and Brown EM (1988) Histochemical study of normal and collapsed tracheas in dogs. *American Journal of Veterinary Research* **49**, 2117–2125

Demetriou JL, Hughes R and Sissener TR (2006) Pullout strength for three suture patterns used for canine tracheal anastomosis. *Veterinary Surgery* **35**, 278–283

Dugas B, Hoover J and Pechman R (2011) Computed tomography of a cat with primary intratracheal lymphosarcoma before and after systemic chemotherapy. *Journal of the American Animal Hospital Association* **47**, 131–137

Fingland RB, Layton CI, Kennedy GA and Galland JC (1995) A comparison of simple continuous *versus* simple interrupted suture patterns for tracheal anastomosis after large segment tracheal resection in dogs. *Veterinary Surgery* **24**, 320–330

Fossum TW (2002) Surgical management of tracheal collapse. In: *Proceedings of the World Small Animal Veterinary Association Congress*. Available at www.vin.com/apputil/content/defaultadv1aspx?id=3846306&pid=11147

Guenther-Yenke CL and Rozanski EA (2007) Tracheostomy in cats: 23 cases (1998–2006). *Journal of Feline Medicine and Surgery* **9**, 451–457

Halfacree ZJ, Wilson AM and Baines SJ (2009) Evaluation of *in vitro* performance of suction drains. *American Journal of Veterinary Research* **70**, 283–289

Hamaide A, Arnoczky SP, Ciarelli MJ and Gardner K (1998) Effects of age and location on the biomechanical and biochemical properties of canine tracheal ring cartilage in dogs. *American Journal of Veterinary Research* **59**, 18–22

Hedlund CS (1984) Tracheal anastomosis in the dog. Comparison of two end to end techniques. *Veterinary Surgery* **13**, 135–142

Hedlund CS, Tangner CH and Montgomery DL (1982) A procedure for permanent tracheostomy and its effects on tracheal mucosa. *Veterinary Surgery* **11**, 13–17

Hedlund CS, Tangner CH, Waldron DR *et al.* (1988) Permanent tracheostomy: perioperative and long-term data from 34 cases. *Journal of the American Animal Hospital Association* **24**, 585–591

Hobson HP (1976) Total ring prosthesis for the surgical correction of collapsed trachea. *Journal of the American Animal Hospital Association* **12**, 822–828

Holt DE and Griffin G (2000) Bite wounds in dogs and cats. *Veterinary Clinics of North America: Small Animal Practice* **30**, 669–679

Jordan CJ, Halfacree ZJ and Tivers MS (2013) Airway injury associated with cervical bite wounds in dogs and cats: 56 cases. *Veterinary and Comparative Orthopaedics and Traumatology* **26**, 89–93

Johnson LR and Fales WH (2001) Clinical and microbiologic findings in dogs with bronchoscopically diagnosed tracheal collapse: 37 cases (1990–1995). *Journal of the American Veterinary Medical Association* **219**, 1247–1250

Lau RE, Schwarz A and Buergelt CD (1980) Tracheal resection and anastomosis in dogs. *Journal of the American Veterinary Medical Association* **176**, 134–139

Maeda M and Grillo H (1973) Effect of tension on tracheal growth after resection and anastomosis in puppies. *Journal of Thoracic and Cardiovascular Surgery* **65**, 658–668

Mahler SP, Mootoo NF, Reece JL *et al.* (2006) Surgical resection of a primary tracheal fibrosarcoma in a dog. *Journal of Small Animal Practice* **47**, 537–540

Mason RA and Johnson LR (2004) Tracheal collapse. In: *Textbook of Respiratory Disease in Dogs and Cats*, ed. L King, pp. 346–355. Saunders, St Louis

Mawby DI, Krahwinkel DJ, Donnell RL *et al.* (2006) Segmental tracheal dysplasia in a mixed breed dog. *Canadian Veterinary Journal* **47**, 1003–1006

McKeown PP, Tsuboi H, Togo T *et al.* (1991) Growth of tracheal anastomoses: advantages of absorbable interrupted sutures. *Annals of Thoracic Surgery* **51**, 636–664

Mitchell SL, McCarthy R, Rudloff E *et al.* (2000) Tracheal rupture associated with intubation in cats: 20 cases (1996–1998). *Journal of the American Veterinary Medical Association* **216**, 1592–1595

Moritz A, Schneider M and Bauer N (2004) Management of advanced tracheal collapse in dogs using intraluminal self-expanding biliary wallstents. *Journal of Veterinary Internal Medicine* **18**, 31–42

Nicholson I and Baines S (2012) Complications associated with temporary tracheostomy tubes in 42 dogs (1998–2007). *Journal of Small Animal Practice* **53**, 108–114

Occhipinti LL and Hauptman JG (2014) Long-term outcome of permanent tracheostomies in dogs: 21 cases (2000–2012). *Canadian Veterinary Journal* **55**, 357–360

Queen EV, Vaughan MA and Johnson LR (2010) Bronchoscopic debulking of tracheal carcinoma in three cats using a wire snare. *Journal of Veterinary Internal Medicine* **24**, 990–993

Radlinsky MG, Fossum TW, Walker MA, Aufdemorte TB and Thompson JA (1997) Evaluation of the Palmaz stent in the trachea and mainstem bronchi of normal dogs. *Veterinary Surgery* **26**, 99–107

Stepnik MW, Mehl ML, Hardie EM *et al.* (2009) Outcome of permanent tracheostomy for treatment of upper airway obstruction in cats: 21 cases (1990–2007). *Journal of the American Veterinary Medical Association* **234**, 638–643

Tinga S, Thieman Mankin KM, Peycke LE and Cohen ND (2015) Comparison of outcome after use of extra-luminal rings and intra-luminal stents for treatment of tracheal collapse in dogs. *Veterinary Surgery* **44**, 858–865

Tivers MS and Hotston Moore A (2006) Tracheal foreign bodies in the cat and the use of fluoroscopy for removal: 12 cases. *Journal of Small Animal Practice* **47**, 155–159

Weisse C (2015) Intraluminal tracheal stenting. In: *Veterinary Image-Guided Interventions*, ed. C Weisse and AC Berent, pp. 73–82. Wiley-Blackwell, Ames

White RAS and Williams JM (1994) Tracheal collapse in the dog – is there really a role for surgery? A survey of 100 cases. *Journal of Small Animal Practice* **35**, 191–196

White RN (1995) Unilateral arytenoid lateralisation and extraluminal polypropylene ring prostheses for correction of tracheal collapse in the dog. *Journal of Small Animal Practice* **36**, 151–158

Yamamoto Y, Ootsuka T, Atoji Y and Suzuki Y (1998) Morphological and quantitative study of the intrinsic nerve plexuses of the canine trachea as revealed by immunohistochemical staining of protein gene product 9.5. *Anatomical Record* **250**, 438–477

Chapter 9

Surgery of the oesophagus

Jennifer Huck and Andrew E. Kyles

Introduction

Oesophageal surgery is performed infrequently in dogs and cats, although there are a number of well defined indications. Surgery on the oesophagus has been associated with a higher prevalence of incisional dehiscence than surgery on other portions of the alimentary tract, however, it can be successfully performed by adhering to certain surgical principles.

Functional anatomy

The oesophagus is a muscular tube that functions as a conduit between the pharynx and stomach, with functional sphincters at the pharyngo-oesophageal and gastro-oesophageal junctions. The 'upper' oesophageal sphincter comprises the cricopharyngeus muscle and circular muscle fibres of the proximal oesophageal wall. The cervical portion of the oesophagus begins dorsal to the cranial trachea and, as the oesophagus runs caudally, inclines to the left of the trachea. The cervical oesophagus is closely associated with the left carotid sheath and left recurrent laryngeal nerve. The thoracic portion of the oesophagus inclines dorsally in the cranial mediastinum to return to its position dorsal to the trachea at the level of the tracheal bifurcation. The oesophagus passes to the right of the aortic arch, and runs through the caudal mediastinum to the oesophageal hiatus of the diaphragm. The 'lower' oesophageal sphincter acts as a high-pressure zone with contributions from the diaphragmatic crural muscles and folds of the gastro-oesophageal mucosa. The short abdominal portion of the oesophagus begins at the oesophageal hiatus and ends at the cardia of the stomach.

The oesophageal wall consists of four layers: mucosa; submucosa; muscularis; and adventitia. The adventitia of the oesophagus blends readily with the fascia of other surrounding structures.

- In dogs, the muscularis layer consists of two obliquely positioned layers of striated muscle throughout the length of the oesophagus, and there are distinct longitudinal folds in the mucosa.
- In cats, the muscularis layer consists of striated muscle cranial to the heart and smooth muscle caudal to the heart. There is an abrupt change in the mucosal pattern at the level of the heart base.

The longitudinal mucosal folds continue and distinct transverse mucosal folds are superimposed. This results in the characteristic 'herringbone' appearance of the feline caudal thoracic oesophagus on positive-contrast oesophagogram.

The blood supply to the oesophagus is considered to be segmental. The arterial supply originates from the cranial and caudal thyroid, broncho-oesophageal, intercostal, diaphragmatic and left gastric arteries. A rich intramural plexus of anastomosing vessels exists in the submucosal layer and can support long segments of the oesophagus.

Branches of the vagal nerves are closely associated with the oesophagus from the level of the heart caudally.

Surgical approaches

The cervical portion of the oesophagus is approached by a ventral midline cervical incision, separating the paired sternohyoid muscles and retracting the trachea to the right. Care should be taken to avoid damage to the left recurrent laryngeal nerve during tracheal retraction. This approach can be extended via a cranial median sternotomy to expose the cranial thoracic oesophagus to the level of the tracheal bifurcation.

The cranial thoracic portion of the oesophagus can also be exposed via a left third or fourth, or a right third, fourth or fifth intercostal thoracotomy. During a left-sided approach, the oesophagus is exposed by ventral retraction of the brachiocephalic trunk and subclavian vessels. On the right side, the oesophagus is exposed by ventral retraction of the trachea, which can be combined with retraction or ligation of the azygos vein to increase the exposure of the oesophagus at the base of the heart.

The caudal thoracic portion of the oesophagus is usually approached via a left-sided seventh, eighth or ninth intercostal thoracotomy in order to avoid the caudal vena cava. The dorsal and ventral vagal nerves should be identified and preserved. The caudal oesophagus and stomach can be approached by a combined ventral midline laparotomy and diaphragmatic incision, or caudal median sternotomy.

Principles of oesophageal surgery

When performing oesophageal surgery, the chance of a successful outcome can be increased by adhering to certain surgical principles, including:

- Gentle tissue handling to prevent damage to the intramural blood supply

- Minimization of contamination
- Appropriate selection and application of suture materials
- Appropriate use of electrocautery
- Accurate apposition of tissues with minimal tension.

Various closing techniques have been described and advocated for closure of the oesophagus, including a double-layer appositional pattern, a single-layer inverting pattern, a single-layer everting pattern, and a single-layer appositional pattern. A single-layer appositional simple interrupted suture pattern has been successfully used in dogs and cats for oesophagotomy closure and oesophageal anastomoses (Shamir *et al.*, 1999). This pattern is generally preferred as it allows for expansion of the oesophageal lumen and minimizes disturbance of the intramural blood supply.

As in the remainder of the gastrointestinal tract, the holding layer of the oesophagus is the submucosa (Dallman, 1988). Regardless of the suture pattern utilized, the submucosa must be incorporated into every bite in at least one layer of sutures. The optimal suture choice is a monofilament, minimally reactive, slowly absorbed suture material such as polydioxanone or polyglyconate. Sutures should be spaced 2–3 mm apart to create a tight seal.

Indications for oesophageal surgery

Oesophageal surgery is infrequently performed in dogs and cats. Indications for oesophageal surgery include:

- Foreign bodies
- Strictures
- Perforation
- Fistulae
- Diverticulae
- Neoplasia
- Vascular ring anomalies (see Chapter 15).

Oesophageal tumours are usually highly invasive and advanced at the time of diagnosis and are therefore rarely amenable to surgery. Benign lesions are occasionally diagnosed. The caudal oesophagus is a site of predilection for leiomyoma, a benign smooth muscle tumour, which can often be successfully 'shelled out' of the oesophageal wall without entering the oesophageal lumen.

Vascular ring anomalies are developmental anomalies of the great vessels that result in the encircling of the oesophagus by a complete or incomplete ring of vessels (see Chapter 15). Vascular ring anomalies produce partial to near-complete oesophageal mechanical obstruction, resulting in regurgitation and failure to thrive at the time of weaning and transition to a solid diet.

Oesophageal foreign bodies

Oesophageal foreign bodies are a common problem in dogs and are occasionally diagnosed in cats. The most common foreign bodies in dogs are ingested bones or bone/cartilage composites. Young small-breed dogs, especially terriers, are over-represented. Most affected dogs are less than 3 years of age. In cats, oesophageal foreign bodies are more likely to be fishhooks or needles and string foreign bodies.

The most common locations for foreign bodies include:

- Caudal thoracic oesophagus, between the heart base and diaphragm
- Cranial cervical oesophagus, just caudal to the pharynx
- Thoracic inlet
- Heart base.

Bony foreign bodies are most commonly located in the caudal thoracic oesophagus, between the heart and diaphragm, cranial to the diaphragmatic oesophageal hiatus. Oesophageal fishhooks most commonly lodge in the pharyngeal oesophagus and at the heart base.

Clinical signs

The duration of clinical signs prior to presentation varies considerably, ranging from a few hours to several months. There may be a history of ingesting bone or rubbish, or of roaming. Most animals present with acute clinical signs associated with complete or severe partial obstruction. The most classic clinical sign is regurgitation of food within a few minutes of eating. Water is frequently retained unless there is a complete obstruction. Other clinical signs include retching, gagging, excessive salivation, exaggerated swallowing, restlessness, lethargy and inappetence. Chronically affected animals may remain bright and alert but show weight loss and periodic bouts of regurgitation and inappetence.

Sharp or chronic foreign bodies can result in oesophageal perforation and secondary pneumomediastinum, pneumothorax, mediastinitis, pleuritis, pyothorax, mediastinal abscessation or broncho-oesophageal, tracheo-oesophageal or aortic-oesophageal fistulae. Signs of oesophageal perforation include pyrexia, depression and respiratory distress. Respiratory distress may also be associated with aspiration pneumonia or impingement of a foreign body on the upper airways.

Diagnosis

Most oesophageal foreign bodies are radiopaque and can be diagnosed with survey cervical and/or thoracic radiography (Figure 9.1). Radiographs should also be examined closely for signs of aspiration pneumonia, mediastinitis, pneumomediastinum, pleural effusion and pneumothorax. Radiolucent foreign bodies are infrequently encountered; diagnosis may require a positive contrast oesophagogram, using a sterile water-soluble low-osmolality iodinated solution. Oesophageal perforation may not be evident on oesophagograms because the foreign body may obstruct leakage of the contrast agent from the oesophagus. Additionally, it has been shown in humans that iodinated contrast material is inferior to barium for detecting smaller perforations (Tanomkiat and Galassi, 2000). Oesophagoscopy can also be useful for identifying foreign bodies and should be considered when dealing with suspicious cases that cannot be confirmed radiographically.

Treatment

Endoscopy

Non-surgical retrieval of oesophageal foreign bodies is usually performed under general anaesthesia with endoscopic guidance. This technique is associated with lower morbidity and mortality than surgical removal. It is the

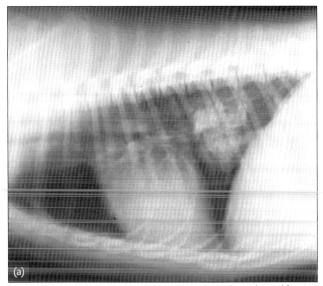

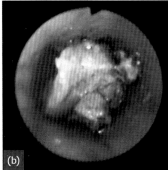

9.1 Oesophageal foreign body. (a) Lateral thoracic radiograph of a 1-year-old Shih-Tzu with a 5-day history of regurgitation, drooling and difficulty swallowing. The radiograph shows an oesophageal foreign body lodged in the caudal thoracic oesophagus. (b) Endoscopic appearance of the oesophageal foreign body (a bone).
(Courtesy of the Veterinary Imaging Database, University of California, Davis)

hook through the tissue such that the barb re-emerges in the lumen. The hook can then be rotated entirely into the lumen and retrieved.

If an oesophageal foreign body cannot be extracted, an attempt should be made to advance it into the stomach if there is little risk of causing a perforation. Bones will be digested in the stomach and do not require a gastrotomy for retrieval, unless they subsequently cause a clinical problem.

If an endoscope is not readily available, similar techniques for the retrieval of oesophageal foreign bodies using fluoroscopic guidance are described (Hotston Moore, 2001).

Non-surgical retrieval of oesophageal foreign bodies can be performed in most cases. In one clinical series of dogs, in which endoscopy was employed, foreign bodies were extracted in 86% of dogs (57 of 66), and pushed into the stomach in 14% (Gianella *et al.*, 2009). Similar results have been reported using fluoroscopic techniques, with foreign bodies being extracted in 84% of dogs (51 of 61) (Hotston Moore, 2001). In another report, fishhooks were successfully extracted endoscopically in 64% of animals (23 of 36) (Michels *et al.*, 1995).

Surgery

Surgical intervention is indicated:

- When retrieval or advancement of the foreign body fails
- When forceps extraction presents a significant risk for laceration of the oesophagus or major vessels
- When the foreign body has perforated the oesophagus.

Oesophagotomy: The surgical site is isolated with moistened laparotomy sponges. An orogastric tube is passed and the oesophagus cranial to the foreign body is suctioned to reduce contamination. Stay sutures can be positioned lateral to the intended oesophagotomy site for ease of tissue manipulation. A stab incision is made into the oesophageal lumen and extended longitudinally or transversely as necessary (Figure 9.2). If the oesophageal wall appears normal, the incision is made directly over the foreign body, whereas if the oesophageal wall appears compromised, the incision should be made caudal to the foreign body. The foreign body is removed with forceps, taking care to avoid further oesophageal trauma. In cases of sharp bone foreign bodies, incremental removal of the foreign body using rongeurs may aid in preventing further trauma to the oesophagus.

The oesophageal lumen is carefully inspected for areas of perforation or necrosis. The oesophagotomy incision can be closed with a single- or two-layer simple interrupted suture pattern (Figure 9.2). With a two-layer pattern, the first layer incorporates the mucosa and submucosa and the knots are placed in the oesophageal lumen. The second layer apposes the muscularis and adventitia, with the knots placed on the external surface of the oesophagus. With a single-layer closure, the suture passes through all layers of the oesophageal wall, with limited penetration of the mucosa, and the knots are placed extraluminally. Sutures should be placed approximately 2 mm from the cut edge and 2–3 mm apart. The integrity of the closure can be tested by distending the oesophagus with saline and placing additional sutures to seal any areas of leakage.

Gastrotomy: Foreign bodies located between the heart and diaphragm can also be removed via a gastrotomy performed through a midline laparotomy (Taylor, 1982). See the *BSAVA Manual of Canine and Feline Abdominal Surgery.*

initial treatment of choice for oesophageal foreign bodies unless perforation is highly suspected. A flexible endoscope is preferred for examining the oesophagus but either a flexible or rigid endoscope can be employed to retrieve the foreign body. The clinician must have the ability to insufflate air through the endoscope to dilate the oesophagus around the foreign body. If oesophageal perforation is suspected, insufflation should be avoided or used sparingly owing to the serious risk of iatrogenic pneumomediastinum and possibly pneumothorax (Gianella *et al.*, 2009). Arterial haemoglobin oxygen saturation, arterial blood pressure and the ease and rate of ventilation should be monitored during oesophagoscopy, because tension pneumothorax can occur during endoscopic oesophageal insufflation if a perforation is present. Periodic suctioning of the insufflated air from the stomach may be required to promote adequate ventilation.

There are various techniques utilized when endoscopically removing an oesophageal foreign body. Most commonly, the foreign body is grasped with rigid forceps passed alongside the endoscope or through an instrument channel. The foreign body is gently rotated to free it, and then withdrawn with the scope, with any sharp points or edges facing caudally. A firmly lodged foreign body should not be forced, as this may induce or enlarge a perforation. An alternative technique described for relatively smooth foreign bodies is to pass a balloon catheter distal to the foreign body, inflate the balloon, and gently apply traction to withdraw the catheter and foreign body.

For the endoscopic retrieval of fishhooks, the neck of the hook is grasped with rigid forceps. The hook is pulled close to the endoscope and then withdrawn with the endoscope. An attempt should be made to dislodge a fishhook embedded in the oesophageal wall by rotating the

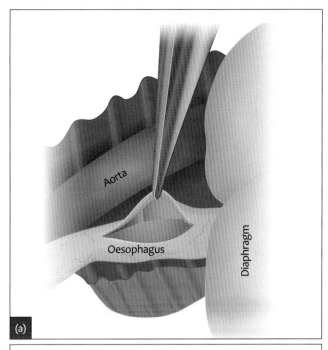

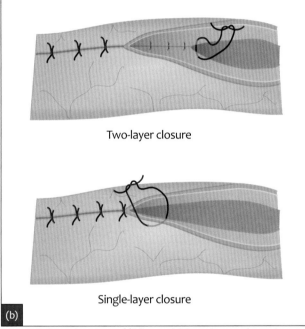

Two-layer closure

Single-layer closure

9.2 Oesophagotomy. (a) The caudal thoracic oesophagus is approached via an intercostal thoracotomy and a longitudinal incision is made into the oesophagus. (b) The oesophagotomy is closed with a single- or two-layer simple interrupted suture pattern (see text for details).

Fishhooks: Penetrating oesophageal fishhooks (Figure 9.3) can be treated by a combination of surgery and endoscopy. The oesophagus is approached through a surgical incision, and the barb is manipulated through the oesophageal wall and cut. The shank of the hook can then be retrieved with the endoscope and forceps.

Debridement, resection and anastomosis: If areas of oesophageal perforation or necrosis are observed, these should be debrided. Up to one quarter of the circumference of the oesophagus can be resected and a primary longitudinal closure performed. Large necrotic areas or extensive perforations are treated by oesophageal resection and anastomosis.

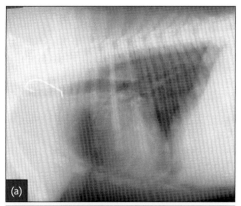

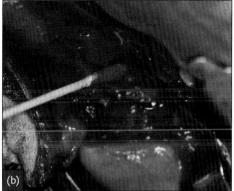

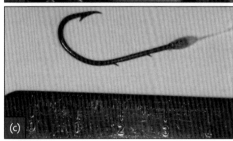

9.3 A 5-year-old Yorkshire Terrier had been observed swallowing a fish with the fishhook and line attached. An attempt had been made to remove the fishhook by applying traction to the fishing line. (a) Lateral thoracic radiograph showing the fishhook lodged in the cranial thoracic oesophagus. Endoscopic retrieval of the fishhook was unsuccessful. (b) A cranial sternotomy revealed a large haematoma and the barb of the fishhook protruding from the oesophagus. The fishhook (c) was removed and the lacerated left subclavian vein ligated.
(Courtesy of the Veterinary Imaging Database, University of California, Davis)

The length of the oesophagus that can be resected without undue risk of dehiscence is limited by anastomotic tension; resection of >3–5 cm of oesophagus has been associated with increased risk of dehiscence. Circumferential partial myotomy may reduce anastomotic tension. The outer longitudinal muscle layer is incised 2–3 cm proximal and/or distal to the anastomosis, leaving the inner circular muscle layer and submucosal blood supply intact (Muangsombut *et al.*, 1974). Separation of the muscle layers may be facilitated by injecting saline into the muscularis.

A small amount of oesophageal mobilization during surgery is necessary, but excessive mobilization should be avoided to prevent compromise to the segmental oesophageal blood supply. The oesophagus is isolated with moistened laparotomy sponges and the lumen occluded with the fingers, umbilical tape or non-crushing clamps. The diseased portion of the oesophagus is resected. Stay sutures are placed to facilitate gentle tissue handling and maintain alignment. The remaining segments are reapposed with a single- or two-layer suture pattern as described for oesophagotomy, with the far oesophageal wall being sutured first. Oesophageal anastomoses can also be performed using surgical stapling instruments; however, there may be an associated increased risk of stricture formation, according to the human medical literature.

Flaps and patches: When there is an increased risk of oesophageal dehiscence due to reduced vascularity or anastomotic tension, the oesophagotomy or oesophagectomy incision can be reinforced with an 'on-lay' patch. Tissues that have been used to patch the oesophagus include omentum, pericardium and muscle flaps. Muscle flaps can be created from the sternothyroid muscles for the cervical oesophagus, from the intercostal muscles for the thoracic oesophagus and from the diaphragm for the caudal thoracic oesophagus. The on-lay patch is sutured over the oesophageal incision to provide structural support, seal the incision and increase vascularity.

Perforations and other complications: If the oesophagus is perforated before or during endoscopic or fluoroscopic retrieval of the foreign body, surgery is generally indicated. Small perforations may seal on their own, particularly if oral intake of food and water is prohibited for 72 hours. Cervical perforations may only require local drainage because of support from local soft tissues. Thoracic perforations are more likely to result in life-threatening consequences, and should be operated upon if peri-oesophageal leakage is present. Samples for culture and sensitivity testing should be obtained and thoracostomy tubes placed intraoperatively in the case of thoracic oesophageal perforation.

Oesophageal perforation can result in mediastinal abscess formation or pyothorax, which should be drained and flushed at the time of surgery. Oesophageal foreign bodies occasionally result in the formation of a secondary oesophageal fistula. Fistulae most commonly form between the oesophagus and a bronchus, but can occasionally communicate with the trachea, lung parenchyma, aorta or skin. Oesophageal fistulae require surgical management. Anaesthesia is a particular challenge as the fistula makes ventilation difficult and inhalant anaesthetics will escape into the oesophagus. The fistulous tract should be excised rather than ligated.

Prognosis

The prognosis after foreign body removal is generally excellent, except in cases of thoracic oesophageal perforation (see above). Complications of oesophageal foreign body removal include oesophagitis, ischaemic necrosis, dehiscence, leakage, infection, and fistula, diverticula or stricture formation. Perforation of the aorta or pulmonary artery by the foreign body before or during retrieval is fatal.

In one study, 10 of 66 dogs (15.2%) that underwent oesophagoscopy for foreign body retrieval experienced complications, with perforation being the most common. Of these 10 dogs, six died or were euthanased as a result of these complications. Bone foreign bodies and a body-weight of <10 kg were found to be significant risk factors for complications (Gianella *et al.*, 2009).

Oesophageal stricture

Oesophageal strictures can be either congenital or acquired. Congenital strictures are rare in dogs and cats. Acquired oesophageal strictures are uncommon, and result from severe circumferential injury to the oesophagus that extends into the muscular layer of the oesophageal wall. The oesophageal injury heals by fibrosis and wound contracture, which results in a narrow lumen and oesophageal obstruction. The most common cause of acquired oesophageal stricture in dogs and cats is oesophageal reflux during anaesthesia.

Clinical signs

Oesophageal strictures can occur in any age, breed or sex of dog or cat. There may be a history of general anaesthesia or oesophageal trauma, generally occurring within a month of presentation. The presenting complaint is usually regurgitation.

Diagnosis

The presence of an oesophageal stricture can be confirmed by positive contrast oesophagography (Figure 9.4) and oesophagoscopy.

- Oesophagography is better for determining the number, location and length of strictures.
- Oesophagoscopy allows direct assessment of the stricture and the mucosal lining of the oesophagus, and treatment by bougienage or balloon dilation. The narrowed oesophageal lumen may prevent passage of the endoscope through the stricture, therefore it may not be possible to evaluate endoscopically the number and length of strictures in certain cases.

Treatment
Dilation

The preferred treatment for oesophageal strictures is bougienage or balloon dilation.

- Bougienage uses conical dilators of increasing diameter to push open the stricture.
- Balloon dilation (Figure 9.5) involves insertion of a balloon catheter through the stricture and inflation of the catheter.

Both techniques can be performed with endoscopic or fluoroscopic guidance. Balloon dilation has the theoretical advantage of exerting a stationary radial stretch force,

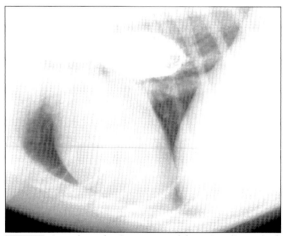

9.4 Oesophageal stricture. Lateral thoracic radiograph of a 6-year-old mixed breed dog that had started regurgitating 1 week after ovariohysterectomy. The radiograph was obtained 30 minutes after administration of a barium meal and demonstrates a caudal oesophageal stricture.
(Courtesy of the Veterinary Imaging Database, University of California, Davis)

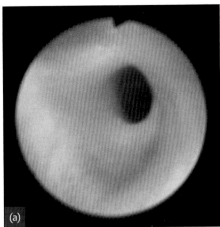 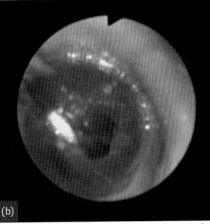 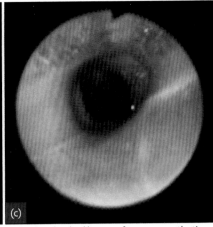

9.5 Oesophageal stricture in a 6-year-old Domestic Shorthaired cat with a 6-month history of regurgitation that had begun after an anaesthetic episode. (a) The endoscopic image shows a stricture in the caudal thoracic oesophagus. (b) Endoscopic view of balloon dilation of the stricture. (c) Endoscopic view immediately following balloon dilation.
(Courtesy of the Veterinary Imaging Database, University of California, Davis)

whereas bougienage exerts longitudinal shearing forces that could predispose to oesophageal perforation. The reported success rates of both techniques are comparable and either technique can result in oesophageal perforation. Most animals will require multiple dilations.

Oesophageal stenting has also been described for treatment of benign oesophageal strictures that were refractory to dilation and medical management. In a case series of 10 dogs, all experienced short-term improvement in dysphagia; however, the complication rate was high (Lam *et al.*, 2013).

Surgery

Surgery is associated with a high incidence of stricture recurrence and oesophageal incisional dehiscence, and is only indicated for the treatment of strictures that fail to respond to dilation or bougienage, or for cases in which perforation occurs during dilation. Surgical options for treatment of strictures include:

- Simple oesophagoplasty
- Oesophageal resection and anastomosis
- Patch oesophagoplasty
- Oesophageal substitution.

Simple oesophagoplasty involves a longitudinal oesophagotomy that is closed transversely. Most oesophageal strictures are too extensive to be treated by oesophagoplasty or oesophageal resection and anastomosis. Oesophageal patching involves a longitudinal oesophagotomy through the stricture and incorporation of an 'in-lay' patch in the closure of the defect to increase the luminal diameter. Tissues that have been used for in-lay patches include pericardium, local muscle flaps (sternothyroid, intercostal or diaphragmatic muscle), stomach and intestine.

Oesophageal substitution can be performed following extensive oesophageal resection, although clinical experience in dogs and cats is very limited. The cervical oesophagus can be replaced in a multistage procedure with an inverse tubed skin graft or an omocervical cutaneous island axial pattern flap. Various muscle grafts have been used experimentally in dogs for complete segmental reconstruction of the oesophagus. The caudal thoracic oesophagus can be replaced by gastric advancement and oesophagogastric anastomosis. Oesophageal replacement with a small intestinal or colonic pedicle graft is hampered by limited mobility of the vascular pedicle. Free microvascular grafts of colon or small intestine can be utilized to replace the cervical oesophagus. In experimental dogs, replacement of the thoracic oesophagus with free grafts has been largely unsuccessful. Numerous biomaterials have been studied in laboratory animal models for use in humans; however, these materials are not commercially available for clinical use.

Prognosis

Most dogs and cats with oesophageal strictures can be improved with repeated bougienage or balloon dilation treatments, although they may continue to regurgitate periodically or have mild dysphagia with an inability to eat dry food. The major complications of stricture dilation are perforation and recurrence of clinical signs.

Intra- and postoperative management of oesophageal surgical cases

After oesophageal surgery, the cervical region or thorax should be lavaged thoroughly. If an oesophageal perforation was present, the surgical site should be swabbed prior to closure and bacteriological culture and antimicrobial sensitivity testing performed. A thoracostomy tube should be placed if the thoracic cavity was entered. Food and water are withheld for a period determined by the extent of the surgery. After oesophagotomy or other less invasive oesophageal procedures, food in the form of a gruel-type diet can be introduced 24–48 hours after surgery as long as the animal is not regurgitating. The diet is gradually returned to normal after 7 days. After oesophageal resection and anastomosis, fluid and nutritional requirements should be provided through a gastrostomy or enterostomy tube for at least a week.

Postoperatively, animals should be observed carefully for 2–3 days for signs of oesophageal leakage, which include cervical pain, swelling, dyspnoea, regurgitation and elevated rectal temperature. Animals can be placed on an H_2 receptor blocker or proton pump inhibitor and a sucralfate slurry to limit gastric fluid acidity and oesophagitis, respectively. Corticosteroids are frequently prescribed to decrease scar tissue formation after oesophageal dilation; however, evidence of therapeutic benefit is lacking. Antibiotics are administered if aspiration pneumonia, mediastinitis, pleuritis or sepsis is present.

References and further reading

Bissett SA, Davis J, Subler K *et al.* (2009) Risk factors and outcome of bougienage for treatment of benign esophageal strictures in dogs and cats: 28 cases (1995–2004). *Journal of the American Veterinary Medical Association* **235**, 844–850

Dallman MJ (1988) Functional suture-holding layer of the esophagus in the dog. *Journal of the American Veterinary Medical Association* **192**, 638–640

Gianella P, Pfammatter NS and Burgener IA (2009) Oesophageal and gastric endoscopic foreign body removal: complications and follow-up of 102 dogs. *Journal of Small Animal Practice* **50**, 649–654

Harai BH, Johnson SE and Sherding RG (1995) Endoscopically guided balloon dilatation of benign esophageal strictures in 6 cats and 7 dogs. *Journal of Veterinary Internal Medicine* **9**, 332–335

Hotston Moore A (2001) Removal of oesophageal foreign bodies in dogs: use of the fluoroscopic methods and outcome. *Journal of Small Animal Practice* **42**, 227–230

Houlton JEF, Herrtage ME, Taylor PM and Watkins SB (1985) Thoracic oesophageal foreign bodies in the dog: a review of ninety cases. *Journal of Small Animal Practice* **26**, 521–536

Kyles AE (2012) Esophagus. In: *Small Animal Veterinary Surgery, 1st edn*, ed. K Tobias and S. Johnston, pp. 1461–1483. Elsevier Saunders, St Louis

Lam N, Weisse C, Berent A *et al.* (2013) Esophageal stenting for treatment of refractory benign esophageal strictures in dogs. *Journal of Veterinary Internal Medicine* **27**, 1064–1070

Michels GM, Jones BD, Huss BT and Wagner-Mann C (1995) Endoscopic and surgical retrieval of fishhooks from the stomach and esophagus in dogs and cats: 75 cases (1977–1993). *Journal of the American Veterinary Medical Association* **207**, 1194–1197

Muangsombut J, Hawkins JR, Mason GR and McLaughlin JS (1974) The use of circular myotomy to facilitate resection and end-to-end anastomosis of the esophagus. An experimental study. *Journal of Thoracic and Cardiovascular Surgery* **68**, 522–529

Orton EC (1995) Esophagus. In: *Small Animal Thoracic Surgery*, ed. EC Orton, pp. 117–131. Williams and Wilkins, Baltimore

Runge JJ and Culp WT (2013) Surgical treatment of esophageal disease. In: *Small Animal Soft Tissue Surgery*, ed. E Monnet, pp. 304–320. Wiley-Blackwell, Oxford

Shamir MH, Shahar R, Johnston DE and Mongil EM (1999) Approaches to esophageal suturing. *Compendium on Continuing Education for the Practicing Veterinarian* **21**, 414–421

Tanomkiat W and Galassi W (2000) Barium sulfate as contrast medium for avaluation of postoperative anastomic leaks. *Acta Radiologica* **41**, 482–485

Taylor RA (1982) Transdiaphragmatic approach to distal esophageal foreign bodies. *Journal of the American Animal Hospital Association* **18**, 749–752

Weyrauch EA and Willard MD (1998) Esophagitis and benign esophageal strictures. *Compendium on Continuing Education for the Practicing Veterinarian* **20**, 203–210

Williams JM and Niles J (2015) *BSAVA Manual of Canine and Feline Abdominal Surgery, 2nd edn*. BSAVA Publications, Gloucester

Chapter 10

Surgery of the thyroid and parathyroid glands

Davina Anderson

Introduction

The thyroid and parathyroid glands are a significant cause of disease in both the dog and the cat. They are intimately related to each other anatomically but the physiological consequences of disease or surgical removal are vastly different. The thyroid gland produces thyroxine, which is involved in metabolic homeostasis; parathyroid hormone (PTH) is pivotal for calcium homeostasis. Both glands can be affected by neoplastic processes that may result in excess secretion of active hormone. Equally, both glands may cease to produce hormones as a result of either iatrogenic damage after surgery or primary inflammatory or autoimmune conditions. The *BSAVA Manual of Canine and Feline Endocrinology* deals with medical aspects of gland disorders; this chapter only covers those conditions that require surgery.

Anatomy and function

Thyroid glands

The thyroid glands are paired ductless glands situated lateral and slightly ventral to the trachea (Figure 10.1). Their size and position varies with species and breed, but they are usually found between the fifth and eighth tracheal rings. Dorsal to the right thyroid gland are the common carotid artery, internal jugular vein, tracheal duct and vagosympathetic nerve trunk. The recurrent laryngeal nerve passes dorsally close to the right thyroid lobe. The left thyroid gland is usually further caudal and adjacent to the oesophagus, so that it is not in contact with the carotid sheath. The caudal laryngeal nerve passes dorsally. In the dog and cat, accessory (ectopic) thyroid tissue is common and can be found anywhere along the midline cervical or thoracic structures. The cranial thyroid artery arises from

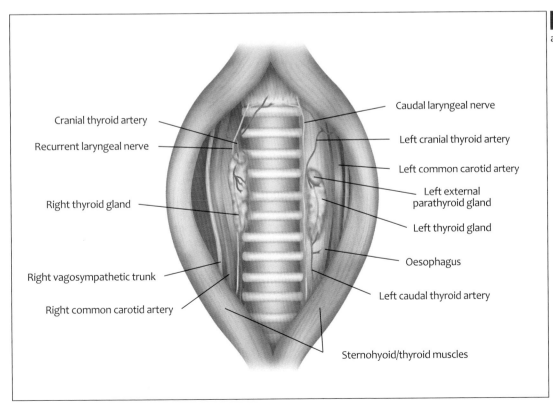

10.1 Anatomy of the thyroid and parathyroid glands.

Labels: Cranial thyroid artery; Recurrent laryngeal nerve; Right thyroid gland; Right vagosympathetic trunk; Right common carotid artery; Caudal laryngeal nerve; Left cranial thyroid artery; Left common carotid artery; Left external parathyroid gland; Left thyroid gland; Oesophagus; Left caudal thyroid artery; Sternohyoid/thyroid muscles

the common carotid artery; it gives a branch to the external parathyroid gland as it enters the cranial pole of the thyroid gland and anastamoses with the caudal thyroid artery on the dorsal surface of the thyroid. The caudal thyroid artery arises from the brachiocephalic trunk and travels up the neck along the trachea, but is not always present in the cat. The cranial and caudal thyroid veins drain into the internal jugular vein. Lymphatic drainage is to the retropharyngeal and deep cervical lymph nodes, but can also occur directly into the cervical lymphatic trunk or internal jugular vein.

The thyroid gland produces and stores thyroglobulin, which is the precursor of active thyroxine. Thyroid-stimulating hormone (TSH) is released from the pituitary gland to stimulate trapping of iodide by the thyroid gland and subsequent formation of triiodothyronine (T3) and thyroxine (T4) from iodination of thyroglobulin. T4 is the predominant hormone secreted and >99% of this is protein-bound. It is deiodinated peripherally to give rise to a more biologically active form, T3. Release of T3 and T4 is stimulated by TSH and results in an increase in the overall metabolic rate and anabolic effects.

Parathyroid glands

The parathyroid glands are smaller, closely related to the thyroid glands (Figure 10.2), and produce parathyroid hormone. There are four parathyroid glands: two are usually well demarcated and located on the outside of the craniodorsal aspect of each thyroid gland; the other two are embedded in the parenchyma of the thyroid gland, usually in the caudal part. However, there are many reported variations in the number and relationships of the thyroid and parathyroid glands. Ectopic parathyroid tissue has been reported in up to 50% of cats and, in various studies, in between 6% and 100% of dogs.

The vascular supply is directly linked to that of the thyroid gland. In cats, the cranial thyroid artery may release a branch to the cranial parathyroid externally, or it may pass through the thyroid parenchyma first, perforating the thyroid capsule to reach the external parathyroid gland. Like ectopic thyroid tissue, the ectopic parathyroid tissue may be found at any point along the ventral neck, thoracic inlet and mediastinum.

PTH maintains blood calcium levels by stimulating resorption of calcium by the renal tubules, mobilizing calcium from bone and augmenting intestinal absorption of calcium. High levels of circulating PTH cause an increase in total and ionized blood calcium. The parathyroid gland responds directly to circulating serum calcium levels, regulating the release of PTH.

Calcitonin is secreted by the thyroid gland and has a minor role in calcium homeostasis. Circulating phosphate levels have no direct effect on PTH release, but they may indirectly cause release of PTH, as high levels of phosphate may depress serum calcium levels. There is also a limited direct response to serum magnesium.

Some of the effects of PTH are mediated by vitamin D. PTH controls the final metabolism of vitamin D in the kidney to 1,25-dihydroxyvitamin D3, which promotes intestinal absorption of calcium and bone calcium resorption. Receptors for 1,25-dihydroxyvitamin D3 in the parathyroid gland provide another negative feedback mechanism, inhibiting PTH synthesis.

Thyroid disorders

Diagnostics

Owing to the superficial location of the thyroid gland, enlarged glands are often palpable in the neck of the conscious animal. Physical examination may reveal other signs suggestive of thyroid hormone abnormalities such as tachy- or bradycardia, restlessness or lethargy, and hair coat abnormalities.

Cervical masses can be assessed using ultrasonography. This also enables determination of uni- or bilateral disease, and the extent of invasion in the case of neoplastic disease. Computed tomographic (CT) scanning is preferable to determine the extent of local disease as well as allowing staging at the same time, assessing regional lymph nodes and pulmonary parenchyma for metastatic disease. Surgical biopsy of large cervical masses may be difficult as thyroid masses in the dog are often extremely vascular; therefore, fine-needle aspiration with ultrasound guidance may be safer. In the cat, confirmation of hyperthyroidism with clinical biochemistry is considered adequate for diagnosis, and thyroid masses are rarely biopsied or aspirated. Scintigraphy using Technetium[-99] can help to identify thyroid masses and may be particularly useful for identification of ectopic thyroid tissue. In the dog, up to 90% of thyroid masses are carcinomas and frequently metastasize. In the cat, carcinomas account for only 1–3% of thyroid masses; adenomatous hyperplasia accounts for the remaining 97–99%. Blood analysis may yield results suggestive of hyper- or hypothyroid disease (see below) but specific tests include T4 and TSH levels, and TSH response.

Specific tests

Hyperthyroidism (thyrotoxicosis) is the most common endocrine disorder in cats and is reported to affect up to 1 in 300 cats. Measurements of serum T3 and T4 vary with species, time of day and levels of circulating binding proteins; measurement of peripheral serum T3 can be unhelpful because most T3 is intracellular. In some non-thyroid diseases total serum T3 decreases, although this does not cause clinical manifestations of hypothyroidism and free T4 is often within normal limits ('sick euthyroid syndrome'). Scintigraphy may be useful to distinguish those cases with true hypothyroidism and those with a falsely low T4.

In older cats that are hyperthyroid, total T4 may fluctuate widely, and repeated tests may be required to confirm

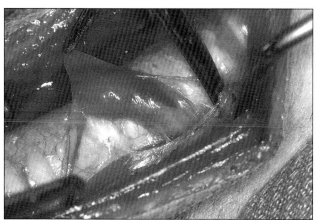

10.2 The left thyroid gland of a dog has been elevated using forceps. The normal parathyroid gland is visible on the cranial pole as a paler flat disc closely associated with the thyroid gland. The caudal thyroid artery is clearly visible.
(© Davina Anderson)

the diagnosis. However, in some cases, total T4 is persistently within the normal range, despite a high index of clinical suspicion for hyperthyroidism. In these cases, measuring the free T4 level may be more sensitive, as this is less affected by non-thyroidal factors. In combination with a total T4 level in the upper half of the normal range, an elevated serum level of free T4 may be considered diagnostic of hyperthyroidism. However, measurements of free T4 alone can still be misleading, and some cats with non-thyroidal disease may have a high free T4 level with normal levels of total T4 and T3. Finally, a T3 suppression test or a thyroid-releasing hormone (TRH) stimulation test may be used to confirm the diagnosis.

Hypothyroidism

Hypothyroidism is the most common thyroid disorder affecting dogs. Most cases are due to primary destruction of thyroid gland tissue due to lymphocytic thyroiditis or primary atrophy, although some animals may present subsequent to thyroidectomy or radiation therapy to the neck. Hypothyroidism is important to surgeons as a cause of delayed wound healing, poor postoperative recovery and wound dehiscence.

Clinical hypothyroidism is rare in cats, even when bilateral thyroidectomy has been performed. It is occasionally seen after radioiodine treatment.

Diagnosis is through confirmation of persistently low total T4 accompanied by high TSH. Dogs with non-thyroid disease or receiving phenobarbital may show decreased T4 that is not associated with clinical hypothyroidism; if there is any suspicion of this the diagnosis should be confirmed with a TRH or TSH stimulation test (Figure 10.3).

Clinical signs of hypothyroidism include: skin and hair coat abnormalities; peripheral neuropathy; bradycardia; obesity; lethargy; dullness; heat-seeking behaviour; infertility; exercise and cold intolerance; normochromic normocytic non-regenerative anaemia; hypercholesterolaemia; delayed recovery from anaesthesia; and delayed wound healing.

Drug therapy
• Phenobarbital
• Corticosteroids
• Propranolol
• Furosemide
• Some non-steroidal anti-inflammatory drugs
• Sulphonamides
Diseases
• Hyperadrenocorticism
• Diabetes mellitus
• Renal disease
• Hypoalbuminaemia

10.3 Circumstances that may give a false result of a low total thyroxine (T4).

Hyperthyroidism

Hyperthyroidism is most commonly associated with thyroid adenoma in the cat; dogs occasionally present with a thyroid carcinoma that is producing active hormone. Clinical signs are secondary to excessive production of T4 and T3, with a slow onset.

Clinical signs

These include: weight loss; polyphagia or anorexia; polydipsia; diarrhoea; vomiting; skin and hair coat abnormalities; cardiac abnormalities (heart murmur, gallop rhythm, tachycardia); hypertension; hyperactivity or lethargy; weakness; and panting. Clinical signs associated with congestive heart failure secondary to hypertrophic cardiomyopathy may be seen in cats, and these animals may decompensate if stressed during examination or blood sampling. Hyperthyroidism also results in an increased glomerular filtration rate (GFR), which may compensate for chronic renal failure in older cats. When these patients are treated for thyrotoxicosis, the GFR drops and renal compromise is unmasked. On initiation of treatment, serial measurements of serum urea and creatinine combined with urine specific gravity and protein:creatinine ratios are therefore recommended. Definitive treatment such as thyroidectomy or radioactive iodine treatment may be contraindicated in patients with concurrent renal disease. Large masses or retropharyngeal metastases may cause: coughing; dysphagia; facial oedema due to lymphatic obstruction; or a neuropathy such as Horner's syndrome or laryngeal paralysis.

Diagnosis

The enlarged thyroid gland is often palpated in the neck. In the cat, it can be felt as a smooth nodule that 'pops' between the fingers as they are slid down the tracheal groove.

Canine thyroid tumours

Thyroid tumours account for up to 3.8% of all tumours in dogs, and whilst up to 50% may be benign adenomas more than 90% of those that present clinically are malignant. Thyroid tumours usually present as a firm painless mass in the neck, often associated with the larynx, but they can be found at any site along the ventral cervical and mandibular region and up to 60% may have bilateral involvement. A small number of thyroid tumours may present as heart-base masses, arising from ectopic thyroid tissue. Only about 6–10% of dogs with thyroid masses show clinical signs of hyperthyroidism. Preoperative staging and screening for other disease is important and up to 40% will have detectable metastases at the time of presentation.

Diagnosis

A minimum database should include: three-view thoracic radiographs (or CT scan); a full haematology and biochemistry blood screen; and ultrasonographic or CT/magnetic resonance imaging examination of the neck mass and regional lymph nodes. Advanced imaging is strongly recommended for preoperative planning in the dog as palpation has been shown to be a poor indicator of invasive behaviour; it also improves the sensitivity for detection of metastatic disease (Taeymans et al., 2013). Ultrasonographic investigation of the liver, spleen and mediastinal lymph nodes may also assist in identifying metastatic disease. The mass should be aspirated, under ultrasound guidance, to confirm the diagnosis, although haemodilution may make aspirates difficult to interpret. Trucut biopsy carries a significant risk due to local coagulopathy and the high vascular component of thyroid tumours. Fine-needle aspirates of regional lymph nodes may be helpful in making a diagnosis and staging.

Treatment

Surgical resection is the treatment of choice for thyroid tumours. However, whilst thyroid tumours that are freely mobile on palpation may be amenable to surgical resection, palpation alone may not be a good indicator of the likelihood of vascular invasion. Tumours that are freely mobile on palpation and also appear well encapsulated on advanced imaging would be considered good candidates for surgical excision, and median survival times of 3 years have been reported. However, most thyroid tumours are highly vascular and fixed to underlying structures, making surgical removal extremely difficult, and considerable haemorrhage is common. Thyroidectomy of invasive tumours is associated with a shorter remission time of 6–12 months (Carver et al., 1995; Klein et al., 1995). Obtaining effective surgical margins may be very challenging and in some cases referral may be appropriate.

Debulking or marginal surgery to remove most of the tumour may be possible by an experienced surgeon and may have some palliative effect, or it can be combined with radiotherapy to improve remission times. Some tumours may be controlled by radiotherapy alone, with palliative radiotherapy achieving a median survival time of 22 months and definitive radiotherapy protocols achieving 72% progression-free survival at 3 years (Brearley et al., 1999; Theon et al., 2000).

Postoperative complications include: hypocalcaemia due to hypoparathyroidism; laryngeal paralysis; Horner's syndrome; and hypothyroidism.

Histopathological features and Ki67 immunohistochemistry of resected tissue may help in determining the prognosis for individual dogs (Campos et al., 2014).

Feline thyroid tumours

Hyperthyroidism is the most common endocrine disease in the cat, affecting both sexes and all breeds, with a mean age at diagnosis of 13 years. Although feline thyroid carcinomas are rare, they are more common in males. They rarely metastasize and the cat nearly always exhibits clinical signs of hyperthyroidism (see above).

Clinical signs

Although there are a wide range of potential clinical signs, the typical picture is of a polyphagic, restless cat over the age of 10 years, with tachycardia and weight loss.

Diagnosis

Physical examination is often rewarding, as these cats may be thin and the enlarged thyroid can be easy to palpate in the jugular groove. Although up to 70% of cats are affected bilaterally, this may not be detected during physical examination because one thyroid gland often slips caudally into the thoracic inlet. Confirmation of diagnosis usually relies on the identification of a raised serum total T4 level (see above). If total T4 is high-normal, testing should be repeated in 1–2 weeks. Free T4 levels should not be used as a screening tool for hyperthyroidism as they can be elevated due to non-thyroidal illness. Pretreatment investigations should include screening for occult renal and cardiac disease; a minimum database should include haematology, biochemistry, urinalysis and blood pressure measurements. Thoracic radiography, renal ultrasonography and echocardiography should be recommended. Thyroid scintigraphy can be useful to identify ectopic thyroid tissue or metastatic disease, although this is not specific to malignant thyroid disease.

Treatment

There are four therapeutic options in the cat (Figure 10.4).

Medical treatment: This is used as a simple long-term or temporary preoperative treatment. It is not curative; lifelong therapy or subsequent treatment by other means is required. Regular biochemical monitoring is necessary to assess total T4 and it is essential that the owner is able to administer the tablets consistently two or three times daily.

There are two available drugs: methimazole and carbimazole. These drugs are not cytotoxic and have no anti-tumour activity. They work by resolving the clinical signs of hyperthyroidism by lowering serum thyroid hormone levels. Side effects are reported for both drugs, although carbimazole (which is converted after administration to methimazole) is better tolerated. Reported side effects include: vomiting; anorexia; depression; eosinophilia; leucopenia; lymphocytosis (5–15%); self-induced excoriation (2%); agranulocytosis; thrombocytopenia (<5%); hepatopathy (<2%); and positive testing for antinuclear

Treatment	Advantages	Disadvantages	Availability
Oral medication	• Simple, inexpensive, low risk • Can be used until other therapy available • Reversible if renal insufficiency becomes evident once thyrotoxicosis resolved	• Daily effective medication is essential • Not curative • Some cats become increasingly difficult to medicate	Prescription-only medication dispensed by veterinary surgeons
Thyroidectomy	• No special equipment required • Curative	• Irreversible • Postoperative complications (hypocalcaemia) may require intensive management and can be life-threatening	Some experience and surgical skill required
Radioiodide therapy	• Curative • Few complications after treatment • Treats bilateral or malignant disease • No risk to parathyroid or normal thyroid tissue • Treats unidentified ectopic thyroid adenomas simultaneously	• Irreversible • Expensive • Requires hospitalization for 2–4 weeks depending on the dose and ionizing radiation protection rules of the centre • Development of any medical disease during isolation cannot be treated	Specialist centres only
Prescription low-iodine diet	• Reversible • Hypothyroidism does not occur	• Owners must be completely compliant and feed the diet exclusively • Not all cats respond: at 4 weeks, 63% of cats had normalized T4. No further improvement after 8 weeks	Widely available

10.4 Treatments available for hyperthyroidism in the cat.

antibody (ANA) (>50%). Most of these are noticed within the first 3 months of therapy and resolve fairly rapidly with dose reduction or drug withdrawal. Some complications should be expected with long-term treatment, although in many cases the cat is elderly and long-term therapy is not expected.

The main limitation is the ability of the owner to dose the cat effectively, particularly in the early stages of treatment when the disease may make the cat more difficult to handle. However, a UK-based owner survey indicated that 79% of owners were willing to medicate their cats twice daily to achieve control of their clinical signs (Caney, 2013).

Medical management is also an extremely important part of preparing a cat for surgical or radioiodine treatment. Temporary resolution of the effects of the hyperthyroidism has a number of advantages.

- Reversal of thyrotoxic hypertrophic cardiomyopathy, resolution of dysrhythmias and desensitization of cardiac muscle to decrease anaesthetic risk. Many cats will recover normal cardiac parameters in the 6 months following resolution of hyperthyroidism. In those cats whose cardiac signs worsen or fail to resolve after treatment, there may be an underlying primary cardiomyopathy or thyroid hormone-induced structural damage.
- Reduction of the GFR allows repeat urinalysis and blood biochemistry to determine whether the cat has occult renal disease. Medical therapy is an important tool as a trial treatment prior to using an irreversible therapy, such as surgery or radioiodine therapy, to monitor the response of the kidneys to a reduction in GFR as the cat becomes euthyroid. The 'development' of biochemical evidence of renal disease should be regarded as an 'unmasking' of the renal disease, and the long-term management of the cat should be reassessed with regard to which of the two diseases is more severe. Medical management may be titrated to keep both diseases under moderate control.
- Cachexic or severely debilitated cats may put on weight and improve condition prior to surgery.

PRACTICAL TIP

Preoperative medical therapy is an important part of assessing the cat's renal status. Some cats will go into overt renal failure if the hyperthyroidism is fully resolved

---

Radioactive iodine treatment: Treatment with ^{131}I is the treatment of choice for functional thyroid tumours and can also be used for those cats with thyroid carcinoma; it is non-invasive and curative in 95% of cases. It will also treat unidentified ectopic adenomas. [131]I emits beta and gamma radiation and is selectively taken up by the most active thyroid tissue (i.e. in the adenoma). Beta particles account for 80% of the radiation and have a very short path length

in tissue (0.4–2 mm); therefore, adjacent thyroid, parathyroid and cervical tissues are not affected during treatment. Normal thyroid tissue is suppressed by the negative feedback, does not take up the ^{131}I and should gradually recover over 3–6 months following treatment of the adenoma. The ^{131}I is administered on licensed premises with a single subcutaneous injection. The cat is then hospitalized until the ^{131}I has decayed and been excreted to acceptable levels, which takes about 10–14 days. The treatment dose of ^{131}I is calculated for each individual cat and clinical hypothyroidism or recurrence of hyperthyroidism are rare complications. Cats that have thyroid carcinomas are treated with a higher dose and may need to be hospitalized for longer before they are considered safe to go home.

Surgical treatment: Adequate preoperative assessment and preparation are important (see Medical treatment, above). Thyroidectomy is a simple, if skilled, surgical procedure, requiring no specialist instruments. Meticulous technique is important, particularly if bilateral surgery is required. There are four reported techniques.

- The **extracapsular** technique involves complete dissection of the enlarged thyroid gland, ligation of the cranial and caudal blood supply, and removal of the parathyroid glands. Hypoparathyroidism is a near certainty with the technique if bilateral thyroidectomy is necessary, even if the procedures are done several weeks apart.
- The **intracapsular** technique dissects all thyroid parenchyma away, leaving the entire capsule and blood supply intact. This technique has a high rate of recurrence of hyperthyroidism due to residual thyroid tissue inside the capsule, but a low rate of hypocalcaemia postoperatively.
- A **modified extracapsular** approach (see Operative Technique 10.1) involves ligation of the caudal blood supply and dissection of the thyroid gland, together with the capsule, up to the level of the external parathyroid gland. At this point, bipolar cautery is used to minimize dissection underneath the external parathyroid gland, and the capsule is released from the parathyroid gland. This technique is difficult in some cats that have a closely attached parathyroid gland.
- With the **modified intracapsular** approach (see Operative Technique 10.2), the thyroid gland is dissected away from inside the capsule and then the thyroid capsule is removed, leaving the capsule intact at the level of the external parathyroid gland.

Prognosis: Postoperative complications after thyroidectomy using different surgical techniques have been compared (Figure 10.5). Bilateral disease has been reported in up to 70% of cats with hyperthyroidism, and bilateral surgery is commonly indicated. Depending on the surgical technique (see Figure 10.5), there may be an increased risk of postoperative hypocalcaemia if bilateral thyroidectomy is carried out, and some surgeons prefer to stage the surgery, with 6 weeks between procedures.

Technique	Mild hypocalcaemia	Severe hypocalcaemia	Long-term hypoparathyroidism	Recurrence of hyperthyroidism (Welches *et al.*, 1989)
Intracapsular	22%	6%	None	Up to 22%
Modified intracapsular	33%	13.3%	None	0
Modified extracapsular	23%	3.8%	None	4% (not statistically significant)

10.5 Postoperative complications associated with different thyroidectomy techniques in the cat.

However, one study (Flanders, 1999) showed that there was no difference in the incidence of hypocalcaemia when the operations were staged by 3–4 weeks, or if bilateral simultaneous thyroidectomy was performed using an intracapsular technique.

PRACTICAL TIPS

- Haemostasis is particularly important in those cats that have received methimazole or carbimazole
- Do not take jugular blood samples in the days preceding thyroid surgery
- Sometimes the cranial thyroid artery travels through the parenchyma of the thyroid gland prior to supplying the parathyroid gland. In this situation, the parathyroid gland is unlikely to be salvaged and there is an increased risk of postoperative hypocalcaemia. Staged thyroidectomy or autotransplantation of parathyroid tissue should be considered
- Examine both thyroid glands closely before deciding which gland to start with. Remove the thyroid on which the parathyroid is most likely to be saved first, and then remove the second thyroid gland if that procedure went well

---

If inadvertent complete parathyroidectomy occurs, resolution of postoperative hypocalcaemia may be quicker if the parathyroid gland is immediately reimplanted into well vascularized tissue such as muscle.

Postoperative complications:

- **Hypoparathyroidism:** Bilateral thyroidectomy can result in iatrogenic damage to the parathyroid glands, resulting in hypoparathyroidism. Anecdotal reports of hypoparathyroidism in cases of unilateral thyroidectomy may be due to over-vigorous retraction of tissues, damaging the contralateral parathyroid gland or its blood supply. Loss of PTH secretion causes increased urinary loss of calcium, reduced mobilization of calcium from bone and decreased intestinal absorption of calcium. Postoperative anorexia may exacerbate this. Secondary effects result from increased phosphate and decreased renal synthesis of calcitriol.

  Clinical signs are related to hypocalcaemia. Low levels of ionized calcium result in increased excitability of neuromuscular tissue and in muscle fasciculations, twitching, irritability and disorientation, leading up to seizures. Facial trembling and pruritus are particularly common signs in cats. Diagnosis is confirmed by measurement of serum calcium (measurement of ionized calcium will detect subtle changes earlier) and serum phosphate.

  It is important to instigate specific treatment as soon as possible to prevent the onset of seizures or, in severe cases, respiratory arrest and death. The aim is to increase calcium levels to physiological levels without causing hypercalcaemia (vitamin D toxicosis), keeping calcium levels at the low end of normal to stimulate compensatory ectopic parathyroid hypertrophy. In cats whose calcium levels are steadily or rapidly declining, or those where there is severe hypocalcaemia but no clinical signs, treatment should be started immediately.

  Frequent measurements (e.g. 2–4 times daily) of serum ionized calcium levels are necessary to keep serum calcium levels on the low end of the reference range to allow recovery of normal homeostatic mechanisms.

Cats with tetany or seizures should be treated to effect with a slow intravenous bolus of calcium. Twitching or panting may take up to an hour to resolve, and the effects of the bolus may last only 1–2 hours. Ongoing management should be instigated as soon as the initial crisis is under control. Multiple intermittent calcium injections are less beneficial than constant rate infusion as the former cause large serum calcium fluctuations and will significantly delay recovery. Oral calcium and vitamin D supplementation should be started and a continuous calcium infusion used until the oral supplementation is able to maintain calcium levels adequately. Oral supplementation of calcium is absorbed through passive mechanisms and is not dependent on the activity of the vitamin D supplementation; it is therefore particularly important in an anorexic cat. As the activity of the vitamin D supplementation takes effect, the calcium supplementation may be tapered or stopped (Figure 10.6).

- **Cardiac or renal disease:** Thyrotoxic cardiac changes will resolve postoperatively; persistent clinical signs usually indicate primary cardiac disease. In cats where hyperthyroidism has masked the presence of renal disease, the urea and creatinine levels will rise postoperatively as the GFR falls. This complication is irreversible, and conventional management of renal failure is instigated (see the *BSAVA Manual of Canine and Feline Nephrology and Urology*).
- **Laryngeal paralysis:** Retraction of the tissues during surgery can cause trauma to the recurrent laryngeal nerve, resulting in laryngeal paralysis. Unilateral paresis may not cause clinical signs, but acute bilateral paresis can cause significant laryngeal obstruction

Drug	Dose rate	Comments
Calcium borogluconate 10% Available elemental calcium 9.3 mg/ml	Slow i.v. 0.5–1.5 ml/kg to effect if seizuring, over 20–30 minutes. 5–15 mg/kg/h elemental calcium i.v.	Monitor heart rate during initial treatment and monitor serum ionized calcium levels regularly
Calcium chloride 10% Available elemental calcium 27.2 mg/ml	Slow i.v. 5–15 mg/kg/h	Vascular irritant – use with caution
Calcium carbonate	Oral treatment 5–22 mg/kg q8h	Other oral calcium supplements may also be used at the same dose
Vitamin D analogues		
Dihydrotachysterol	0.02–0.03 mg/kg q24h initially, reduce to 0.01–0.02 mg/kg every 1–2 days	Onset 1–7 days Discontinuation time of 1–3 weeks for serum calcium levels to normalize Overdosing may result in hypercalcaemia
1,25-Dihydroxy-cholecalciferol	10–15 ng/kg orally q12h for 3–4 days then reduce to 2.5–7.5 ng q12h for 2–3 days, then give q24h. Higher doses have also been reported	Quicker onset, 1–2 days; short half-life, reduces risk of overdose and iatrogenic hypercalcaemia

10.6 Treatments for hypocalcaemia following parathyroid gland damage or removal. Obtain owner consent to use drugs not licensed for veterinary use.

(Data from the *BSAVA Small Animal Formulary, 9th edn, Part A: Canine and Feline*)

necessitating an emergency tracheostomy. Tracheostomy in the cat requires intensive management and has a high complication rate (see Chapters 2 and 8). Laryngeal function usually recovers over a period of 5–7 days postoperatively.

- **Recurrence of hyperthyroidism:** Intracapsular techniques have a higher incidence of recurrence of hyperthyroidism, subsequent to regeneration of the thyroid adenoma from fragments left behind on the capsule. Clinical signs tend to be similar to the initial presentation, and diagnosis is confirmed in the same manner. Some cats may develop adenomas in ectopic thyroid tissue. Scintigraphy may be required to detect the site of the ectopic thyroid tissue. Radioactive iodine therapy is the preferred treatment for intrathoracic ectopic thyroid tissue.

Parathyroid disorders

Diagnostics

Diagnosis of primary parathyroid disease relies largely on the measurement of serum PTH levels, although a thorough examination of the animal is necessary to rule out other causes of hypercalcaemia (Figure 10.7). Currently there is no feline-specific PTH assay, which creates additional challenges to confirming the diagnosis in cats. Rarely, parathyroid tumours may be part of a syndrome involving multiple endocrine neoplasms such as thyroid carcinoma, phaeochromocytoma and thymoma. Although scintigraphy has been described for the identification of enlarged parathyroid glands, it is not very sensitive or specific, and is not recommended as a means of identifying parathyroid disease in animals with hypercalcaemia. High-resolution ultrasonography is much more useful; guidelines for dogs indicate that parathyroid glands >4 mm across should rouse suspicion of neoplastic disease, whereas enlarged glands <4 mm are more likely to be hyperplastic (due to other diseases). Parathyroid glands are symmetrically enlarged in animals with chronic, although not acute, renal failure.

Hyperparathyroidism

Parathyroid tumours are uncommon in dogs and rare in cats. Dogs usually present at older than 6 years, and a breed predisposition in the Keeshond with autosomal dominant inheritance has been reported (Goldstein *et al.*, 2007). The most important clinical sign is consistent hypercalcaemia, causing polydipsia and polyuria. Hypercalcaemia due to primary hyperparathyroidism is less common than that from other causes, and a full investigation to rule out other causes should always be completed (Figure 10.7).

Parathyroid adenomas are far more common than carcinomas and are usually functional. Rarely, carcinoma may be diagnosed on the basis of histopathological criteria, but these tumours usually behave in a benign manner and are non-metastatic. Adenomas usually affect a single parathyroid gland (Figure 10.8), but in predisposed breeds bilateral adenomas may be present or an adenoma may develop *de novo* in the contralateral gland at a later date.

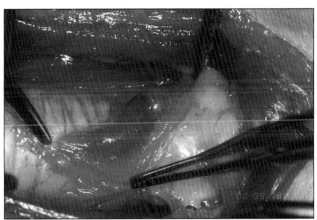

10.8 Right parathyroid adenoma in the dog shown in Figure 10.2. The adenoma is visible as a pale nodule on the cranial pole of the thyroid gland.
(© Davina Anderson)

Clinical signs

Elevation of the serum ionized calcium occurs gradually and often clinical signs are subtle. Clinical signs may include: lethargy; inappetence; weakness; polydipsia; polyuria; hypercalcaemia (with associated renal damage); pathological fractures; vomiting; constipation; and urolithiasis (calcium phosphate or oxalate). Dogs with hypercalcaemia due to primary hyperparathyroidism will have a decreased phosphorus level, resulting in a normal calcium x phosphorus product. This means that the risk of renal mineralization and renal failure is low. In one study, 95% of dogs with primary hyperparathyroidism had blood urea nitrogen and serum creatinine within or below the normal range (Feldman *et al.*, 2005).

Diagnosis	Recommended investigations
Hypercalcaemia of malignancy (lymphosarcoma, apocrine gland carcinomas of the anal sac, multiple myeloma, other carcinomas)	Complete physical examination for evidence of neoplasia, including diagnostic imaging of the chest and abdomen. Aspirate lymph nodes and masses
Granulomatous or severe inflammatory disease (including pancreatitis and inflammatory bowel disease)	Other blood analysis findings and clinical history may be suggestive
Primary hyperparathyroidism	Confirm with parathyroid hormone (PTH) assay
Secondary nutritional hyperparathyroidism	Clinical history, age
Secondary renal hyperparathyroidism	Blood and urine analysis confirm renal failure. Radiography confirms decalcification of bones
Destructive disease of bone (e.g. systemic mycosis)	Radiography
Vitamin D intoxication	Clinical history (e.g. on therapy for hypoparathyroidism, consumption of rat bait)
Hypoadrenocorticism	Blood analysis, age, history, bradycardia associated with hyperkalaemia
Hypoalbuminaemia	Blood analysis, clinical history

10.7 Differential diagnosis for serum hypercalcaemia.

Diagnosis

A full blood analysis and urinalysis, as well as radiography of the abdomen and thorax and ultrasonographic examination of the abdomen and neck, should be performed. Ultrasound examination is useful to identify the location of the tumour and to rule out the 10% of cases that have masses in more than one gland. Occasionally, advanced imaging is indicated when the parathyroid glands appear to be normal and an ectopic parathyroid tumour is suspected. It is essential to rule out other causes of hypercalcaemia, such as granulomatous disease, vitamin D toxicosis, anal sac carcinoma and lymphosarcoma, and to investigate for other concurrent diseases. Hypercalcaemia should be confirmed by measuring serum ionized calcium, and diagnosis of primary hyperparathyroidism is confirmed by documentation of an inappropriately normal or high serum PTH in the face of a concurrent hypercalcaemia.

PRACTICAL TIPS

- Lymphoma may be very difficult to rule out in some dogs. Where diagnosis is equivocal, referral to a specialist centre would be advisable
- Be sure to distinguish between hypercalcaemic renal failure and primary hyperparathyroidism

Treatment

Progression of clinical signs associated with primary hyperparathyroidism is slow and the hypercalcaemia in these patients is no longer thought to be associated with renal failure. However, the treatment of choice remains surgical removal of the adenoma (Figure 10.9). Preoperative diuresis with intravenous 0.9% saline may help reduce serum ionized calcium levels to decrease the risk of cardiac dysrhythmias and reduce negative feedback on the normal parathyroid gland. However, preoperative ionized calcium levels and serum PTH levels have not been shown to be predictive of postoperative hypocalcaemia (Arbaugh *et al.*, 2012). After successful parathyroidectomy, ionized calcium should drop to within the normal range within 24 hours. If the normal parathyroid tissue does not resume homeostatic function, clinical signs of hypocalcaemia may develop 24–48 hours after surgery. This effect can be attenuated if the animal is prepared preoperatively by administering vitamin D analogues; given that it usually takes a few days for the vitamin D to affect serum calcium levels, this should be started the day before surgery. The

prognosis should be excellent for complete resolution of the disease after surgery.

The parathyroidectomy procedure is described in Operative Technique 10.3.

Postoperative complications

Hypocalcaemia: Over 50% of dogs will develop some degree of hypocalcaemia postoperatively, and there is no way to accurately predict those dogs at increased risk. Intravenous soluble calcium is given to treat acute hypocalcaemia and oral vitamin D analogues and oral calcium supplementation are given until the animal is able to maintain normal calcium homeostasis; 1,25-dihydroxyvitamin D (calcitriol) has the most rapid onset of action and a short half-life (see Figure 10.6). This helps with dose adjustments and prevention of vitamin D toxicosis and hypercalcaemia. Ionized calcium should be measured daily and the dose adjusted to maintain the calcium just below the normal range, allowing stimulation of the normal parathyroid tissue to regain control of homeostasis. In some cases, hypocalcaemia is very resistant to treatment, and medication and blood tests may be required for some weeks.

Laryngeal paralysis: Rough retraction of tissues during examination and surgery of the parathyroid glands or excessive use of monopolar diathermy may cause bruising or damage to the recurrent laryngeal nerve. In cases where the damage is not reversible over 2–4 weeks postoperatively, arytenoid lateralization may be necessary (see Chapter 7).

Recurrence of hyperparathyroidism: The blood calcium level should immediately respond to surgery, becoming normal or low. Where there is no response, there may be multiple parathyroid tumours, the wrong parathyroid gland may have been removed or the diagnosis was incorrect. In a small number of cases, the surgeon may find no abnormal parathyroid tissue at surgery, and the disease is due to an ectopic parathyroid tumour. In this situation, referral for advanced imaging and further investigations would be appropriate. Predisposed breeds may present months to years later with a second tumour.

Hypoparathyroidism

Hypoparathyroidism is most commonly associated with parathyroidectomy or devascularization of the parathyroid glands during thyroidectomy. It rarely occurs as a primary disorder; see above under postoperative complications of thyroidectomy.

References and further reading

Arbaugh M, Smeak D and Monnet E (2012) Evaluation of preoperative serum concentrations of ionized calcium and parathyroid hormone as predictors of hypocalcaemia following parathyroidectomy in dogs with primary hyperparathyroidism: 17 cases (2001–2009). *Journal of the American Veterinary Medical Association* **241**, 233–236

Brearley MJ, Hayes AM and Murphy S (1999) Hypofractionated radiation therapy for invasive thyroid carcinoma in dogs: a retrospective analysis of survival. *Journal of Small Animal Practice* **40**, 206–210

Campos M, Ducatelle R, Rutteman *et al.* (2014) Clinical, pathologic and immunohistochemical prognostic factors in dogs with thyroid carcinoma. *Journal of Veterinary Internal Medicine* **28**, 1805–1813

Caney SMA (2013) An online survey to determine owner experiences and opinions of the management of their hyperthyroid cats using anti-thyroid medication. *Journal of Feline Medicine and Surgery* **15**, 494–502

Carver JR, Kapatkin A and Patnaik AK (1995) A comparison of medullary thyroid carcinoma and thyroid adenocarcinoma in dogs: a retrospective study of 38 cases. *Veterinary Surgery* **24**, 315–319

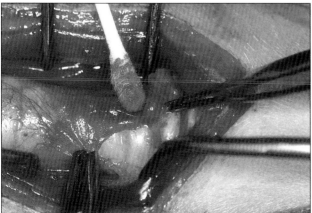

10.9 Removal of the adenoma shown in Figure 10.8.
(© Davina Anderson)

Dobson J and Lascelles D (ed.) (2011) *BSAVA Manual of Canine and Feline Oncology, 3rd edn*. BSAVA Publications, Gloucester

Elliott J, Grauer G and Westropp J (2017) *BSAVA Manual of Canine and Feline Nephrology and Urology, 3rd edn*. BSAVA Publications, Gloucester

Feldman EC, Hoar B, Pollard R *et al.* (2005) Pretreatment clinical and laboratory findings in dogs with primary hyperparathyroidism: 210 cases (1987–2004). *Journal of the American Veterinary Medical Association* **227**, 756–761

Feldman EC and Nelson RW (2014) Hypercalcaemia and primary hyperparathyroidism in dogs. In: *Kirk's Current Veterinary Therapy XV: Small Animal Practice*, ed. JD Bonagura and DC Twedt, Web Chapter 11, pp. e69–e73. WB Saunders, St Louis

Flanders JA (1999) Surgical options for treatment of hyperthyroidism in the cat. *Journal of Feline Medicine and Surgery* **1**, 127–134

Flanders JA and Harvey HJ (1987) Feline thyroidectomy. A comparison of postoperative hypocalcaemia associated with three different surgical techniques. *Veterinary Surgery* **16**, 362–366

Fritsch DA, Allen TA, Dodd CE *et al.* (2014) A restricted iodine food reduces circulating thyroxine concentrations in cats with hyperthyroidism. *International Journal of Applied Research in Veterinary Medicine* **12**, 24–32

Galvao JF, Chew DJ, Nagode LA and Schenck PA (2014) Treatment of hypoparathyroidism. In: *Kirk's Current Veterinary Therapy XV: Small Animal Practice*, ed. JD Bonagura and DC Twedt, Web Chapter 22, pp. e22–e129. WB Saunders, Missouri

Goldstein RE, Atwater DZ, Cazolli DM *et al.* (2007) Inheritance, mode of inheritance and candidate genes for primary hyperparathyroidism in Keeshonden. *Journal of Veterinary Internal Medicine* **21**, 199–203

Kemppainen RJ and Behrend EN (2000) CVT update: interpretation of endocrine diagnostic test results for adrenal and thyroid disease. In: *Kirk's Current Veterinary Therapy XIII: Small Animal Practice*, ed. JD Bonagura, pp. 322–324. WB Saunders, St Louis

Klein MK, Powers BE, Withrow SJ *et al.* (1995) Treatment of thyroid carcinoma in dogs by surgical resection alone: 20 cases. *Journal of the American Veterinary Medical Association* **206**, 1007–1009

Lunn KF and Page RL (2013) Tumors of the endocrine system. In: *Small Animal Clinical Oncology*, ed. SJ Withrow, DM Vail and RL Page, pp. 513–531. WB Saunders, St Louis

Milovancev M and Schmiedt CW (2013) Preoperative factors associated with postoperative hypocalcaemia in dogs with primary hyperparathyroidism that underwent parathyroidectomy: 62 cases (2004–2009). *Journal of the American Veterinary Medical Association* **242**, 507–515

Mooney CT and Peterson M (2012) *BSAVA Manual of Canine and Feline Endocrinology, 4th edn*. BSAVA Publications, Gloucester

Parker VJ, Gilor C and Chew DJ (2015) Feline hyperparathyroidism: pathophysiology, diagnosis and treatment of primary and secondary disease. *Journal of Feline Medicine and Surgery* **17**, 427–439

Peterson ME (2012) Hyperthyroidism in cats: what's causing this epidemic of thyroid disease and can we prevent it? *Journal of Feline Medicine and Surgery* **14**, 804–818

Peterson ME and Broome MR (2014) Radioiodine for feline hyperthyroidism. In: *Kirk's Current Veterinary Therapy XV*, ed. JD Bonagura and DC Twedt, Web Chapter 21, pp. e112–e121. WB Saunders, St Louis

Peterson ME, Melian C and Nichols R (2001) Measurement of serum concentrations of free thyroxine, total thyroxine and total triiodothyronine in cats with hyperthyroidism and cats with nonthyroidal disease. *Journal of the American Veterinary Medical Association* **218**, 529–536

Ramsey IK (2017) *BSAVA Small Animal Formulary, 9th edn – Part A: Canine and Feline*. BSAVA Publications, Gloucester

Seguin B and Brownlee L (2012) Thyroid and parathyroid glands. In: *Veterinary Surgery: Small Animal*, ed. KM Tobias and SA Johnston, pp. 2043–2058. WB Saunders, St Louis

Slater MR, Geller S and Rogers K (2001) Long-term health and predictors of survival for hyperthyroid cats treated with iodine 131. *Journal of Veterinary Internal Medicine* **15**, 47–51

Syme HM (2014) Feline hyperthyroidism and renal function. In: *Kirk's Current Veterinary Therapy XV*, ed. JD Bonagura and DC Twedt, pp. 185–189. WB Saunders, St Louis

Taeymans O, Penninck DG and Peters RM (2013) Comparison between clinical, ultrasound, CT, MRI and pathology findings in dogs presented for suspected thyroid carcinoma. *Veterinary Radiology and Ultrasound* **54**, 61–70

Theon AP, Marks SL, Feldman ES and Griffey S (2000) Prognostic factors and patterns of treatment failure in dogs with unresectable differentiated thyroid carcinomas treated with megavoltage irradiation. *Journal of the American Veterinary Medical Association* **216**, 1775–1779

Trepanier LA (2014) Medical treatment of feline hyperthyroidism. In: *Kirk's Current Veterinary Therapy XV*, ed. JD Bonagura and DC Twedt, Web Chapter 19, pp. e102–e106. WB Saunders, St Louis

van der Kooij M, Becvarova I, Meyer HP *et al.* (2013) Effects of an iodine-restricted food on client-owned cats with hyperthyroidism. *Journal of Feline Medicine and Surgery* **16**, 491–498

Welches CD, Scavelli TD, Matthiesen DT and Peterson ME (1989) Occurrence of problems after three techniques of bilateral thyroidectomy in cats. *Veterinary Surgery* **18**, 392–396

Wisner ER, Penninck D, Biller DS *et al.* (1997) High resolution parathyroid sonography. *Veterinary Radiology and Ultrasound* **38**, 462–466

Wright KN, Breitschwerdt EB, Feldman JM *et al.* (1995) Diagnostic and therapeutic considerations in a hypercalcaemic dog with multiple endocrine neoplasia. *Journal of the American Animal Hospital Association* **31**, 156–162

Wucherer KL and Wilke V (2010) Thyroid cancer in dogs: an update based on 638 cases (1995–2005). *Journal of the American Animal Hospital Association* **46**, 249–254

OPERATIVE TECHNIQUE 10.1

Feline thyroidectomy (modified extracapsular)

PATIENT POSITIONING

Dorsal recumbency, with equal retraction of the forelimbs caudally to ensure that the neck is symmetrical.

PRACTICAL TIP

It is helpful to place the neck over a small sandbag or bandage roll to hyperextend the cervical vertebrae. This exposes more of the thoracic inlet and brings the trachea (and thyroid glands) to a more superficial position

ASSISTANT

Not necessary if good self-retaining retractors are available.

ADDITIONAL INSTRUMENTS

Very fine forceps; fine scissors (e.g. Stevens tenotomy scissors); small self-retaining retractors (Gelpi, sternomastoid); sterile cotton tips can be helpful for fine dissection; bipolar diathermy. *It is essential to have in-house serum calcium measurement, ideally ionized calcium.*

→

→ **OPERATIVE TECHNIQUE 10.1 CONTINUED**

Approach

Palpate the neck to confirm clinical findings of enlarged thyroid glands in the conscious patient. Make a midline skin incision at about the level of the palpated glands extending from the caudal edge of the larynx down to the manubrium.

Surgical manipulations

1 Continue the dissection in the midline, separating the sternohyoid and sternothyroid muscles. Place retractors to hold the muscles apart.

2 Expose the ventral trachea and identify the thyroid glands on the lateral and ventral aspects of the trachea. Identify and avoid the caudal laryngeal nerves. Inspect both glands carefully to identify disease as well as to identify the parathyroid glands and the pattern of vascularization in the individual patient. *Note: If the contralateral gland is normal, it should be atrophied; if the contralateral gland is a 'normal' size, then the cat probably has bilateral disease.*

3 Ligate the caudal blood supply and gently lift the thyroid gland (by the caudal pole) out of the tracheal fascia. Continue meticulous dissection cranially up to the level of the parathyroid gland.

4 The parathyroid gland is to be preserved. Make an incision into the capsule around the extrathyroid parathyroid gland. Some texts describe using bipolar cautery to cut the capsule around the parathyroid gland. Lift the parathyroid gland off the underlying thyroid gland, retaining the cranial blood supply and its attachment to the capsule.

Closure

The site is observed closely for haemostasis prior to closure. The sternohyoid and sternothyroid muscles are reapposed using a simple continuous suture. Most hyperthyroid cats are too thin to require subcutaneous tissue closure and the skin is closed with a continuous subcuticular suture, or simple interrupted skin sutures.

Modified extracapsular thyroidectomy in a cat.

Cats should be hospitalized to watch closely for clinical signs of hypocalcaemia, including weakness and muscle tremors, often first recognized as twitching of the ears and face.

OPERATIVE TECHNIQUE 10.2

Feline thyroidectomy (modified intracapsular)

Dorsal recumbency, with equal retraction of the forelimbs caudally to ensure that the neck is symmetrical.

It is helpful to place the neck over a small sandbag or bandage roll to hyperextend the cervical vertebrae. This exposes more of the thoracic inlet and brings the trachea (and thyroid glands) to a more superficial position

→ **OPERATIVE TECHNIQUE 10.2 CONTINUED**

ASSISTANT

Not necessary if good self-retaining retractors are available.

ADDITIONAL INSTRUMENTS

Very fine forceps; fine scissors (e.g. Stevens tenotomy scissors); small self-retaining retractors (Gelpi, sternomastoid); sterile cotton-tipped applicators can be helpful for fine dissection; bipolar diathermy. *It is essential to have in-house serum calcium measurement.*

SURGICAL TECHNIQUE

Approach

Palpate the neck to confirm clinical findings of enlarged thyroid glands in the conscious patient. Make a midline skin incision at about the level of the palpated glands, extending from the caudal edge of the larynx down to the manubrium.

Surgical manipulations

1 Continue the dissection in the midline, separating the sternohyoid and sternothyroid muscles. Place retractors to hold the muscles apart.

2 Expose the ventral trachea and identify the thyroid glands on the lateral and ventral aspects of the trachea. Identify and avoid the caudal laryngeal nerves. Inspect both glands carefully to identify disease as well as to identify the parathyroid glands and the pattern of vascularization in the individual patient. *Note: If the contralateral gland is normal, it should be atrophied; if the contralateral gland is a 'normal' size, then the cat probably has bilateral disease.*

3 Make a small, very superficial incision in the caudoventral gland and carefully peel away the thyroid gland from the capsule.

4 Ligate the caudal vessels with very fine suture material or cauterize them.

5 Continue the dissection, meticulously removing all traces of thyroid tissue within the capsule.

6 Separate the capsule and remove it, but leave the part of the capsule underneath the cranial (extrathyroid) parathyroid gland intact. It is also important to preserve the blood vessels entering the cranial aspect of the thyroid gland capsule because this will maintain blood supply to the external parathyroid gland.

Closure

The site is observed closely for haemostasis prior to closure. The sternohyoid and sternothyroid muscles are reapposed using a simple continuous suture. Most hyperthyroid cats are too thin to require subcutaneous tissue closure and the skin is closed with a continuous subcuticular suture, or simple interrupted skin sutures.

POSTOPERATIVE CARE

Fluid therapy should be continued until the cat is eating and drinking normally. Signs of hypocalcaemia are usually seen between 24 and 72 hours postoperatively and owners should expect a period of postoperative hospitalization, even when there are no complications.

OPERATIVE TECHNIQUE 10.3

Canine parathyroidectomy

PATIENT POSITIONING

Dorsal recumbency with a small sandbag or bandage roll under the neck to hyperextend the cervical vertebrae.

ASSISTANT

Not necessary if good self-retaining retractors are available.

ADDITIONAL INSTRUMENTS

Fine self-retaining retractors; fine scissors (e.g. Stevens tenotomy scissors); sterile cotton-tipped applicators are useful. *In-house serum calcium measurement is essential; ionized calcium is preferred.*

L THYROID

Ultrasound image of a parathyroid mass on the left thyroid.
(© Davina Anderson)

SURGICAL TECHNIQUE

Approach

A standard midline cervical approach is used.

Surgical manipulations

1   Make an incision extending from just caudal to the larynx to about two-thirds of the distance to the manubrium. Split the sternohyoid and sternothyroid muscles and expose the trachea. Cautiously expose the thyroid glands on each side of the trachea, taking care not to damage the recurrent laryngeal nerves, and the carotid/jugular bundle.

2   Examine the cranial poles of both thyroid glands closely and palpate them, if necessary. The parathyroid gland should be of smooth texture, with a lighter colour, on the cranial aspect of the gland. Adenomas tend to be variable in colour but have a definite nodular appearance and texture. Sometimes it is necessary to palpate both parathyroid glands simultaneously to determine which has a more nodular texture. Preoperative high-definition ultrasonography is useful to avoid doubt as to which gland is abnormal.

3   Examine the caudal pole of the thyroid gland carefully for involvement of the internal parathyroid gland.

4   Assess the blood supply to the thyroid gland carefully prior to removal of the nodule.

5   The affected gland/nodule can be sharply dissected off the cranial pole of the thyroid, disturbing adjacent structures as little as possible. If the internal parathyroid gland is involved, a small portion of thyroid tissue may be removed to ensure adequate margins are obtained.

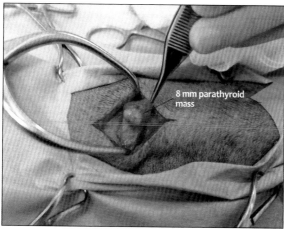

Intraoperative view of identified parathyroid mass in the left thyroid.
(© Davina Anderson)

8 mm parathyroid mass

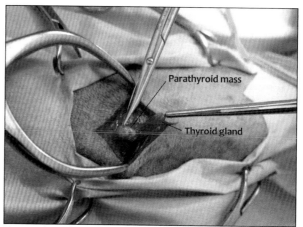

The parathyroid mass has been dissected free of the thyroid. Note the Stevens tenotomy scissors, which are very useful for this procedure.
(© Davina Anderson)

Parathyroid mass

Thyroid gland

→

➔ **OPERATIVE TECHNIQUE 10.3 CONTINUED**

Closure

Muscle layers are closed with a simple continuous suture and fat in a separate layer if necessary. Skin can be closed with skin sutures or a continuous subcuticular layer.

POSTOPERATIVE CARE

Monitor serum ionized calcium closely for several days. If the calcium level does not drop within 12–24 hours postoperatively, consider multiple adenomas, removal of the wrong parathyroid gland or an incorrect diagnosis. Maintain oral medication with vitamin D analogues and calcium (see Figure 10.6). If the dog is eating normally, oral calcium supplements are often not necessary, and vitamin D supplements are gradually tapered over the 4–8 weeks following surgery. Serum calcium and phosphate should be measured weekly as medications are reduced.

Chapter 11

Thoracic wall anatomy and surgical approaches

Zoë J. Halfacree and Julius M. Liptak

Introduction

Surgery is required to manage pathology of the thoracic wall, including neoplasia and trauma, and to access the thoracic cavity. Knowledge of anatomy is important to guide selection of an appropriate surgical approach and to ensure that vital structures are not inadvertently damaged. Thorough patient assessment, stabilization and careful attention to anaesthesia and analgesia regimens are essential.

Thoracic wall anatomy

Skeleton and anatomical boundaries

The thoracic wall is composed of 13 paired ribs (Figure 11.1). The most cranial nine ribs join the sternum ventrally, via the costal cartilages, while the last four ribs create the costal arch. The sternum is composed of eight sternebrae joined by fibrocartilage articulations; the most cranial sternebra is the manubrium and the most caudal sternebra is the xiphoid. The costal cartilages articulate with the intersternebral cartilages, apart from the first rib, which articulates directly with the manubrium. The sternum is laterally flattened, creating a narrow midline to follow when performing a median sternotomy.

The first ribs delineate the cranial extent of the thoracic cavity: the thoracic inlet. There is no dividing structure at this anatomical boundary and the cervical tissue planes are continuous with the cranial mediastinum; disease processes within the neck may readily extend into the thoracic cavity via this route. The caudal boundary of the thoracic cavity is delineated by the diaphragm.

Muscles

Muscular attachments to the thoracic skeleton create respiratory movement and contribute to thoracic limb locomotion, in addition to creating a robust thoracic wall and origins for the muscular abdominal wall. The manubrium serves as an attachment for the sternocephalic muscles, whilst the xiphoid provides diaphragmatic insertion and the origin of the linea alba, which merges with the tendinous sheath of the rectus abdominis muscles. The ribs are connected by the internal and external intercostal muscles. Internally, the transversus thoracis muscle runs ventrally between the sternum and the

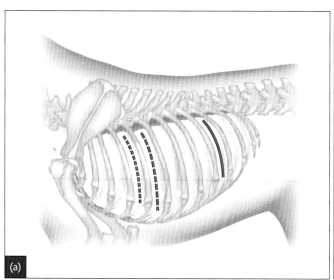

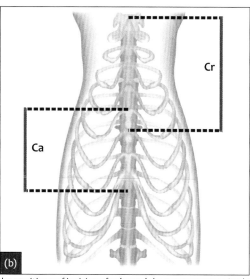

11.1 Skeletal anatomy of the thorax. (a) The left thorax, demonstrating the positions of incisions for lateral thoracotomy required to perform, for example, patent ductus arteriosus ligation (fourth), lung lobectomy or pericardectomy (fifth) or thoracic duct ligation (ninth; left in the cat, right in the dog). (b) Anatomy of the sternum, showing the extent of sternotomy incisions for procedures such as resection of a cranial (Cr) or caudal (Ca) mediastinal mass.
(Redrawn after Evans, 1993)

costal cartilages, marking the path of the internal thoracic artery along its dorsal border. Externally, several muscles create a robust thoracic wall (Figure 11.2). The scalenus is a multipartite muscle originating from the caudal cervical vertebrae and inserting on the lateral aspect of the more cranial ribs. The most caudal portion inserts over the fifth rib, providing a useful anatomical landmark. The serratus ventralis muscle is a fan-like muscle that originates from the thoracic vertebrae and inserts on the lateral aspects of the ribs; separate serrations of the muscle can be preserved by dissecting between them when performing an intercostal thoracotomy. These muscles are overlain by the robust latissimus dorsi, a triangular muscle originating from the dorsal thoracolumbar fascia and inserting on the aponeurosis of the triceps muscle. The dominant blood supply of this muscle arises from the thoracodorsal artery and the muscle can be transposed to achieve thoracic wall reconstruction. The external abdominal oblique is a large sheet-like muscle that covers the ventral half of the lateral thoracic wall (costal portion) before extending caudally to provide the lateral portion of the composite abdominal wall (lumbar portion); the costal part of the external abdominal oblique originates from the fourth or fifth to the 13th ribs. The ventral aspect of the sternum serves as the insertion for the pectoral muscles; the superficial pectoral muscles insert only on the cranial portion of the sternum, whilst the deep pectoral muscle spans more widely along the length of the sternum.

Neurovascular structures of the thoracic wall

Each intercostal space contains a neurovascular bundle running caudal to each rib. The intercostal nerves are ventral branches of the thoracic spinal nerves. The intercostal nerves maintain a caudal position behind each rib and continue to reach the lateral aspect of the sternum, sending a ventral cutaneous branch to ramify in the skin; the dorsal cutaneous branch of each nerve passes caudally to overlie the more caudal adjacent rib proximally. It is recommended that, prior to intercostal thoracotomy, nerve blocks should be performed caudal and cranial to the rib of the appropriate intercostal space and for both ribs either side. The first three or four intercostal arteries are branches of the thoracic vertebral artery and the last eight or nine are direct branches from the aorta.

The internal thoracic artery runs in a subpleural position on the inside of the ventral chest wall. It may be inadvertently lacerated during intercostal thoracotomy, at the ventral extent of the incision, or at the cranial extent of a median sternotomy where the vessels converge towards the midline as they arise bilaterally as branches from the subclavian arteries. The left and right subclavian veins and external jugular veins are the major veins converging at the thoracic inlet, draining via the brachiocephalic veins into the cranial vena cava. These large veins are separated from the cranial sternum only by thin mediastinal tissue and care must be taken to avoid laceration during median sternotomy.

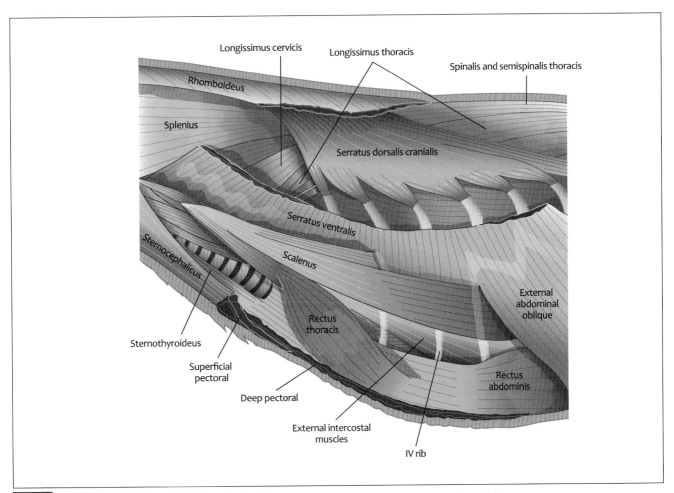

11.2 Diagram showing the external muscular anatomy of the thoracic wall relevant to performing a lateral thoracotomy.

Skin

The skin overlying the thorax is relatively loose laterally, therefore facilitating closure of skin wounds. A robust axial pattern flap based upon the thoracodorsal artery lies caudal to the scapula and can be used for reconstruction of proximal thoracic limb or axillary wounds and large thoracic wall skin defects. The axillary flank fold flap can be used to reconstruct sternal or ventral thoracic skin defects. The skin overlying the pectoral muscles is tightly tethered, meaning that minimal skin recruitment is achieved following undermining at this site.

Anaesthetic management, analgesia and postoperative care

Anaesthesia

A high level of anaesthetic knowledge, skills and monitoring are required to meet the anaesthetic, oxygen and analgesic requirements of thoracic surgery patients. Prior to anaesthesia, general health status should be assessed. A minimum database should include a complete blood count, biochemistry, urinalysis and thoracic radiographs. Ideally, an electrocardiogram (ECG), blood pressure measurement and pulse oximetry should also be performed.

Thoracic surgery patients are frequently hypoxaemic prior to surgery and each patient needs to be assessed to determine whether premedication is appropriate. Advantages of premedication include a calmer patient, less need for general anaesthetic during induction, potentially less initial hypotension, easier administration of pre-anaesthetic oxygen, less struggling during intravenous catheter placement and increased ability to place monitoring equipment prior to induction. Disadvantages of premedication include respiratory depression, worsened hypoxaemia and potentially decreased cardiac output or hypotension. Preoxygenation is required for 5 minutes prior to anaesthesia induction.

Basic anaesthesia monitoring, which should be performed in all thoracic surgery patients, includes an ECG, indirect (Doppler or oscillometric) blood pressure measurement, capnography, pulse oximetry and audible pulse monitoring (Doppler or oesophageal stethoscope). Direct blood pressure and in-house blood gas analysis should also be available for most thoracic surgeries. It is safest to have a specific person dedicated to monitoring the animal, as the patient's status can change quickly and dramatically. In addition, an anaesthetic record should be kept and, at an absolute minimum, the pulse rate, respiratory rate, blood pressure and temperature should be recorded every 5 minutes.

Supportive care measures, which should be routinely used or readily available, include fluid therapy (crystalloids and colloids), analgesia, allogeneic blood products (fresh frozen plasma, packed red blood cells, whole blood and/or albumin), supplemental oxygen, inotropes, vasopressors, anti-arrhythmics, ventilatory therapy and emergency drugs and equipment for cardiopulmonary–cerebral resuscitation.

Please refer to the *BSAVA Manual of Canine and Feline Anaesthesia and Analgesia* for further information.

Analgesia

Thoracic surgery is very painful and multimodal analgesia is essential to decrease the doses of anaesthetic drugs, ameliorate the negative effects of pain on ventilation and wound healing, improve recovery and decrease hospitalization times. Analgesia should be started prior to surgery. Analgesic protocols should include pre-, intra- and postoperative bolus or constant rate infusion (CRI) administration of an opioid, either alone or in combination with ketamine and/or lidocaine CRIs. Mild sedation may be required postoperatively, in particular following thoracic wall reconstruction, but careful attention must be paid to avoiding hypoventilation. The administration of intercostal nerve blocks perioperatively and local anaesthesia via the thoracostomy tube postoperatively (Conzemius *et al.*, 1994) may aid in postoperative analgesia. A subcutaneously implanted wound diffusion catheter is useful for the administration of local anaesthesia for 24–48 hours postoperatively. Postoperative pain should be monitored closely using a standardized pain score.

A non-steroidal anti-inflammatory drug should be administered for a minimum of 10–14 days postoperatively, when not contraindicated, and this should be combined with a stronger oral analgesic for a minimum of 5–7 days.

Postoperative care

A smooth and calm recovery from anaesthesia is important, and it may be necessary for someone to sit with the patient to ensure they wake up quietly. This is particularly important following chest wall reconstruction, as these patients do not have the normal protective barrier present between the skin and internal thoracic organs. Postoperative flailing or aggressive handling can disrupt the surgical site or potentially cause thoracic visceral damage. Adequately thick bedding is essential for postoperative comfort.

Heart rate, ECG, temperature and blood pressure should be monitored in the immediate postoperative period and this is frequently continued on a regular basis for 24–48 hours. Animals seem to recover quickly once the thoracostomy tube is removed, which is usually determined by the degree of fluid or air production. If the thoracostomy tube is negative for air over 6–8 hours and is producing minimal fluid, it is removed.

Animals recovering from any thoracic surgery should receive supplemental oxygen until they can maintain adequate oxygenation on 21% oxygen (P_aO_2 >60 mmHg, S_aO_2 >90%) at sea level, or an alveolar–arterial oxygen gradient <25 mmHg. Two hours of postoperative oxygen supplementation has been shown to decrease wound infection and improve tissue oxygen levels in humans (Greif *et al.*, 2000). Oxygen supplementation is beneficial for a minimum of 12–24 hours following open thoracic surgery. It is important to keep the F_iO_2 <60% during this time to prevent oxygen toxicity (Lodato, 2006).

Animals that have chronic lung atelectasis (e.g. due to chest wall tumours that have been slow growing or chronic diaphragmatic rupture) are susceptible to re-expansion pulmonary oedema. The risk of oedema developing can be mitigated by applying a conservative ventilation strategy intraoperatively (low tidal volume with a higher respiratory rate) and gradually evacuating air from the pleural space postoperatively, whilst carefully monitoring respiratory parameters. Pulmonary crackles on auscultation, respiratory distress and hypoxaemia are all indications that re-expansion pulmonary oedema may be occurring. This is not a furosemide-responsive oedema and supportive care with oxygen is the best treatment. In severe situations, mechanical ventilation with positive end-expiratory pressure may be necessary.

Ventilation should be taken into consideration for all thoracic surgery patients and, although it has not seemingly been a problem in animals with six or fewer ribs resected, the potential for hypoventilation may be greater following chest wall resection as the animal adapts to new chest wall dynamics. The P_aCO_2 should ideally be <45 mmHg, although most animals do not need mechanical ventilation unless the P_aCO_2 is >55–60 mmHg or there is severe respiratory acidosis. Partial reversal of pure opioids with low-dose butorphanol or low-dose naloxone can help with opioid-induced hypoventilation whilst maintaining analgesia. Arterial blood gases should be measured every 2–6 hours initially until the animal is adequately oxygenated and ventilating; every 6–12 hours thereafter is usually adequate. Pulse oximetry may be useful to monitor oxygenation, but can be difficult in the awake patient.

Surgical approaches

Lateral or intercostal thoracotomy

A lateral or intercostal thoracotomy is the standard approach for many intrathoracic diseases and provides good exposure for a specifically defined region (Figure 11.3). See Operative Technique 11.1 for a step-by-step guide to performing a lateral thoracotomy.

Access to structures not in the immediate area of the thoracotomy is limited and, as a general rule, an intercostal thoracotomy allows access to approximately one-third of the ipsilateral thoracic cavity (Orton, 2003; Moores *et al.*, 2007). Although rarely required, exposure can be increased by approximately 33% with dorsal and ventral osteotomies of the rib either cranial or caudal to the intercostal incision. Closure of the intercostal thoracotomy is achieved by placement of circumcostal (see Operative Technique 11.1) or transcostal sutures (Figure 11.4). In one study, the intercostal nerve was entrapped by circumcostal sutures in 70% and 100% of cases when the blunt and the sharp end, respectively, of the needle was passed around the caudal rib. In the same study, it was shown that dogs whose intercostal thoracotomies were closed with circumcostal sutures showed significantly more pain and had significantly greater requirements for fentanyl in the first 24 hours postoperatively than dogs whose ribs were closed using a transcostal technique (Rooney *et al.*, 2004).

Access required	Surgical approach
Trachea	Right 3rd to 4th intercostal space
Patent ductus arteriosus	Left 4th intercostal space
Ligamentum arteriosum	Left 4th intercostal space
Lung lobectomy	Right or left 5th or 6th intercostal space
Pericardectomy	Right or left 5th intercostal space
Pulmonic stenosis	Left 5th intercostal space
Oesophagus: • Cranial • Caudal	Left 4th intercostal space Left 9th intercostal space
Thoracic duct: • Dog • Cat	Right 9th intercostal space Left 9th intercostal space
Caudal mediastinal mass	Left or right 9th intercostal space
Cranial mediastinal mass	Cranial sternotomy
Hepatic surgery	Caudal sternotomy

11.3 Recommended surgical approach for a defined surgical procedure or to reach a specific anatomical location.

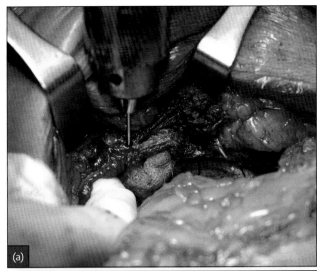
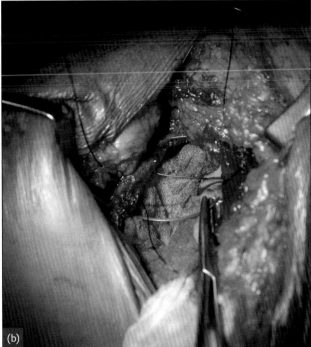

11.4 Intercostal thoracotomy closure using a transcostal technique. (a) Holes are drilled into the mid-body of the caudal rib with a small intramedullary pin or large Kirschner wire. Note that the underlying lungs are being protected from iatrogenic trauma with a moistened laparotomy sponge. (b) Once the hole is drilled in the caudal rib, suture material is passed around the cranial rib and through the hole in the caudal rib. Following preplacement of the transcostal sutures, the sutures are used to approximate the ribs by an assistant while the surgeon ties the knots.

Complications

Short-term complications are reported in up to 47% of cats and dogs following lateral intercostal thoracotomy (Moores *et al.*, 2007). Haemorrhage, pain, air leakage, seroma, infection, wound dehiscence, thoracic limb lameness and re-expansion pulmonary oedema are all potential complications. Haemorrhage is most often caused by inadvertent trauma to the internal thoracic artery during the approach or closure of an intercostal thoracotomy (Bonath, 1996). Postoperative air leakage, which can manifest as pneumothorax, pneumomediastinum or subcutaneous emphysema, is caused by problems with either the thoracotomy closure (such as failure to achieve an airtight closure, incisional dehiscence, infection or self-mutilation) or the thoracostomy tube (leakage from either the stoma or the seals between the thoracostomy tube and three-way stopcock). Pneumomediastinum is most commonly seen as a result of barotrauma causing marginal alveolar rupture. Re-expansion pulmonary oedema can occur following forcible or excessive re-expansion of chronically collapsed lung lobes. The pathogenesis is complex and multifactorial, with proposed mechanisms including mechanical disruption of vessels during re-expansion of collapsed lung lobes, surfactant abnormalities, changes in pulmonary artery pressures as a result of lung re-expansion, release of free radicals and a direct effect of hypoxia on vascular permeability. To minimize the risk of re-expansion pulmonary oedema, chronically atelectatic lungs should be reinflated with gradual re-expansion and airway pressure should not exceed 15 cmH$_2$O, or the lungs should be allowed to re-expand with normal respiration during recovery (Worth and Machon, 2006).

Median sternotomy

A median sternotomy is the only approach that provides exposure to the entire thoracic cavity and is recommended for diseases involving both hemithoraces (e.g. cranial mediastinal tumours, pyothorax and penetrating thoracic injuries) and for exploratory thoracotomies (e.g. spontaneous pneumothorax). Access to structures in the dorsal thoracic cavity, such as the great vessels and bronchial hilus, can be difficult, particularly in deep-chested dogs. If required, a median sternotomy can be combined with a ventral midline cervical incision, coeliotomy or lateral thoracotomy.

Surgical technique

Animals are positioned in dorsal recumbency. The skin and subcutaneous tissues are incised along the ventral midline over the sternum (Figure 11.5a). The pectoral muscles are sharply incised along the sternal midline (Figure 11.5b). Some surgeons bluntly elevate the pectoral muscles from the sternebrae, whilst others prefer to incise but not elevate the muscles. A sternotomy is then performed along the midline with an oscillating saw (Figure 11.5c), although an osteotome and mallet, Lebsche sternum knife or No. 10 scalpel blade can also be used, depending on the size of the animal. Care should be taken to avoid iatrogenic

damage to the lungs and heart during the sternal osteotomy by limiting penetration of the saw blade. Once a segment of the sternotomy has been completed, a malleable retractor can be inserted into the thorax to protect the intrathoracic structures during completion of the remainder of the sternotomy. The manubrium and/or xiphoid should be preserved if possible, but occasionally a complete median sternotomy is required, such as when excising a large cranial mediastinal mass. Some surgeons have expressed concerns that complete median sternotomy results in sternal instability and an increased risk of postoperative complications, but these are not supported by the findings of other investigators provided that the median sternotomy is closed appropriately (Burton and White, 1996). The edges of the sternotomy incision should be protected with moistened laparotomy sponges, and Finochietto rib retractors are recommended to maintain retraction and maximize exposure of the thoracic cavity (Figure 11.5d).

Following completion of the surgical procedure, a thoracostomy tube should be inserted into one or both hemithoraces. The thoracostomy tube should be kept open to the atmosphere during closure to prevent tension pneumothorax. Once an airtight closure is achieved, air and fluid are evacuated from the pleural space, subatmospheric intrathoracic pressure is re-established and the thoracostomy tube is then closed. Stable closure of the median sternotomy is imperative to avoid postoperative pain, pneumothorax and sternal non-union. A figure-of-eight technique over the sternal synchondrosis is preferred, using heavy-gauge suture material (Figure 11.5e), sternal wire or orthopaedic wire (Figure 11.5fg) passed around each sternebra so that each costosternal junction is incorporated in the closure. Sternal wire can be more convenient to place as it has greater malleability than orthopaedic wire and is manufactured with swaged-on needles. A figure-of-eight pattern can be performed with orthopaedic wire using either one twist (i.e. one wire in a figure-of-eight pattern around the sternal synchondrosis) or two twists (i.e. one wire each side of the sternal synchondrosis and the wires twisted together). One- and two-twist figure-of-eight orthopaedic wire closure of the median sternotomy is significantly less likely to fail than one or two cerclage wires around the body of each sternebra (Davis et al., 2006). Figure-of-eight patterns will re-inforce abaxial sternal segments and also prevent direct perpendicular shearing forces being exerted by the orthopaedic wire (Burton and White, 1996; Davis et al., 2006).

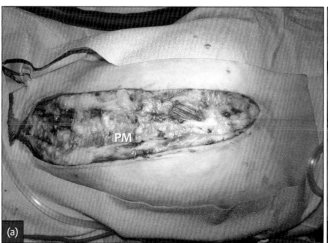
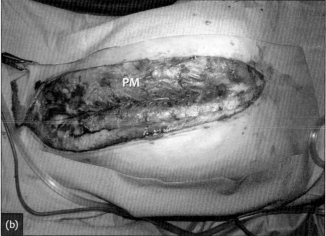

11.5 The steps involved in performing a median sternotomy. (a) A skin incision is made along the ventral midline over the length of the sternum. The incision is continued through the subcutaneous tissues to expose the pectoral muscles (PM). (b) The pectoral muscles (PM) are sharply incised along the ventral midline. (continues)

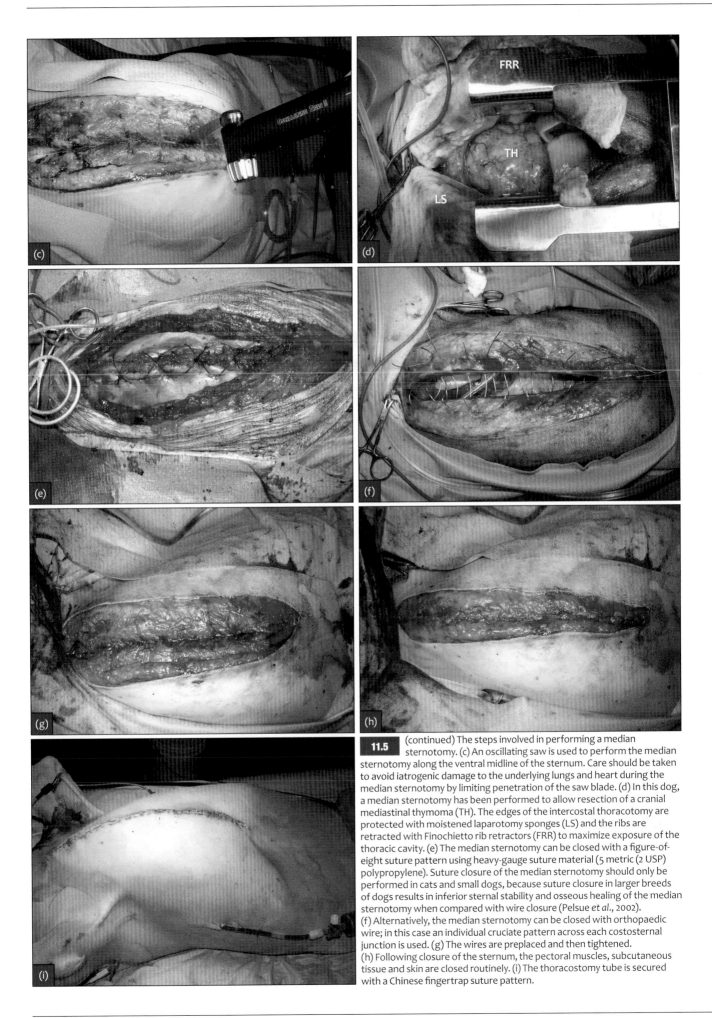

11.5 (continued) The steps involved in performing a median sternotomy. (c) An oscillating saw is used to perform the median sternotomy along the ventral midline of the sternum. Care should be taken to avoid iatrogenic damage to the underlying lungs and heart during the median sternotomy by limiting penetration of the saw blade. (d) In this dog, a median sternotomy has been performed to allow resection of a cranial mediastinal thymoma (TH). The edges of the intercostal thoracotomy are protected with moistened laparotomy sponges (LS) and the ribs are retracted with Finochietto rib retractors (FRR) to maximize exposure of the thoracic cavity. (e) The median sternotomy can be closed with a figure-of-eight suture pattern using heavy-gauge suture material (5 metric (2 USP) polypropylene). Suture closure of the median sternotomy should only be performed in cats and small dogs, because suture closure in larger breeds of dogs results in inferior sternal stability and osseous healing of the median sternotomy when compared with wire closure (Pelsue *et al.*, 2002). (f) Alternatively, the median sternotomy can be closed with orthopaedic wire; in this case an individual cruciate pattern across each costosternal junction is used. (g) The wires are preplaced and then tightened. (h) Following closure of the sternum, the pectoral muscles, subcutaneous tissue and skin are closed routinely. (i) The thoracostomy tube is secured with a Chinese fingertrap suture pattern.

There are no significant differences in either postoperative pain or wound complication rates between suture and wire sternotomy closure. Closure with suture material is significantly faster than orthopaedic wire closure, but orthopaedic wire closure is recommended for large dogs because sternal stability and osseous healing are superior. Closure with orthopaedic wire results in less radiographic evidence of displacement of sternebrae 28 days post sternotomy. Furthermore, closure with orthopaedic wire results in better sternal stability because of chondral or osteochondral union between the osteotomized sternebrae, whereas suture closure only results in fibrous union (Pelsue *et al.*, 2002). Following closure of the sternotomy, the pectoral muscles, subcutaneous tissue and skin are closed routinely in separate layers (Figure 11.5h). The thoracostomy tube is secured with a Chinese fingertrap suture pattern (Figure 11.5i) and the thoracic cavity is evacuated to re-establish negative intrathoracic pressure.

Complications

Overall, complications are reported in 0–78% of cats and dogs following median sternotomy. Complications are rare in cats surviving more than 14 days after surgery (Burton and White, 1996), and are more common in cats and dogs with pyothorax (Tattersall and Welsh, 2006). Short-term complications are reported in 19–40% of dogs surviving longer than 14 days, including haemorrhage, incisional seroma, wound infection (Figure 11.6), thoracic limb neurological deficits and excessive postoperative pain (Burton and White, 1996; Pelsue *et al.*, 2002; Tattersall and Welsh, 2006). Heavier dogs are predisposed to short-term complications, but not long-term complications (Burton and White, 1996). Wound complications are significantly more likely in dogs treated with a median sternotomy compared with a lateral intercostal thoracotomy (Tattersall and Welsh, 2006). Long-term complications occur in 22% of dogs and include haemorrhage, sternal fracture, sternal osteomyelitis and delayed wound healing (Burton and White, 1996). Sternal osteomyelitis is the most common long-term complication and causes sternal discomfort, bilateral thoracic limb lameness, recurrent ventral thoracic oedema, pyrexia, inappetence and depression. Other reported complications include unstable sternebrae repair, transient iatrogenic chylothorax, incisional oedema and incisional dehiscence (Burton and White, 1996).

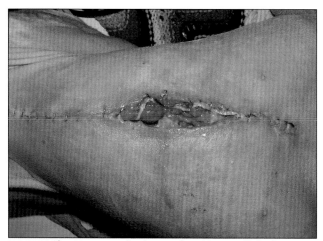

11.6 Short-term complications, such as this wound infection, are reported in up to 40% of cases in dogs following median sternotomy.

Thoracic wall resection and reconstruction

Thoracic wall tumours

Thoracic wall resection is most commonly performed in dogs for the management of rib tumours and in cats for the management of injection-site sarcomas. The majority of rib tumours in dogs are primary malignant sarcomas, with osteosarcoma (OSA) and chondrosarcoma (CSA) being the two most common rib tumours (Baines *et al.*, 2002; Liptak *et al.*, 2008b).

Computed tomography (CT) scans are recommended for both local and distant staging of chest wall tumours. Local staging assists in surgical planning by determining the size and location of the tumour, the extent of rib involvement (both the number of ribs and the dorsal and ventral extent of the tumour), and whether there is adhesion or invasion of the tumour into adjacent structures such as the lungs, pericardium, sternum and vertebrae (Incarbone and Pastorino, 2001); however, CT is not always sufficiently sensitive for differentiating between true adhesion and just contact. Helical CT scans are significantly more sensitive for the detection of metastatic pulmonary lesions than survey radiographs, and this may be more pertinent in dogs with rib tumours because superimposition of the lungs by the chest wall mass and pleural effusion can make the detection of pulmonary metastasis difficult (Nemanic *et al.*, 2006). There is a relatively high incidence of bone metastasis in dogs with primary rib OSA (16%) and, similar to appendicular OSA in dogs (Jankowski *et al.*, 2003), whole-body bone scans are recommended for the detection of occult synchronous or metastatic disease and possibly determination of dorsal and ventral surgical margins for rib resection.

Preoperative incisional biopsy should be considered if a knowledge of the tumour type will change the willingness of the owner to proceed with surgery, because the prognosis is significantly worse for dogs with primary rib OSA (median survival times of 90–120 days with surgery alone and 240–290 days with surgery and adjuvant chemotherapy) than for dogs with primary rib CSA (median survival times of 1080 to >3820 days) (Pirkey-Ehrhart *et al.*, 1995; Baines *et al.*, 2002; Waltman *et al.*, 2007; Liptak *et al.*, 2008b).

Chest wall resection

Surgical technique: Surgical excision of rib tumours should include one rib cranial and one caudal to the tumour, 3 cm of grossly normal bone dorsal and ventral to the tumour in the affected rib(s), and 3 cm lateral margins around all contiguous soft tissues, including biopsy tracts, pleura, muscle and fascia (Figure 11.7ab). Non-involved muscle should be preserved for autogenous reconstruction. The caudal intercostal thoracotomy incision should be performed first, one rib caudal to the tumour based on preoperative imaging, to assist in determining ventral and dorsal margins (Figure 11.7cd). The intercostal vessels are ligated dorsally, either individually or with a heavy-gauge circumcostal ligature (Figure 11.7e). The internal thoracic artery should be identified and ligated. The ribs are ostectomized dorsally and ventrally with bone cutters (Figure 11.7fg), a sagittal saw or an oscillating saw. An oscillating saw is preferred if a partial sternectomy is required to achieve adequate ventral margins (Figure 11.8). In some human and veterinary reports, excision of the entire affected rib has been recommended for treatment of primary malignant sarcomas because of intramedullary spread of the tumour (Figure 11.9; Incarbone and Pastorino, 2001; Halfacree *et al.*, 2007). If

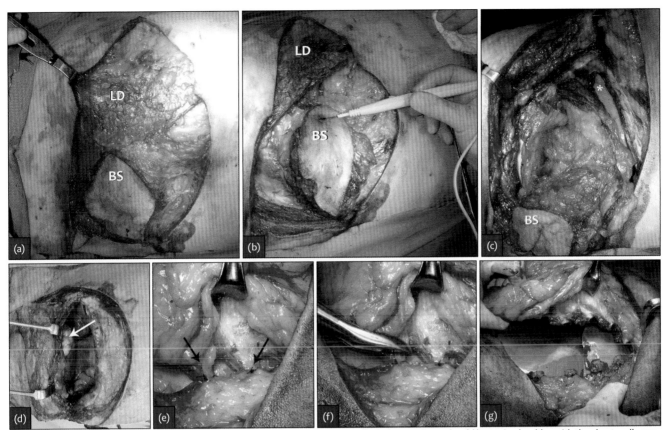

11.7 Thoracic wall resection in a dog. (a) When resecting chest wall masses, all contiguous tissue should be excised *en bloc* with the chest wall mass, including biopsy sites (BS). LD = latissimus dorsi muscle. (b) The biopsy tract excision is continued deeply through all soft tissues. The latissimus dorsi muscle was able to be preserved in this case for autogenous reconstruction of the chest wall defect, but these soft tissue structures should be excised if required to achieve adequate surgical margins for complete resection of the tumour. (c) Once the soft tissue resection has been performed to the level of the ribs, an intercostal thoracotomy (*) is performed one rib caudal to the tumour (as determined from preoperative imaging). (d) Visualization of the rib tumour (arrowed) permits visual assessment of the mass, determination of ventral and dorsal surgical margins in combination with preoperative imaging, and preparation of the ribs for ostectomy. (e) The intercostal vessels are ligated on the dorsal aspect of each rib to be resected either individually or, as depicted, with heavy-gauge circumcostal ligatures (arrowed). (f) The ribs are ostectomized immediately ventral to the ligated intercostal vessels with bone cutters or power saws. (g) The ribs are progressively ostectomized along their dorsal borders until the cranial aspect of the excision is identified, one rib cranial to the rib tumour. The excision can then be continued either ventrally or with the cranial intercostal thoracotomy.

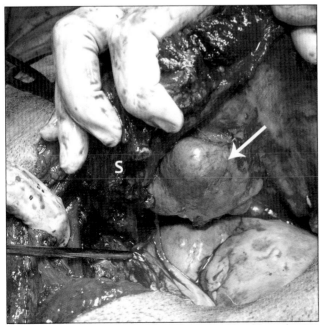

11.8 A partial sternectomy (S) may be required to achieve adequate ventral margins for tumours located at or ventral to the costochondral junction (arrowed). The costosternal junction should provide a barrier to tumour extension, but part of the sternum should be excised to ensure complete surgical excision.

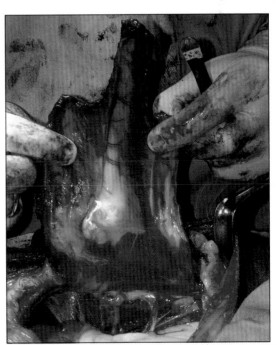

11.9 Resection of the entire affected rib(s) has been recommended because of the possibility of intramedullary extension of the rib tumour and resultant incomplete excision if margins were based on the palpable limits of the tumour.

there is evidence of either adhesion or invasion of the rib tumour into adjacent structures, such as the lungs, pericardium, diaphragm or vertebrae, then these should be resected *en bloc* with the rib tumour (Figures 11.10 and 11.11). Adhesions should be excised *en bloc* rather than broken down because 57% of tumour-associated adhesions in humans have histological evidence of invasion (Nogueras and Jagelman, 1993). In one series of chest wall resections for rib tumours in dogs, *en bloc* partial lung lobectomy was reported in 25.6% of dogs and partial pericardectomy in 7.7% of dogs (Liptak *et al.*, 2008a). Concurrent resection of any volume of lung is associated with a significantly higher risk of respiratory complications and perioperative mortality in humans (Weyant *et al.*, 2006). However, respiratory complications are rare in dogs following chest wall resection, and *en bloc* partial lung lobectomy is not associated with an increased risk of postoperative complications in dogs (Liptak *et al.*, 2008a).

Number of ribs resected: The maximum number of ribs that can be safely resected in cats and dogs is unknown. Six ribs can be safely resected in dogs without the need for rigid reconstruction of the thoracic wall. Furthermore, the number of ribs resected does not significantly increase the risk of postoperative complications (Pirkey-Ehrhart *et al.*, 1995; Liptak *et al.*, 2008a).

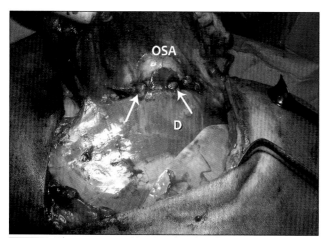

11.10 Rib tumours can either invade or be adherent to adjacent structures such as lung lobes, pericardium or diaphragm. In this dog with a rib osteosarcoma (OSA), the tumour has invaded the diaphragm (D) (arrowed). The diaphragm should be excised with 3 cm margins *en bloc* with the rib tumour.

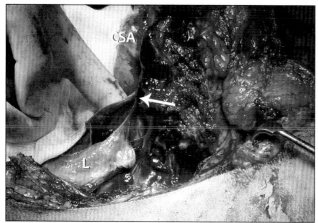

11.11 In this dog with a primary rib chondrosarcoma (CSA), a lung lobe (L) has adhered to the tumour (arrowed). A lung lobectomy was performed with a thoracoabdominal stapler *en bloc* with the rib tumour to minimize the risk of incomplete tumour excision and local tumour recurrence.

Excision of rib tumours with incomplete histological margins is the most important risk factor for local tumour recurrence and survival in both dogs and humans (Pirkey-Ehrhart *et al.*, 1995), hence chest wall resection should not be compromised by either the location of the affected rib(s) or the number of ribs that require resection.

Sternal tumours and resections: Sternal resection and reconstruction presents a greater challenge than rib resection and reconstruction because of the role of the sternum in chest wall stability and the increased risk of complications following sternal reconstruction with standard autogenous and prosthetic techniques in dogs (Liptak *et al.*, 2008a). Sternal defects should be reconstructed with autogenous muscle flaps, composite techniques such as prosthetic mesh with either autogenous muscle flaps or omental pedicle flaps, or more rigid prosthetic techniques such as mesh–methylmethacrylate sandwiches (Liptak *et al.*, 2008a).

Chest wall reconstruction

Surgical technique: Primary repair of chest wall defects involves suturing of the ribs without supplemental reconstruction and is only possible following resection of a small number of ribs (Pirkey-Ehrhart *et al.*, 1995). Primary suturing is acceptable if wide excision of the tumour is possible with minimal rib resection, but wide excision of the tumour should not be compromised because of concerns regarding closure. Primary repair of chest wall defects is rarely possible because of their large size (Figures 11.12–11.14). As a result, a number of autogenous and prosthetic techniques have been reported for the reconstruction of chest wall defects. The aim of chest wall reconstruction is to fill the defect and reduce dead space, establish an airtight seal of the pleural cavity and provide sufficient rigidity to prevent respiratory compromise and protect intrathoracic structures.

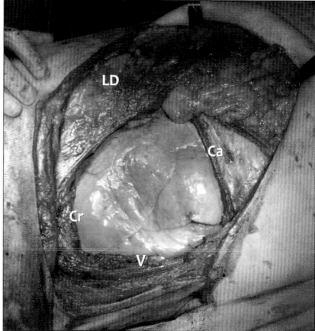

11.12 A typical chest wall defect following resection of a primary rib osteosarcoma with five ribs. These defects are too large for primary repair and require reconstruction with autogenous and/or prosthetic techniques. Ca = caudal extent of the chest wall defect; Cr = cranial extent of the chest wall defect; LD = latissimus dorsi muscle; V = ventral extent of the chest wall defect.

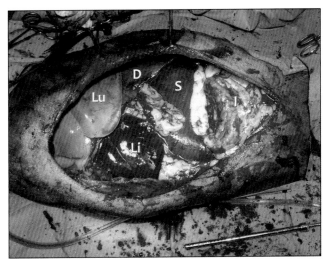

11.13 A typical chest wall defect following resection of a caudal rib osteosarcoma. Note the exposure of the abdominal cavity. In such cases, the thoracic cavity can be reconstructed by advancing the diaphragm and then the abdominal wall is reconstructed with autogenous and/or prosthetic techniques. D = diaphragm; I = intestines; Li = liver; Lu = lungs; S = spleen.

In dogs, the selection of a chest wall reconstructive technique depends on the size and location of the defect. Surgical techniques to reconstruct chest wall defects in dogs include: autogenous latissimus dorsi muscle and myocutaneous flaps; deep pectoral muscle flap; external abdominal oblique muscle flap; omental pedicle flap; diaphragmatic advancement; using prosthetic mesh; a mesh–methylmethacrylate sandwich; and rib replacement with rib grafts or spinal plates.

Latissimus dorsi muscle flap: Pedicled muscle flaps are ideal for reconstruction of chest wall defects because of their large size and good survival rates. The latissimus dorsi muscle is the most common autogenous flap used for reconstruction of chest wall defects in both dogs and humans (Liptak *et al.*, 2008a) because of its location relative to the chest wall, large size, good arc of rotation to permit coverage of the majority of chest wall defects and excellent flap survival based on the thoracodorsal artery and extensive anastomoses between its intercostal and thoracodorsal pedicles. The latissimus dorsi flap can be harvested either as a muscle alone or as a myocutaneous flap (Halfacree *et al.*, 2007); it is a type V muscle flap based on the thoracodorsal artery arising at the level of the caudal depression of the shoulder (Purinton *et al.*, 1992). The dorsal border of the flap extends from ventral to the acromion and the caudal border of the triceps muscle to the head of the 13th rib. The ventral border is either the ventral border of the muscle, if intact, or the incised edge if part of the latissimus dorsi is excised *en bloc* with the rib tumour (Figure 11.15a). Perforating intercostal vessels are ligated and divided, allowing elevation of the flap and rotation into the chest wall defect (Figure 11.15b). The muscle flap is sutured to the cranial and caudal ribs of the chest wall defect and the ventral pectoral musculature with an interrupted or continuous suture pattern using monofilament absorbable suture material (Figure 11.15c). Chest wall defects of up to six ribs have been reconstructed with latissimus dorsi muscle flaps in dogs. For larger defects, the latissimus dorsi muscle flap can be used to reconstruct part of the defect and a prosthetic mesh used for the remainder of the defect (see Figure 11.14bc).

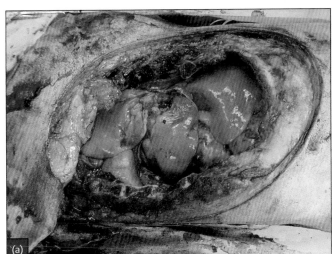

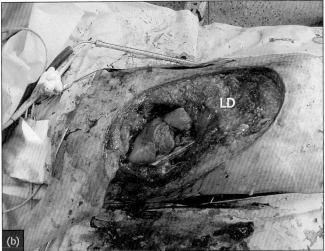

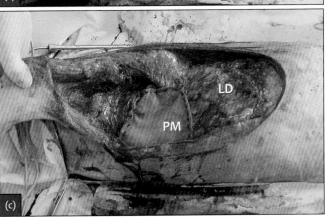

11.14 (a) A large chest wall defect and cutaneous defect following the resection of six ribs for a primary rib chondrosarcoma, including *en bloc* excision of an adhered lung lobe (see Figure 11.11) and pericardium. The cutaneous defect was larger than normal because of combined excision of both the biopsy tract and a concurrent grade II mast cell tumour with 3 cm lateral margins. The cutaneous defect was closed primarily. Note the partial sternectomy to achieve adequate ventral margins. (b) A latissimus dorsi muscle flap (LD) can be used to reconstruct chest wall defects resulting from the resection of up to six ribs, but occasionally this muscle flap will not be sufficient to reconstruct the chest wall defect if part of the muscle has been excised *en bloc* with the tumour, if the chest wall defect is not within the arc of rotation of the muscle flap, or if the chest wall defect is too large, such as with this chest wall defect resulting from the excision of a primary rib chondrosarcoma with six ribs and a portion of the latissimus dorsi muscle. (c) If the latissimus dorsi muscle flap (LD) is not sufficient for reconstruction of the entire chest wall defect, then autogenous reconstruction can be supplemented with a prosthetic mesh (PM).

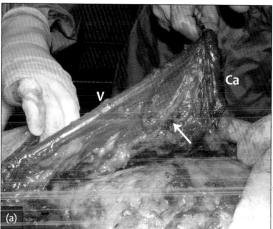
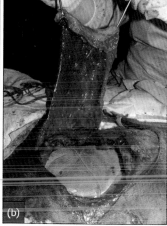
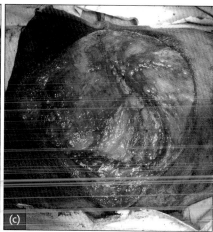

11.15 (a) The latissimus dorsi muscle is being prepared. The ventral border (V) is the ventral aspect of the muscle, which borders the edge of the chest wall resection. The caudal border (Ca) has been incised from the 13th rib. Perforating intercostal vessels (arrowed) are ligated or cauterized and transected. (b) Following elevation of the caudal border, the dorsal border of the flap is incised parallel to the ventral border from the head of the 13th rib to the caudal border of the triceps muscle. (c) The latissimus dorsi muscle flap is sutured into the chest wall defect with either an interrupted or a continuous (depicted) suture pattern to the cranial and caudal ribs and ventrally to the pectoral musculature.

Latissimus dorsi myocutaneous flap: The latissimus dorsi myocutaneous flap has been advocated for reconstruction of chest wall defects (Halfacree *et al.*, 2007) because of the observation that the distal aspect of the muscle flap can undergo necrosis. The thoracodorsal artery is the dominant pedicle of the latissimus dorsi muscle, but the lateral thoracic, intercostal and subscapular arteries also provide minor contributions to the vascular supply of the latissimus dorsi muscle (Purinton *et al.*, 1992). Furthermore, perfusion of the middle segment of the latissimus dorsi muscle is significantly better when the perforating artery from the fifth intercostal space and thoracodorsal artery were preserved, compared with the thoracodorsal artery alone (Monnet *et al.*, 2003). The extensive choke anastomoses between the latissimus dorsi muscle and overlying skin may increase the likelihood of survival of the muscle flap. Failure of the muscle flap was not reported in one series of five dogs whose chest wall defects were reconstructed with a latissimus dorsi myocutaneous flap (Halfacree *et al.*, 2007).

Deep pectoral muscle flap: The deep pectoral muscle is a suitable muscle flap for reconstruction of ventral chest wall and sternal defects in dogs because of its accessibility and favourable vascular pattern (Liptak *et al.*, 2008a). The deep pectoral muscle is a type V muscle, which can be rotated cranially and dorsally based on its lateral thoracic pedicle or ventrally across the midline based on segmental branches of the internal thoracic artery (Purinton *et al.*, 1992). The latter is more commonly used for reconstruction of chest wall defects. In such cases, the muscle flap is elevated by incising its sternal attachment, undermining the muscle belly whilst preserving the cranial portion of the sternal attachment and as many branches of the internal thoracic artery as possible, and rotating the muscle flap across the ventral midline into the contralateral chest wall or sternal defect.

External abdominal oblique muscle flap: The external abdominal oblique muscle (lumbar portion) has been suggested as an autogenous muscle flap for caudal thoracic wall reconstruction. The external abdominal oblique muscle is supplied by the cranial branch of the cranial abdominal artery, which supplies the middle zone of the lateral wall, and the deep branch of the deep circumflex artery, which anastomoses with the cranial and caudal abdominal arteries and supplies the caudodorsal abdominal wall. The fascial edges of the lumbar portion of the external abdominal oblique muscle are divided ventrally and caudally, leaving a 0.5 cm margin of fascia along the muscular edge. The muscle is then undermined and the neurovascular pedicle (cranial abdominal artery, cranial hypogastric nerve and satellite vein) is identified craniodorsal to the 13th rib and preserved. The dorsal fascial attachment is divided and the lumbar part of the external abdominal oblique muscle is severed at the level of the 13th rib. The lumbar external abdominal oblique musculofascial island flap, tethered by its neurovascular pedicle, can be rotated into caudal thoracic wall defects.

Omental pedicle flap: The omental pedicle flap is a supplementary technique to other autogenous or prosthetic reconstructions (Figure 11.16ab). It should not be used for primary reconstruction of chest wall defects. In humans, omental pedicle flaps are used to cover the pleural surface of the mesh to minimize mesh-induced pleuritis, by promoting local healing and enhancing neovascularity, and to provide an airtight seal.

The omentum is composed of the greater and lesser omenta. The lesser omentum arises from the ventral mesogastria and extends between the lesser curvature of the stomach and the duodenum. The greater omentum arises from the dorsal mesogastria and is composed of a large bursal portion and smaller splenic and veil portions. The bursal portion is the most significant and attaches to the cranioventral aspect of the stomach, extends as far caudally as the urinary bladder and then reflects back on itself to the dorsal region of the stomach to cover the intestines with visceral and parietal leaves. The epiploic branches of the right and left gastroepiploic arteries supply the greater omentum. The right and left omental arteries arise from the right gastroepiploic artery and splenic artery, respectively, and course caudally along the right and left borders of the parietal and visceral leaves of the greater omentum.

Preparation of the omental pedicle graft involves lengthening the bursal portion of the greater omentum, based on either the left or right gastroepiploic arteries. The omentum and spleen are exteriorized and the visceral leaf of the greater omentum is retracted cranially to identify and transect its pancreatic attachments to the level of the spleen. Omental vessels originating from the splenic artery

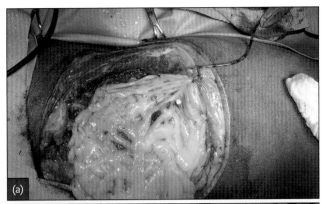

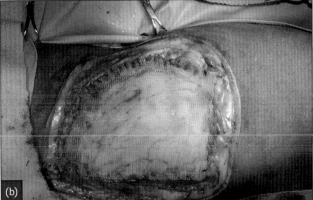

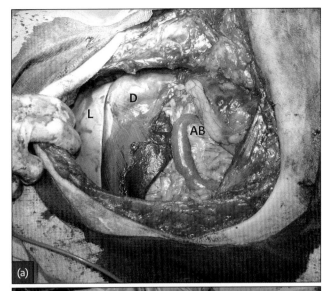

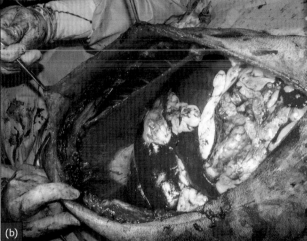

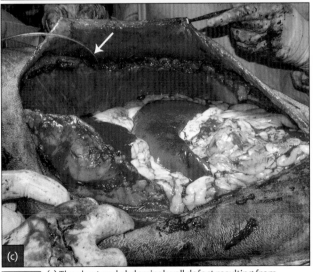

11.16 (a) A caudal rib tumour has been excised and the chest wall has been reconstructed by advancing the diaphragm. The resultant abdominal wall defect has initially been reconstructed with an omental pedicle graft with the omentum sutured to the edges of the abdominal and chest wall defect. Omentum should not be used for primary reconstruction of chest wall defects. In this case, the omentum will cover the peritoneal aspect of the prosthetic mesh reconstruction of the abdominal and chest wall defect.
(b) Reconstruction of the chest and abdominal wall defect is completed by suturing prosthetic mesh into the defect with a simple continuous suture pattern over the omental pedicle graft. The omental pedicle graft should reduce pleural and peritoneal inflammation and promote healing and incorporation of the prosthetic mesh.

are ligated and transected to allow caudal retraction of the visceral leaf. An inverted L-shaped incision is then made. Omental vessels are ligated along the left border of the greater omentum caudal to the gastrosplenic ligament and the omental incision is then continued caudally parallel to the remaining omental vessels for two-thirds of its length. The epiploic branches to the greater curvature of the stomach and the opposite gastroepiploic artery are ligated and divided. The omental pedicle graft can then be extended into the thoracic cavity, either through the diaphragm if a median sternotomy has been performed or through a subcutaneous tunnel via a paracostal incision if a lateral intercostal thoracotomy has been performed. The abdominal exit site should be as close as possible to the origin of the omental pedicle graft and large enough to prevent vascular compromise of the omental pedicle graft (Ross and Pardo, 1993).

Diaphragmatic advancement: Chest wall defects involving the ninth to 13th ribs do not necessarily require reconstruction as normal thoracic physiology and function can be restored by advancing the diaphragm cranially. Following resection of a caudal chest wall tumour, the free edge of the diaphragm is sutured to the ribs and chest wall defect with absorbable suture material in either a continuous or interrupted suture pattern (Figure 11.17). Rarely, caudal lung lobectomy may be required to allow sufficient intrathoracic

11.17 (a) The chest and abdominal wall defect resulting from resection of a caudal rib osteosarcoma. Following caudal rib resections, the thoracic cavity can be restored by advancing the diaphragm (D) rather than reconstruction of the chest wall. (b) The free edge of the diaphragm is advanced and sutured to the edge of the chest wall resection with a simple interrupted (depicted) or continuous suture pattern. (c) The diaphragm has been advanced to restore normal thoracic function and physiology. Note the temporary thoracostomy tube (arrowed), which is used to evacuate air and fluid from the thoracic cavity intraoperatively and is removed once negative intrathoracic pressure has been established. The resultant abdominal wall defect is then reconstructed using autogenous and/or prosthetic techniques (see Figure 11.16). AB = abdominal cavity; L = lungs.

volume for lung expansion following diaphragmatic advancement (Figure 11.18). The resultant abdominal wall defect can be repaired primarily, or reconstructed with autogenous muscle flaps (e.g. latissimus dorsi and/or external abdominal oblique muscle flaps) or prosthetic mesh (see Figure 11.16).

Prosthetic mesh: Prosthetic meshes are commonly used to reconstruct chest wall defects, either alone or in combination with muscle flaps and/or omental pedicle flaps. Composite autogenous–prosthetic reconstruction techniques are used if the chest wall defect is too large to be reconstructed with an autogenous muscle flap alone or to decrease the perceived risks of complications associated with prosthetic meshes, such as infection (see Figure 11.14bc). Prosthetic meshes are used for reconstruction of larger chest wall defects in humans because they provide additional rigidity when sutured under tension and as a result are associated with a significantly decreased rate of respiratory complications and shorter hospital stays when compared with autogenous muscle flap reconstructions (Losken *et al.*, 2004).

Non-absorbable polypropylene mesh (Marlex) is the most commonly used mesh for chest wall reconstruction in dogs, but Prolene, polytetrafluoroethylene (PTFE), and Vicryl meshes are also used in humans (Skoracki and Chang, 2006). The ideal material characteristics for chest wall reconstruction include rigidity, malleability, inertness, radiolucency and resistance to infection. Marlex mesh is constructed of knitted non-absorbable monofilament polypropylene; it has a high tensile strength and low permeability to liquids and gases. The pore size of 200–800 μm permits rapid ingrowth of vascularized tissue and, by 6 weeks, Marlex mesh is infiltrated with 3–4 mm thick fibrous tissue (Trostle and Rosin, 1994); by 6 months it is incorporated, with no loss of tensile strength or fragmentation. Prolene mesh is often preferred to Marlex mesh in humans, despite both being constructed from polypropylene, because Prolene mesh is constructed from double-knitted polypropylene and thus resists stretching in all directions. Vicryl is an absorbable mesh and is indicated for reconstruction of contaminated wounds (Skoracki and Chang, 2006). PTFE is strong, resistant to infection and impervious to air and fluids, and therefore

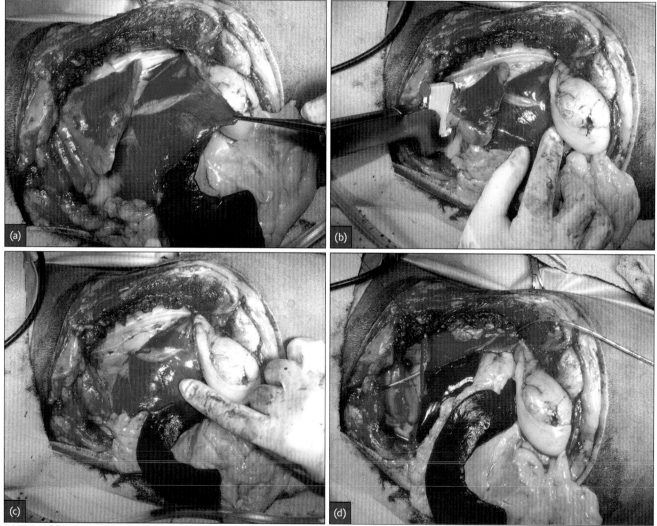

11.18 (a) A chest wall defect following resection of seven ribs (ribs 7–13) for excision of an injection-site sarcoma in a cat. The diaphragm will be advanced to reconstruct the thoracic cavity, but it is likely that diaphragmatic advancement will decrease intrathoracic volume and restrict lung expansion, resulting in hypoxaemia and respiratory distress. In these cases, lobectomy of the caudal lung lobe should be considered. (b) A caudal lung lobectomy is being performed with a thoracoabdominal stapler to permit sufficient intrathoracic volume for normal expansion of the remaining lung lobes following diaphragmatic advancement. (c) Following caudal lung lobectomy, there is sufficient intrathoracic volume for normal expansion of the remaining lung lobes. (d) The diaphragm is being advanced to restore normal thoracic function and physiology. Note the temporary thoracostomy tube, which is used to evacuate air and fluid from the thoracic cavity intraoperatively and is removed once negative intrathoracic pressure has been established. The resultant abdominal wall defect is then reconstructed using autogenous and/or prosthetic techniques (see Figure 11.16).

has ideal characteristics; however, it is very expensive. Marlex and Prolene meshes, whilst not impervious to air and fluids, are just as effective as PTFE for chest wall reconstruction (Incarbone and Pastorino, 2001).

When performing chest wall reconstruction, the size of the prosthetic mesh is tailored to the size of the chest wall defect so that the edges are doubled over to provide a double layer for suturing to adjacent host tissue. The mesh is sutured under mild tension to either the pleural or the lateral surface of the defect using either absorbable or non-absorbable monofilament suture material (Figure 11.19). If possible, the mesh should be sutured to the ribs. Although it is rarely required, prosthetic mesh can be supported with autogenous split rib grafts, allogeneic free rib grafts or plastic spinal plates between the ends of the resected ribs following extensive resections. If a composite reconstruction is planned, then omental pedicle grafts should cover the pleural surface of the mesh and autogenous muscle flaps should be sutured over the lateral surface of the mesh (see Figure 11.16).

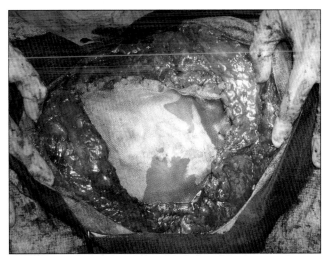

11.19 Prosthetic polypropylene (Marlex) mesh has been used to reconstruct a chest wall defect following resection of a primary rib osteosarcoma. The edges of the mesh are doubled over and sutured to the chest wall defect using either an interrupted (depicted) or continuous suture pattern under mild tension.

Complications: Complications following chest wall resection and reconstruction are reported in up to 50% of dogs; however, the majority of these complications are minor and require no to minimal intervention. Respiratory complications are common in humans and include prolonged mechanical ventilation, pneumonia, acute respiratory distress syndrome and pulmonary hypofunction. In contrast, respiratory complications are very rare in dogs (Halfacree *et al.*, 2007; Liptak *et al.*, 2008a). Pulmonary function is normal, respiratory pattern and blood gas analyses are typical of dogs treated with any type of open-chest surgical procedure (including thoracotomy), and no dog has been reported to require postoperative mechanical ventilation following chest wall resection and reconstruction (Halfacree *et al.*, 2007; Liptak *et al.*, 2008a). Paradoxical motion of the reconstructed chest wall is common for 3–7 days post surgery, but paradoxical motion in the absence of underlying pulmonary trauma does not result in pulmonary hypofunction in dogs in either experimental or clinical studies (Halfacree *et al.*, 2007; Liptak *et al.*, 2008a). As a result, more rigid chest wall reconstruction techniques, such as mesh–methylmethacrylate sandwiches and rib replacement with spinal Lubra plates, are probably unnecessary.

Wound problems are the most common complications following chest wall resection in dogs. Incisional seromas are reported in up to 40% of dogs; seromas are common because of the aggressive resection and the amount of dead space following reconstruction. Seroma formation may also indicate partial failure of the latissimus dorsi muscle flap, and distal flap necrosis should be suspected if the seroma does not resolve spontaneously within 2 weeks (Liptak *et al.*, 2008a). The incidence of incisional seromas may be decreased with the use of either active or passive drains, and bandaging the chest postoperatively. Early wound infection, incisional wound dehiscence and muscle flap necrosis and failure are rare (Figure 11.20).

Some surgeons avoid the use of non-absorbable meshes because of the perception that the risk of infection is increased with prosthetic material. However, Marlex mesh is considered an ideal material for chest wall reconstruction partly because of its resistance to infections and this is supported by retrospective clinical studies in dogs and humans, which show that prosthetic meshes used for chest wall reconstruction are associated with very low rates of infection. Infection rates of 0% and 2.3% have been reported in two retrospective studies with long-term follow-up of chest wall reconstruction with prosthetic mesh (Liptak *et al.*, 2008a). The majority of these infections are deep seated and they usually occur late in the postoperative period, with infection reported in one dog 767 days postoperatively (Liptak *et al.*, 2008a). In humans, infected meshes are managed with surgical removal and culture-directed antimicrobial therapy. Fibrous ingrowth into Marlex mesh results in a stable fibrous wall within 6 weeks, and removal of the mesh does not compromise the integrity or strength of the reconstructed chest wall (Skoracki and Chang, 2006).

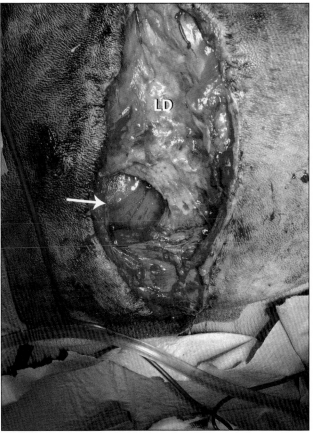

11.20 Distal necrosis of a latissimus dorsi (LD) muscle flap resulting in a chest wall defect (arrowed).

Postoperative pleural effusion and peripheral oedema are uncommon complications. These complications were reported in five of 54 dogs in one retrospective series (9.3%), but resolved without specific treatment in all five dogs (Pirkey-Erhart *et al.*, 1995). In contrast, three of 42 dogs (7.1%) developed pleural effusion in another study, and these did not resolve spontaneously (Liptak *et al.*, 2008a). One dog died as a result of haemothorax secondary to disruption of the internal thoracic artery, and two dogs developed a serosanguineous pleural effusion secondary to pleuritis because of a large surface area of contact between the lungs and Marlex mesh following large sternal reconstructions (Figure 11.21) (Liptak *et al.*, 2008a). Furthermore, these dogs also developed subcutaneous oedema because Marlex mesh is not impervious to fluids and the accumulation of large amounts of pleural fluid early in the postoperative period resulted in the flow of pleural fluid through the mesh into dependent subcutaneous spaces (Liptak *et al.*, 2008a). For dogs in which large sternal resections are planned, composite reconstructions are recommended with prosthetic mesh and well vascularized autogenous tissue, such as omental pedicle grafts on the pleural surface or muscle flaps on either the pleural or lateral surface of the mesh (Liptak *et al.*, 2008a).

Thoracic wall trauma

Thoracic wall injury may be caused by blunt trauma in a road traffic accident or a fall from a height, impalement injuries or, most commonly, bite wounds from a larger dog (Figure 11.22). Blunt trauma may result in rib fracture, pneumothorax, haemothorax, pulmonary contusions and diaphragmatic rupture. If multiple rib fractures are present a flail chest may occur, in which a segment of the chest wall is drawn in during inspiration, thereby reducing thoracic volume and efficiency of ventilation (see **Flail chest in a dog** video clip). Pseudo-flail chest occurs when there is one or more sites of intercostal muscle avulsion, without multiple segmental rib fractures. Whilst the paradoxical movement of the thoracic wall in either flail or pseudo flail chest does not alone substantially compromise ventilation, concurrent hypoventilation associated with pain and ventilation–perfusion mismatch from associated pulmonary contusions can cause hypoxia (Cappello *et al.*, 1995). Patient stabilization is a priority, with provision of supplemental oxygen, analgesia, intravenous fluid therapy or transfusion of blood products as required, and thoracocentesis. In severe cases, it may be necessary to perform emergency intubation to obtain control of ventilation.

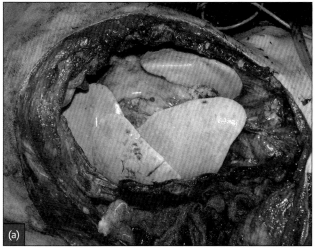

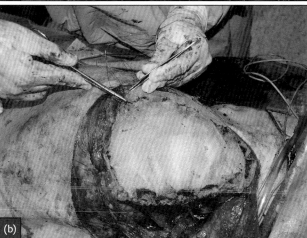

11.21 (a) A chest wall defect following resection of a sternal haemangiosarcoma, which included six sternebrae and approximately 50% of the associated six ribs left and right of the sternum. (b) This large chest wall and sternal defect was reconstructed with a prosthetic Marlex mesh because autogenous reconstruction was not possible. However, the large surface area of the lungs in contact with the prosthetic mesh resulted in pleuritis and subsequent pleural effusion. To minimize the risk of this complication, an omental pedicle graft should be considered on the pleural surface of the mesh (see Figure 11.16).

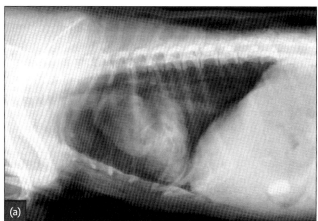

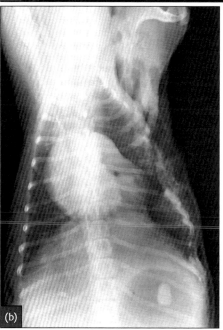

11.22 Bite wounds to the chest following an attack on a Chihuahua by a larger dog. (a) Lateral thoracic view and (b) dorsoventral view of the thorax. These radiographs of a Chihuahua reveal fracture of the fifth and sixth ribs, pneumothorax and subcutaneous emphysema.

Stabilization of a flail chest segment is most simply achieved by placement of an external splint with transcutaneous sutures encircling the 'floating' rib segments and stabilizing them to the surrounding chest wall (McAnulty, 1995). However, specific treatment of a flail chest is not always required, and it is essential that adequate drainage of the pleural space has been performed and that the patient has received adequate analgesia; one study failed to demonstrate any difference in outcome in patients with or without stabilization of the chest wall (Olsen et al., 2002).

Bite wounds produce a combination of penetrating wounds, allowing inoculation of bacteria into the wound, and deep tissue trauma, with extensive crushing injury compromising muscle viability. The appearance of a small bite mark on the skin surface often belies extensive injury beneath; therefore, it is important that bite wounds, in particular those over the thoracic cavity, are thoroughly investigated, which requires surgical exploration (Scheepens et al., 2006). Surgical exploration is performed by extending the skin wound at the site of the injury. This approach will often reveal more extensive injury to underlying muscle; an intercostal thoracotomy can be performed by extending the muscle incisions at this level, therefore allowing inspection of the thoracic cavity, debridement and lavage. Samples must be obtained for bacteriological culture prior to closure of the wound, and a thoracostomy tube and wound drain should be placed (Figure 11.23). In some circumstances, extensive trauma to the thoracic wall may have created a defect necessitating thoracic wall reconstruction; owing to the risk of infection, use of autogenous tissue is preferred.

Pectus excavatum

Pectus excavatum refers to a developmental abnormality in which the caudal sternum is deviated dorsally, therefore reducing the volume of the thoracic cavity and sometimes compressing the heart. This condition is seen rarely; it affects cats more often than dogs. When this deformity is marked, significant compromise of ventilatory function may be present and surgical correction may be warranted. Surgical correction is achieved by placement of an external splint (Yoon et al., 2008; Figure 11.24), under

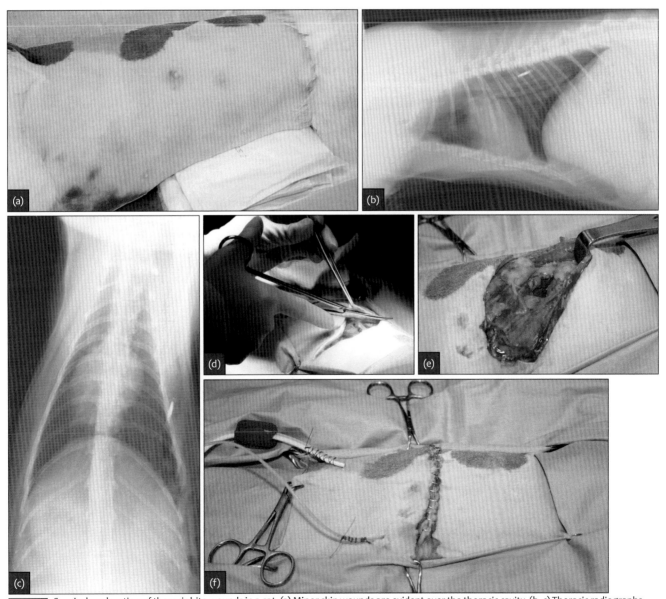

11.23 Surgical exploration of thoracic bite wounds in a cat. (a) Minor skin wounds are evident over the thoracic cavity. (b, c) Thoracic radiographs reveal subcutaneous emphysema and mild pneumothorax. (d) Surgical exploration is performed by extending the skin incision dorsoventrally. (e) Intercostal muscle laceration and penetration of the thoracic cavity are revealed. (f) Following lavage, debridement and repair, the wound is closed with a thoracostomy tube and wound drain in place.

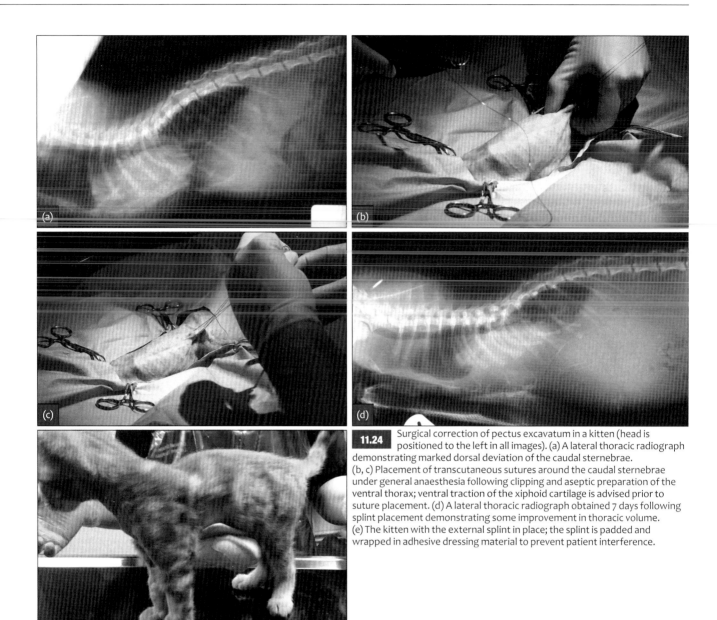

11.24 Surgical correction of pectus excavatum in a kitten (head is positioned to the left in all images). (a) A lateral thoracic radiograph demonstrating marked dorsal deviation of the caudal sternebrae. (b, c) Placement of transcutaneous sutures around the caudal sternebrae under general anaesthesia following clipping and aseptic preparation of the ventral thorax; ventral traction of the xiphoid cartilage is advised prior to suture placement. (d) A lateral thoracic radiograph obtained 7 days following splint placement demonstrating some improvement in thoracic volume. (e) The kitten with the external splint in place; the splint is padded and wrapped in adhesive dressing material to prevent patient interference.

general anaesthesia. Transcutaneous sutures are placed, encircling the caudal sternebrae. These sutures are passed through holes drilled in a custom-made external splint, therefore exerting ventral traction, which both repositions the caudal sternum and corrects the deformity during growth.

Possible complications include haemorrhage from inadvertent laceration of an intercostal vessel or even the heart; it is recommended that the sternum is elevated away from the chest by ventral retraction of the xiphoid before transcutaneous sutures are placed. A dorsoventral thoracic radiograph obtained preoperatively allows the position of the heart to be determined and the encircling sutures are then placed from the side on which the heart is resting, to avoid directing the needle towards the heart. The skin–splint interface is ideally protected with a padded dressing material that can be changed as necessary; the animal, splint placement and skin–splint interface should be checked regularly. The splint remains in place for approximately 3–6 weeks.

References and further reading

Baines SJ, Lewis S and White RA (2002) Primary thoracic wall tumours of mesenchymal origin in dogs: a retrospective study of 46 cases. *Veterinary Record* **150**, 335–339

Bonath KH (1996) Thoracic wall closure. In: *Complications in Small Animal Surgery, 1st edn*, ed. AJ Lipowitz, pp. 229–239. Williams and Wilkins, Baltimore

Burton CA and White RN (1996) Review of the technique and complications of median sternotomy in the dog and cat. *Journal of Small Animal Practice* **37**, 516–522

Cappello M, Yuehua C and De Troyer A (1995) Rib cage distortion in a canine model of flail chest. *American Journal of Respiratory and Critical Care Medicine* **151**, 1481–1485

Conzemius MG, Brockman DJ, King LG et al. (1994) Analgesia in dogs after intercostal thoracotomy: a clinical trial comparing intravenous buprenorphine and interpleural bupivacaine. *Veterinary Surgery* **23**, 291–298

Davis KM, Roe RC, Mathews KG et al. (2006) Median sternotomy closure in dogs: a mechanical comparison of technique stability. *Veterinary Surgery* **35**, 271–277

Duke-Novakovski T, de Vries M and Seymour C (2016) *BSAVA Manual of Canine and Feline Anaesthesia and Analgesia, 3rd edn*. BSAVA Publications, Gloucester

Evans HE (1993) *Miller's Anatomy of the Dog, 3rd edn*. Saunders, Philadelphia

Greif R, Akça O, Horn EP et al. (2000) Supplemental perioperative oxygen to reduce the incidence of surgical-wound infection. *New England Journal of Medicine* **342**, 161–167

Halfacree ZJ, Baines SJ, Lipscomb VJ *et al.* (2007) Use of a latissimus dorsi myocutaneous flap for one-stage reconstruction of the thoracic wall after *en bloc* resection of primary rib chondrosarcoma in five dogs. *Veterinary Surgery* **36**, 587–592

Incarbone M and Pastorino U (2001) Surgical treatment of chest wall tumors. *World Journal of Surgery* **25**, 218–230

Jankowski MK, Steyn PJ, Lana SE *et al.* (2003) Nuclear scanning with 99mTc-HDP for the initial evaluation of osseous metastasis in canine osteosarcoma. *Veterinary and Comparative Oncology* **1**, 152–158

Liptak JM, Dernell WS, Rizzo SA *et al.* (2008a) Reconstruction of chest wall defects following rib tumor resection: a comparison of autogenous, prosthetic, and composite techniques in 44 dogs. *Veterinary Surgery* **37**, 479–487

Liptak JM, Kamstock DA, Dernell WS *et al.* (2008b) Oncologic outcome after curative-intent treatment in 39 dogs with primary chest wall tumors (1992–2005). *Veterinary Surgery* **37**, 488–496

Lodato RF (2006) Oxygen toxicity. In: *Principles and Practice of Mechanical Ventilation, 2nd edn*, ed. MJ Tobin, pp. 1065–1090 McGraw-Hill, New York

Losken A, Thourani VH, Carlson GW *et al.* (2004) A reconstructive algorithm for plastic surgery following extensive chest wall resection. *British Journal of Plastic Surgery* **57**, 295–302

McAnulty JF (1995) A simplified method for stabilisation of flail chest injuries in small animals. *Journal of the American Animal Hospital Association* **31**, 137–141

Monnet E, Rooney MB and Chachques JC (2003) *In vitro* evaluation of the distribution of blood flow within a canine bipedicled latissimus dorsi muscle flap. *American Journal of Veterinary Research* **64**, 1255–1259

Moores AL, Halfacree ZJ, Baines SJ *et al.* (2007) Indications, outcomes and complications following lateral thoracotomy in dogs and cats. *Journal of Small Animal Practice* **48**, 695–698

Nemanic S, London CA and Wisner ER (2006) Comparison of thoracic radiographs and single breath-hold helical CT for detection of pulmonary nodules in dogs with metastatic neoplasia. *Journal of Veterinary Internal Medicine* **20**, 508–515

Nogueras JJ and Jagelman DG (1993) Principles of surgical resection. Influence of surgical technique on treatment outcome. *Surgical Clinics of North America* **73**, 103–116

Olsen D, Renberg W, Perrett J *et al.* (2002) Clinical management of flail chest in dogs and cats: a retrospective study of 24 cases (1989–1999). *Journal of the American Animal Hospital Association* **38**, 315–320

Orton EC (2003) Thoracic wall. In: *Textbook of Small Animal Surgery, 3rd edn*, ed. DH Slatter, pp. 373–387. Saunders, Philadelphia

Pelsue DH, Monnet E, Gaynor JS *et al.* (2002) Closure of median sternotomy in dogs: suture *versus* wire. *Journal of the American Animal Hospital Association* **38**, 569–576

Pirkey-Ehrhart N, Withrow SJ, Straw RC *et al.* (1995) Primary rib tumours in 54 dogs. *Journal of the American Animal Hospital Association* **31**, 65–69

Purinton PT, Chambers JN and Moore JL (1992) Identification and categorization of the vascular patterns to muscles of the thoracic limb, thorax, and neck of dogs. *American Journal of Veterinary Research* **53**, 1435–1445

Rooney MB, Mehl M and Monnet E (2004) Intercostal thoracotomy closure: transcostal sutures as a less painful alternative to circumcostal suture placement. *Veterinary Surgery* **33**, 209–213

Ross WE and Pardo AD (1993) Evaluation of an omental pedicle extension technique in the dog. *Veterinary Surgery* **22**, 37–43

Scheepens ET, Peeters ME, L'Eplanttenier HF *et al.* (2006) Thoracic bite trauma in dogs: a comparison of clinical and radiological parameters with surgical results. *Journal of Small Animal Practice* **47**, 721–726

Skoracki RJ and Chang DW (2006) Reconstruction of the chest wall and thorax. *Journal of Surgical Oncology* **94**, 455–465

Tattersall JA and Welsh E (2006) Factors influencing the short-term outcome following thoracic surgery in 98 dogs. *Journal of Small Animal Practice* **47**, 715–720

Trostle SS and Rosin E (1994) Selection of prosthetic mesh implants. *Compendium on Continuing Education for the Practicing Veterinarian* **16**, 1147–1154

Waltman SS, Seguin B, Cooper BJ *et al.* (2007) Clinical outcome of nonnasal chondrosarcoma in dogs: 31 cases (1986–2003). *Veterinary Surgery* **36**, 266–271

Weyant MJ, Bains MS, Venkatraman E *et al* (2006). Results of chest wall resection and reconstruction with and without rigid prosthesis. *Annals of Thoracic Surgery* **81**, 279–285

Worth AJ and Machon RG (2006) Prevention of reexpansion pulmonary edema and ischemia–reperfusion injury in the management of diaphragmatic herniation. *Compendium on the Continuing Education for the Practicing Veterinarian* **28**, 531–540

Yoon H-Y, Mann FA and Jeong S-W (2008) Surgical correction of pectus excavatum in two cats. *Journal of Veterinary Science* **9**, 335–337

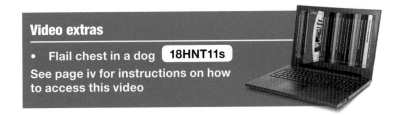

Video extras

- **Flail chest in a dog** `18HNT11s`

See page iv for instructions on how to access this video

OPERATIVE TECHNIQUE 11.1

Lateral or intercostal thoracotomy

PATIENT PREPARATION AND POSITIONING

The patient is clipped and prepared over the entire lateral thoracic cavity, extending just beyond the midline dorsally and ventrally and from the thoracic inlet to the mid-abdomen. The proximal thoracic limb should also be clipped and prepared to the level of the elbow.

The patient is positioned in lateral recumbency. Positioning a sandbag beneath the thorax, just behind the scapula, spreads the intercostal spaces, facilitating access within the thoracic cavity. The thoracic limb is secured in extension.

ASSISTANT

Ideally.

ADDITIONAL INSTRUMENTS

Finochietto rib retractors; laparotomy sponges; thoracostomy tube or alternative tube, such as an infant feeding tube or urinary catheter.

→ **OPERATIVE TECHNIQUE 11.1 CONTINUED**

SURGICAL TECHNIQUE

1   An incision is made through the skin, subcutaneous tissue and cutaneous trunci muscle from the costovertebral junction dorsally to the sternum ventrally and running parallel to the ribs over the desired intercostal space.

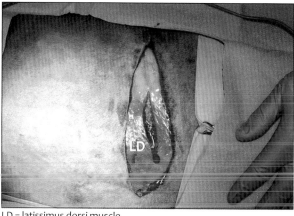

LD = latissimus dorsi muscle.

2   The latissimus dorsi and pectoral muscles are incised parallel to the skin incision across their muscle fibres. The desired intercostal space for the thoracotomy is identified by either counting ribs and intercostal spaces, usually from the first rib caudally, and/or identifying the fifth rib. The external abdominal oblique muscle originates from the fifth rib and the scalenus muscle inserts on the fifth rib.

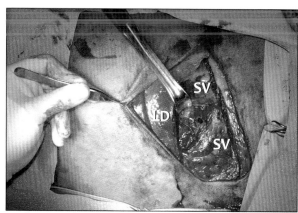

LD = latissimus dorsi muscle; SV = serratus ventralis muscle.

3   One of these muscles is incised, depending on whether the intercostal thoracotomy is cranial (scalenus muscle) or caudal (external abdominal oblique muscle) to the fifth rib. The serratus ventralis muscle is separated between its muscle bellies or incised parallel to its fibres to expose the intercostal space.

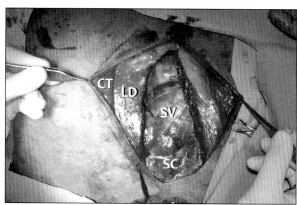

CT = cutaneous trunci muscle; LD = latissimus dorsi muscle; SC = scalenus muscle; SV = serratus ventralis muscle.

4   The external and internal intercostal muscles are then incised in the middle of the intercostal space to avoid iatrogenic trauma to the intercostal vessels coursing over the caudal aspect of the ribs.

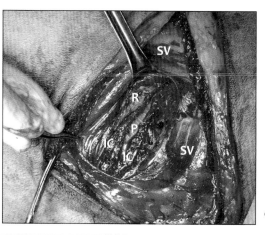

IC = intercostal muscles; P = pleura; R = rib; SV = serratus ventralis muscle.

→ **OPERATIVE TECHNIQUE 11.1 CONTINUED**

5 The pleura is a distinct structure and is penetrated by blunt puncture and then opened to the extent of the thoracotomy using scissors. The edges of the intercostal thoracotomy incision should be protected with moistened laparotomy sponges, and Finochietto rib retractors are recommended to maintain retraction of the ribs and maximize exposure of the thoracic cavity.

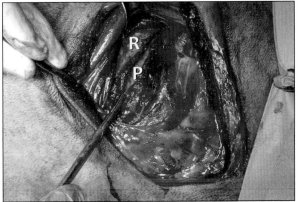

P = pleura; R = rib.

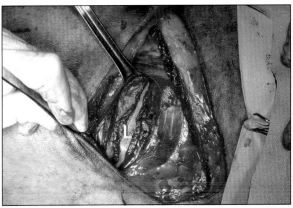

L = lungs.

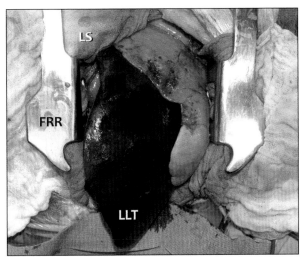

This dog has lung lobe torsion (LLT).
FRR = Finochietto rib retractors;
LS = laparotomy sponge.

6 Following completion of the surgical procedure, a thoracostomy tube can be inserted into the ipsilateral hemithorax, depending on the disease and whether further fluid or air accumulation is anticipated in the postoperative period. For diseases in which this is unlikely, a temporary thoracostomy tube, such as an 8 Fr urinary catheter or infant feeding tube, can be placed through the intercostal thoracotomy incision. Regardless, the thoracostomy tube should be kept open to the atmosphere during closure of the thoracotomy to prevent tension pneumothorax. Once an airtight closure is achieved, air and fluid are evacuated from the pleural space, negative intrathoracic pressure is re-established, and the thoracostomy tube is then closed.

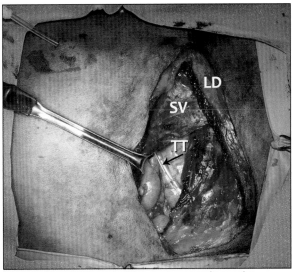

LD = latissimus dorsi muscle; SV = serratus ventralis muscle;
TT = thoracostomy tube (arrowed).

→ **OPERATIVE TECHNIQUE 11.1 CONTINUED**

7 The intercostal thoracotomy incision is closed with either circumcostal or transcostal sutures. The traditional circumcostal suture technique involves preplacing large-gauge (3 to 5 metric (2/0 to 2 USP) depending on the size of the animal) absorbable or non-absorbable suture material around the cranial and caudal ribs in either a simple interrupted or cruciate suture pattern. The needle should be passed as close as possible to the ribs to avoid entrapping soft tissues between the suture material and the ribs. For the transcostal technique, holes are drilled in the mid-body of the caudal rib (see Figure 11.4a) so that the suture material is passed through the rib rather than around the rib, thus avoiding entrapment of the intercostal nerve (see Figure 11.4b). Regardless of whether a circumcostal or transcostal technique is used, the preplaced sutures are used by an assistant to approximate the ribs while the surgeon ties the sutures.

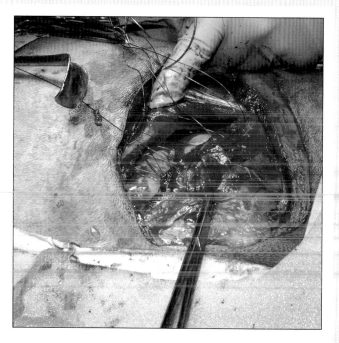

8 The serratus ventralis, scalenus, external abdominal oblique, latissimus dorsi and cutaneous trunci muscles are closed individually with either interrupted or continuous suture patterns to prevent air leakage postoperatively. Following routine closure of the subcutaneous layer and skin, the thoracostomy tube is secured with a Chinese fingertrap suture pattern.

POSTOPERATIVE CARE

The thoracic cavity can be bandaged to minimize the risk of seroma formation and premature removal of the thoracostomy tube, but care should be taken to ensure that the bandage is not applied so tightly that thoracic wall excursion is restricted. If a temporary thoracostomy tube has been used, the thoracic cavity should be evacuated until negative intrathoracic pressure has been re-established and the tube is then removed.

Thoracic surgery is painful and multimodal analgesia is an important consideration to decrease the doses of anaesthetic drugs, improve recovery and decrease hospitalization times. Analgesia should be started prior to surgery. Analgesic protocols should include pre-, intra- and postoperative CRIs of an opioid (fentanyl or morphine) either alone or in combination with ketamine and/or lidocaine CRIs. The administration of intercostal nerve blocks may aid postoperative analgesia. A subcutaneously implanted wound diffusion catheter is useful for the administration of local anaesthesia (ropivacaine and/or lidocaine) for 24–48 hours postoperatively. A non-steroidal anti-inflammatory drug should be administered for a minimum of 10–14 days postoperatively and this should be combined with a stronger oral analgesic (such as tramadol) for a minimum of 5–7 days.

Chapter 12

Pleural drainage techniques

Victoria Lipscomb, David E. Holt and Lori S. Waddell

Anatomy and physiology

A thin serous membrane, the pleura, lines all surfaces within the thoracic cavity.

- The parietal pleura covers the chest wall, diaphragm and mediastinal structures.
- The visceral pleura covers the lungs, including the interlobar fissures.
- The pleural cavity is the potential space between the parietal and visceral pleura, which are normally directly apposed.

The vascular supply to the parietal pleura is via the intercostal, pericardial and diaphragmatic vessels, whereas the visceral pleura is supplied by the pulmonary vasculature.

A small amount of fluid is normally present within the pleural space and lubricates the pleural surfaces, enabling frictionless lung movement. The overall balance of hydrostatic and colloid osmotic pressures in the pleural space under normal physiological conditions results in pleural fluid being produced by the systemic capillaries of the parietal pleura and absorbed by the pulmonary capillaries of the visceral pleura. An important route for pleural fluid removal is via cellular transport mechanisms associated with metabolically active mesothelial cells. The other major drainage route for the pleural cavity is via the rich lymphatic network in the parietal pleura, which empties into the thoracic duct system (TDS).

Inflammation, infection or neoplasia affecting the pleura tends to result in increased pleural fluid production. Drainage of the pleural cavity via the lymphatics is inhibited by thickening of the pleura by neoplastic lymphatic obstruction and by lymphatic hypertension associated with increased venous pressures.

The pressure within the pleural space is approximately 4–6 mmHg below atmospheric pressure. This relatively small pressure difference is sufficient to maintain adequate lung expansion throughout the respiratory cycle. The pressure gradient is greatest during inspiration.

Pleural drainage techniques

Indications for pleural drainage include any situation where fluid or air has accumulated, or is likely to accumulate, in the pleural cavity. The amount of fluid and/or air retrieved is always recorded. The pleural fluid is submitted for laboratory analysis and culture, and this is repeated as required during treatment of the underlying condition.

Thoracocentesis

The simplest and quickest way to remove fluid or air from the pleural cavity is by needle thoracocentesis (see Operative Technique 12.1). Thoracocentesis helps rapid stabilization of an animal in immediate respiratory distress due to pleural space disease and enables diagnostic evaluation of pleural fluid. Butterfly cannulae are well suited for thoracocentesis because they are available in a variety of needle sizes and lengths, are easy to hold and manipulate, and come with pre-attached extension tubing. Over-the-needle catheters may also be used; once the inner stylet is removed, the tip (residing in the pleural cavity) is relatively atraumatic compared with a needle. However, catheters are very flexible and often kink, obstructing drainage.

If possible, a dorsoventral (DV) radiograph or quick thoracic ultrasound examination is recommended prior to thoracocentesis to document the presence of fluid or air and to determine which side might be the most suitable to aspirate first. The stress of radiography can be life-threatening in animals with significant respiratory compromise and in such cases a decision should be made to perform thoracocentesis first on the basis of the clinical findings. A ventrodorsal (VD) position for radiography should not be attempted in these animals as it dramatically reduces the ability to cope with respiratory compromise.

Radiographs are taken after thoracocentesis to document successful aspiration of the pleural cavity and to try to identify an underlying cause, which may have been obscured by the presence of fluid and collapse of the lung lobes.

Complications of thoracocentesis include lung laceration, iatrogenic pneumothorax and haemorrhage, but with attention to careful technique the risks are small (especially when compared with the substantial respiratory relief afforded to the animal). If an animal remains dyspnoeic after successful aspiration of pleural fluid, concurrent lung disease (e.g. neoplasia, pulmonary contusions, pulmonary oedema, pneumonia) or development of a pneumothorax must be suspected.

Chest drains

Placement of a chest drain is indicated when frequent or repeated drainage is required because of ongoing accumulation of fluid or air in the pleural cavity. A chest drain may form part of the definitive treatment plan for a condition such as simple pyothorax. Alternatively, a chest drain may be used for stabilization of an animal prior to definitive surgical treatment, for example in cases of spontaneous pneumothorax (see Chapter 14). Chest drains are also placed at the end of all thoracotomy procedures to enable the lungs to re-expand and allow removal of residual fluid or air in the postoperative period (see Chapter 11).

Three main types of chest drain are available:

- Small-bore, 20 cm long, multi-fenestrated 14 G wire-guided chest drains made of polyurethane can be placed in a closed chest using a modified Seldinger technique under light sedation (with or without the addition of local anaesthetic infiltration and/or a local intercostal nerve block)
- Polyvinylchloride (PVC) chest drains (16–30 Fr) can be used for closed chest insertion. General anaesthesia is recommended for insertion using the trochar or a 'mini-thoracotomy' approach. General anaesthesia removes the stress of manual restraint for these more invasive chest drain placements, allows intubation of the animal (and therefore direct provision of oxygen) and enables manual positive pressure ventilation
- Silicone chest drains (16–30 Fr) are soft and flexible, and are introduced into the open chest using forceps during a thoracotomy procedure. Three to five side holes must be created in the end of the tube with sterile scissors before insertion. The holes should not exceed one-third of the tube diameter or the drain may fracture at the site of the hole.

The optimal size of chest drain is unknown because there have been no studies directly comparing large- and small-bore chest drains. A study evaluating placement of 29 small-bore wire-guided drains into a closed chest for management of pleural disease in dogs and cats showed that they were easy and quick (<10 minutes) to place, were associated with only minor complications and the performance of the chest drain was satisfactory (Valtolina and Adamantos, 2009). It therefore seems sensible to select a small-bore wire-guided chest drain for closed chest insertion unless a specific reason exists (e.g. a chest drain >20 cm in length is needed for a large- or giant-breed dog, or the viscosity of the fluid is expected to be extremely high) to justify the increased pain and invasiveness of placing a large-bore chest drain.

Whichever method of chest drain placement is used, careful preparation of the equipment that may be needed is essential to eliminate delays. Appropriate monitoring of the patient under sedation or anaesthesia is critical. Needle thoracocentesis just prior to sedation or anaesthesia for chest drain placement will minimize respiratory compromise caused by pleural space disease. All chest drains should have a radiopaque marker strip running along their length so that thoracic radiographs taken following placement can document their position. If the most distal side hole includes a portion of the radiopaque marker strip its position can be visualized on the radiograph.

Techniques for placing a closed chest drain are compared in the *BSAVA Manual of Canine and Feline Surgical Principles*. Techniques for placing a 14 G wire-guided tube in a closed chest and a silicone larger-bore tube into an open chest are detailed in Operative Techniques 12.2 and 12.3, respectively.

Intermittent drainage

In most situations intermittent thoracic drainage with a syringe is sufficient. The chest is drained at regular intervals, usually every 1–4 hours, but more frequently if necessary. Minimizing the risk of nosocomial infection is very important and chest drainage is performed using gloves and a sterile syringe. The ends of the bungs are kept sterile during drainage and replaced regularly. A dressing over the chest drain insertion site is changed daily and the thorax is bandaged. The personnel involved in these tasks must wash their hands thoroughly before and after dealing with the patient. Prophylactic antibiotics are not routinely prescribed following placement of a chest drain because this does not reduce the incidence of infection. However, a sample of chest fluid and/or the tip of the chest drain can be submitted for culture at the time of drain removal and any infection identified is treated with an antibiotic course based on the results of sensitivity testing.

Continuous drainage

Continuous drainage of the pleural space is indicated if the rate of fluid or air accumulation is so rapid that frequent intermittent drainage cannot alleviate the animal's respiratory signs. It is also used when continuous subatmospheric pressure is required within the pleural space to enable sealing of a small airway leak. Continuous drainage is best provided by means of an underwater seal, which may be attached to a suction device. Various commercial systems are available that comprise three connected chambers (Figure 12.1):

- The collection chamber acts as a reservoir for suctioned chest fluid
- The underwater seal chamber (water trap) enables unidirectional removal of air from the chest
- The vacuum regulator chamber (suction control) limits the amount of pressure that can be generated by the suction device. Negative pressure exerted on the pleural cavity by the suction device is limited to <10–20 cmH$_2$O.

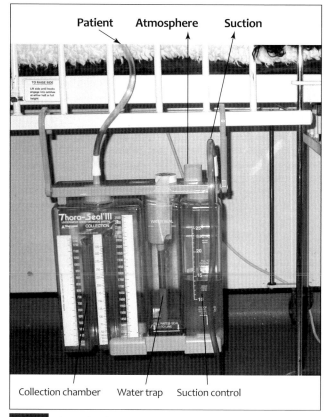

12.1 Three-chamber underwater seal system.

Continuous monitoring of the animal is mandatory when using a continuous drainage system because unnoticed disconnection of the system could rapidly lead to a life-threatening pneumothorax.

Drain removal

Chest drains may be removed when there is no air leakage and the amount of fluid being produced has reduced to a consistently small volume (ideally <2 ml fluid/kg/day). In practice the amount of fluid produced is highly variable and the presence of a chest drain provokes an inflammatory response, which means that fluid in the pleural space rarely resolves completely until the chest drain is removed. In animals that have undergone a simple thoracotomy procedure, this may mean that the chest drain is removed within hours of placement, but in other situations chest drains may remain in place for several days.

Complications

Common complications associated with chest drains include:

- Leaks around the tube due to a wide subcutaneous tunnel
- Leaks at improperly secured connectors
- Backing out of the tube due to a poorly placed Chinese fingertrap suture.

Inadequate drainage can also be a problem and may require slight repositioning of the tube (commonly the tip of the tube is too far cranial in the chest and is obstructed by mediastinal tissues), or the tube may be blocked and require flushing. The longer a chest drain is in place, the greater is the risk of ascending nosocomial infection (pyothorax); everything possible must be done to keep the bandage, tube connections and the animal's environment clean. Lung injury is possible if excessive negative pressure is exerted via the chest drain (using either a syringe or a suction device). No more than 5–10 ml of vacuum in a syringe is recommended when draining the thorax. Re-expansion pulmonary oedema may occur in chronic disease conditions when the lungs are adapted to a contracted state and are unable to cope with rapid and complete evacuation of the pleural cavity. If re-expansion oedema is considered a possibility, the chest should be drained in small incremental stages over at least 24 hours. Occasionally, the presence of the chest drain can cause phrenic nerve irritation, Horner's syndrome or cardiac arrhythmias.

Pleural disease

Pathological or traumatic conditions affecting the pleural space produce respiratory compromise through the accumulation of air (*pneumothorax*), fluid (*pleural effusion*) or both. Soft tissue can also occupy the pleural space, such as abdominal organs protruding through a diaphragmatic rupture. Although unilateral pleural effusion or pneumothorax is occasionally seen, both are commonly bilateral in dogs and cats, suggesting that the mediastinum is easily disrupted or functionally incomplete. By extension, it is often assumed that drainage of one hemithorax also provides drainage of the other side, but this is not always the case.

Clinical signs

The respiratory signs caused by pleural disease are all secondary to reduced lung expansion (and tidal volume), which initially results in rapid shallow breathing. The dyspnoea may also be characterized by prolonged inspiration and increased abdominal effort. Ultimately, the animal may exhibit a 'sprung' or distended chest and position itself with the elbows abducted and neck extended to minimize any resistance to breathing. If hypoxia becomes severe the mucous membranes can become cyanotic.

Thoracic auscultation reveals diminished lung and heart sounds. With pleural effusion, lung sounds are absent ventrally but often still present dorsally. Percussion of the thorax produces a dull hyporesonant sound in the presence of pleural fluid and a hyper-resonant 'ping' if pleural air is present. In a series of 81 dogs with pleural and mediastinal effusions, tachypnoea and/or dyspnoea was present in 91% and muffled heart sounds in 41% (Mellanby *et al.*, 2002).

The degree of respiratory compromise is generally proportional to the volume of fluid or air within the pleural cavity and the rate of accumulation. Fluid that accumulates gradually may reach a large volume and produce only subtle clinical signs. Once a certain volume is exceeded, critical respiratory compromise exists and rapid decompensation can occur if the patient is not handled extremely cautiously. In a series of 82 cats with pleural effusion, most were presented with acute disease but the duration of clinical signs ranged from <12 hours to >12 months (mean 11.2 days) (Davies and Forrester, 1996).

Depending on the underlying cause, additional findings in patients with pleural disease may include coughing, pyrexia, depression, anorexia, weight loss, arrhythmias, murmurs, ascites, lymphadenopathy, pale mucous membranes and chorioretinitis.

Pneumothorax

Pneumothorax may develop following rupture of the oesophagus, chest wall, lung, bronchi or trachea. As air enters the pleural space it prevents normal lung expansion during inspiration. If the site of air leakage acts as a one-way valve, a tension pneumothorax develops, creating supraphysiological pleural pressures that dramatically compress the lungs and great veins. Causes of pneumothorax may be grouped into those of traumatic origin and those arising spontaneously; the aetiology and management of these conditions is discussed in Chapter 14.

Diagnostic imaging

The radiographic appearance of pneumothorax is characterized by retraction of the lungs away from the thoracic wall, resulting in a radiolucent space between the lung and thoracic wall that does not contain lung markings. The lungs have increased opacity because they are compressed by pleural air. Separation of the heart from the sternum is commonly seen on a lateral radiograph and is due to lack of underlying inflated lungs, which results in displacement of the heart from its normal ventral position into the dependent hemithorax (Figure 12.2).

With tension pneumothorax, the increased pleural pressure results in progressive caudal displacement of the diaphragm, and the lungs may become dramatically compressed against the midline. On a lateral radiograph the diaphragm appears 'flattened'; on DV views the costal attachments of the diaphragm may become visible. In unilateral tension pneumothorax the mediastinum is shifted towards the unaffected side (Figure 12.3).

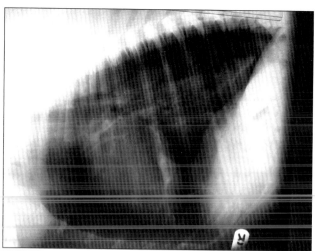

12.2 Pneumothorax in a dog. This lateral radiograph demonstrates elevation of the heart from the sternum. The lungs are retracted away from the thoracic wall and partially collapsed.

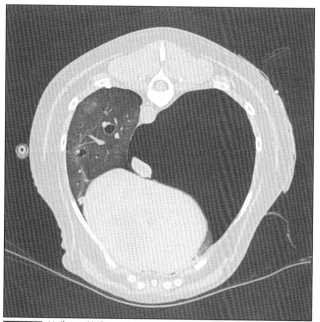

12.3 Unilateral left tension pneumothorax in a dog. This transverse computed tomographic image demonstrates a large volume of air in the left pleural cavity causing almost complete collapse of the left lung lobes, a right mediastinal shift and caudal displacement of the diaphragm: 1.5 litres of air was subsequently drained by thoracocentesis from the left pleural cavity.

It is important to be able to differentiate quickly between varying degrees of simple pneumothorax and tension pneumothorax because the latter is rapidly fatal if left untreated and warrants immediate thoracocentesis.

Recently, the use of thoracic ultrasonography for the diagnosis of pneumothorax has become more common. The tFAST (thoracic focused assessment with sonography for trauma) technique can be used to assess the presence of either pleural effusion or a pneumothorax. Pneumothorax is diagnosed by the absence of the 'glide sign', defined as the lack of the normal dynamic interface between lung margins gliding along the thoracic wall during respiration. Concurrent thoracic trauma can be diagnosed by the presence of pleural or pericardial fluid or the presence of a 'step sign', defined as an abnormal glide sign. A step sign is a glide sign that has deviated from the normal linear continuity of the pulmonary–pleural interface, and is assumed to represent concurrent thoracic injury (Lisciandro et al., 2008).

An underlying cause for the pneumothorax (e.g. a pulmonary mass) is most easily seen on radiographs after drainage of the pleural air and re-expansion of the lungs. Other imaging modalities, such as computed tomography (CT) or magnetic resonance imaging (MRI), may be useful for identifying an underlying cause that is not apparent on radiographs. CT or MRI can help construct a surgical plan by demonstrating the location and extent of a lesion, as well as the involvement of other important structures. However, a retrospective study in which dogs with spontaneous pneumothorax were investigated by CT found that the sensitivity and positive predictive value of CT for bulla detection were low, and CT was of questionable utility (Reetz et al., 2013).

Pleural effusions

Pleural effusions develop if the rate of pleural fluid production increases and/or the rate of pleural drainage decreases or is overwhelmed. The fluid that accumulates is not necessarily of pleural origin, for example, haemorrhage, chylothorax or an effusion across the capsule of an incarcerated or twisted organ. Regardless of underlying aetiology, pleural effusion inhibits lung expansion.

Diagnostic imaging

Thoracic radiography is a useful method of visualizing pleural fluid and can demonstrate smaller amounts of pleural fluid than can be detected clinically. A DV view is appropriate for initial 'screening' of the dyspnoeic patient; this view can be supplemented with lateral views as necessary. Both right and left lateral views may be useful. Although a VD radiograph is more sensitive than a DV radiograph for small volumes of pleural fluid, positioning an animal that has a large amount of pleural fluid for this view can cause decompensation and respiratory arrest.

Free pleural fluid is seen surrounding lung lobes that have retracted from the chest wall, outlining the ventral borders of the lungs and producing a 'scalloped' appearance on a lateral radiograph (Figure 12.4). Pleural fluid may also obscure the cardiac silhouette and the diaphragmatic outline. The cause of the pleural effusion (e.g. mass, lung lobe torsion, diaphragmatic rupture, congestive heart failure) may be apparent on initial radiography, but such lesions are more likely to be appreciated on radiographs taken following removal of the pleural fluid.

Ultrasound imaging can detect small amounts of pleural fluid and is useful for evaluating underlying heart disease and mediastinal masses. Pleural fluid acts as an acoustic

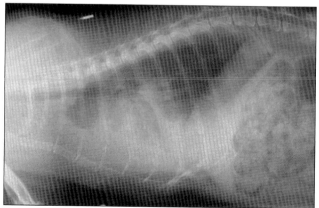

12.4 Pleural effusion in a cat. This lateral radiograph demonstrates outlining of the ventral lung borders by fluid. The cardiac silhouette is also partially obscured.

window, enhancing the visualization of intrathoracic structures. Ultrasonography requires minimal restraint and is particularly useful for patients that are likely to decompensate during positioning for radiography. Ultrasonography can be used to guide thoracocentesis, as well as aspiration of an underlying intrathoracic mass or pericardial effusion.

CT, as for pneumothorax, is extremely useful for investigation of the underlying aetiology, staging neoplasia and/or informing the surgical plan.

Types and causes

Pleural effusions are classified into categories based on the gross appearance, protein content, specific gravity, total nucleated cell count, cytological characteristics of the cells and culture results (see the *BSAVA Manual of Canine and Feline Clinical Pathology*). Pleural fluid should be submitted for both aerobic and anaerobic culture. Analysis of biochemical parameters, such as levels of triglyceride and cholesterol, is also indicated if the effusion is suspected to be chylous. These categories give a useful indication of possible aetiologies for the effusion, although in practice there is considerable overlap (Figure 12.5).

A wide range of diseases may be associated with pleural effusions. In dogs with pleural and mediastinal effusions, the most common underlying disease identified was pyothorax (Mellanby *et al.*, 2002). Other common conditions included idiopathic pericardial effusion, cranial mediastinal mass, idiopathic chylothorax, secondary lung metastases and dilated cardiomyopathy. In cats, the most common underlying diseases associated with pleural effusions have been suggested to be pyothorax, mediastinal lymphoma, hypertrophic cardiomyopathy and feline infectious peritonitis (FIP) (Davies and Forrester, 1996).

The presence of a peritoneal effusion in conjunction with a pleural effusion is relatively rare. In a study that looked at aspects of simultaneous pleural and peritoneal effusions in 48 cases, the presence of a double effusion, irrespective of the underlying disease condition, indicated a poor prognosis and was associated with a greater risk of death when compared with a similar condition without a double effusion (Steyn and Wittum, 1993).

Transudates: These are the result of a disturbance in the overall balance of hydrostatic and colloid osmotic forces governing the formation and absorption of fluid in the pleural space. A major cause of a true transudate is hypoalbuminaemia that results in a decreased intravascular oncotic pressure. Usually the albumin level must be <0.15 g/l to result in transudation (Hackett, 1999). Hypoalbuminaemia may be caused by a protein-losing enteropathy or nephropathy, hepatic disease or marked loss of inflammatory fluid through a wound or into a body cavity. Animals with hypoalbuminaemia may also have ascites or subcutaneous oedema.

Cardiac disease can affect the formation and absorption of fluid in the pleural space by altering pulmonary and systemic capillary pressures. Systemic venous hypertension resulting from right-sided or bilateral congestive heart failure may result in accumulation of pleural transudate and is accompanied by other signs of cardiac disease.

Lung lobe torsion or a diaphragmatic rupture (see Chapter 17) can obstruct venous and lymphatic drainage, resulting in leakage of variable types of fluid through the organ capsule into the pleural space. Lung lobe torsion is not common in dogs, although Afghan Hounds and Pugs appear to be predisposed. Lung lobe torsion may occur as a primary entity, particularly in deep-chested dogs, but may also occur secondarily in any animal with a pleural effusion. Therefore, it may be difficult to determine whether the pleural effusion or the lung lobe torsion occurred first. Other underlying causes for the pleural effusion should be ruled out. Lung lobe torsion has been associated with trauma, chylothorax, pulmonary neoplasia, respiratory disease and thoracic surgery. The right middle lung lobe and the right cranial lung lobe are most frequently affected. Radiography after pleural drainage usually reveals diffuse consolidation of a lung lobe and possibly altered orientation or abrupt termination of the lobar bronchi. Complete lobectomy of the involved lobe is indicated and the pedicle is clamped before the lobe is untwisted (see Chapter 14). The prognosis for dogs with lung lobe torsion following surgery is fair to guarded (Neath *et al.*, 2000).

Effusion category	Gross appearance	Protein content (g/l)	Total nucleated cell count (x 10⁹/l)	Cell cytology	Possible aetiologies
Transudate	Colourless or very pale yellow	<10	<1	Mesothelial cells, macrophages, lymphocytes	Hypoalbuminaemia, heart failure
Modified transudate	Clear or slightly turbid; yellow/pink to orange/reddish	<30	<5	Mesothelial cells, macrophages, lymphocytes, non-degenerate neutrophils	Right-sided heart disease, lung lobe torsion, diaphragmatic rupture, neoplasia
Non-septic exudate	Clear or turbid; yellow to orange/reddish	>30	>25	Mesothelial cells, macrophages, lymphocytes, neutrophils	Feline infectious peritonitis, neoplasia, diaphragmatic rupture, lung lobe torsion
Septic exudate	Turbid, granular; yellow/orange to brown/green; may be foul smelling	>30	>50	Degenerate neutrophils with intracellular bacteria, macrophages, mesothelial cells	Pyothorax
Neoplastic	Variable	30–80	Variable	Possible exfoliated neoplastic cells, mesothelial cells, macrophages, neutrophils	Primary and metastatic thoracic neoplasia
Haemorrhagic	Dark red blood	40–80	>3	Red blood cells, white blood cells (similar to peripheral blood)	Trauma, coagulopathy, lung lobe torsion, neoplasia
Chylous	Milky/opaque; white or pink	30–85	Variable	Small lymphocytes, ± non-degenerate neutrophils, macrophages	Chylothorax (idiopathic or associated with trauma, neoplasia, heart disease, vena cava thrombosis, lung lobe torsion)

12.5 Common causes of pleural effusions in dogs and cats, categorized by fluid characteristics.

Non-septic exudates: These are characterized by high protein levels. A major cause of this type of effusion is FIP; both pleural and peritoneal effusions often occur in this condition. A diagnosis of FIP is strongly supported by finding a globulin concentration >32% of the total protein (TP) concentration in the effusion. If the albumin component is >48% or the albumin:globulin ratio of the effusion is >0.81, FIP is unlikely (Lappin, 1998). Serum hyperproteinaemia, with or without hypoalbuminaemia, is also a common finding.

Septic exudates: These may be caused by: penetrating thoracic injury; perforation of mediastinal structures or a lung abscess; migrating foreign bodies; haematogenous spread; or iatrogenic contamination (see Pyothorax).

Haemorrhagic effusion: A major cause of haemorrhage into the pleural cavity is thoracic trauma, such as fractured ribs or pulmonary parenchymal lacerations. A small amount of haemorrhage is common after thoracic surgery and this may be marked if an intercostal vessel has been punctured during closure. An intrathoracic tumour or a coagulopathy (e.g. anticoagulant rodenticide toxicity) may result in spontaneous haemorrhage into the pleural cavity. Dyspnoea is usually relieved by thoracocentesis. Depending on the severity of blood loss, patients may require supportive treatment with fluid therapy and possibly a blood transfusion. Animals that have anticoagulant rodenticide toxicity also require treatment with vitamin K as well as active clotting factors from fresh whole blood or fresh frozen plasma.

Chylous effusions: These are the result of leakage of chyle from an abnormal TDS and may be primary idiopathic or secondary to mediastinal neoplasia, heart disease, diaphragmatic rupture, lung lobe torsion or other conditions. Chylothorax is a very challenging condition to manage (see below).

Neoplasia: Primary and metastatic thoracic neoplasia may produce variable types of pleural effusion by a number of different mechanisms, such as inflammation of the pleura, haemorrhage and obstruction of lymphatic drainage. Cytological examination will reveal neoplastic cells in approximately 50% of animals with a neoplastic pleural effusion; thus, an absence of neoplastic cells on cytology does not rule out neoplastic disease. Mediastinal lymphosarcoma may exfoliate lymphoblasts into pleural fluid. Mesothelioma (neoplasia of the pleura) is usually characterized by a severe pleural effusion and may also affect the pericardium, causing a pericardial effusion. It is particularly difficult to differentiate between reactive and malignant mesothelial cells on cytology. Thoracoscopic exploration and mediastinal/pleural biopsy is a reliable and effective means of diagnosing mesothelioma that avoids an unnecessary thoracotomy.

Pyothorax

Pyothorax is characterized by the accumulation of septic purulent fluid within the pleural space. Other terms that have been used to describe pyothorax include empyema and purulent pleuritis. It has been described in both dogs and cats, but is more common in cats.

Aetiology

Dogs: The most common bacterial isolates from dogs with pyothorax are the anaerobes *Peptostreptococcus*,

Bacteroides, *Fusobacterium* and *Porphyromonas* and the aerobes *Actinomyces*, *Pasteurella*, *Escherichia coli* and *Streptococcus* (Walker *et al.*, 2000). These bacterial isolates are similar to those identified from cats, with the addition of *Streptococcus* and the enteric *E. coli*. In dogs, reported causes of infection include migrating foreign bodies such as grass awns, penetrating wounds to the chest, neck or mediastinum, oesophageal perforations, lung parasites, bacterial pneumonia with abscessation and rupture, haematogenous or lymphatic spread from other septic foci, spread from cervical or lumbar discospondylitis, neoplasia with secondary abscessation and iatrogenic contamination from thoracocentesis or thoracotomy. The hunting and working breeds of dogs are over-represented in most retrospective studies, and aspiration of grass awns with subsequent migration through the respiratory tract is thought to play an important role in the development of pyothorax in these breeds.

Cats: The most common bacterial isolates from cats with pyothorax are the anaerobes *Peptostreptococcus*, *Bacteroides*, *Fusobacterium*, *Porphyromonas* and *Prevotella* and the aerobes *Pasteurella* and *Actinomyces* (Walker *et al.*, 2000). Mixed populations of bacteria are often cultured from both cats and dogs. The most likely sources of the bacteria that cause pyothorax in cats are from the oral cavity of other cats, transmitted through bite wounds to the chest, or environmental contamination from penetrating thoracic injuries. Other possibilities include bacterial pneumonia leading to lung abscessation and rupture, rupture or perforation of the oesophagus, trachea or bronchi, migrating foreign bodies (grass awns) or lung parasites, or iatrogenic contamination from thoracocentesis or thoracotomy. Cats from multi-cat households have been found to be at an increased risk for the development of pyothorax (Waddell *et al.*, 2002).

Once bacterial infection enters the pleural cavity, the release of inflammatory mediators causes increased permeability of the endothelial lining of the pleural capillaries and impairment of lymphatic outflow. This results in accumulation of fluid, protein and inflammatory cells in the pleural space. Increased protein concentration in the pleural fluid causes an increased oncotic pressure, favouring additional fluid movement out of the capillaries and into the pleural space.

Clinical signs

Presentation of the cat or dog with pyothorax is often delayed for weeks to months after the inciting incident. Penetrating thoracic injuries, such as bite wounds, are often healed by the time respiratory compromise develops, making diagnosis of the underlying cause difficult or impossible. Common clinical signs in cats include respiratory distress, depression, lethargy, pallor, anorexia and pain. In dogs, exercise intolerance, respiratory distress, reluctance to lie down, anorexia, lethargy and cough are common. Clinical presentation can vary widely, from mild respiratory signs to collapse from severe septic shock.

Physical examination

Findings usually include varying degrees of respiratory distress: increased respiratory effort, tachypnoea, dull lung sounds ventrally with harsh sounds dorsally and orthopnoea (breathing with the head and neck extended and elbows abducted, and remaining standing or in sternal recumbency) may all be present. Signs of septic shock, such as hyperthermia or hypothermia, tachycardia (or, in cats, bradycardia), injected or pale mucous membranes and bounding or weak pulses may be present. Recent weight loss may be reported by the owner and a poor body condition may be noted. Additional findings may include depression and dehydration. Hypersalivation has been reported in cats and was found to be associated with a poorer outcome (Waddell *et al.*, 2002).

Diagnostic imaging

Radiography: Thoracic radiography is very useful for confirming the presence of pleural effusion (see above), but care must be taken with patients in respiratory distress. If respiratory compromise is severe, the patient will not be able to tolerate restraint in lateral or dorsal recumbency for thoracic radiography, and thoracocentesis should be performed as both a diagnostic test and immediate stabilizing therapy. Thoracic ultrasonography can be used instead to confirm the presence of fluid and help guide thoracocentesis. Thoracic radiography is often more helpful in searching for underlying causes once the pleural effusion has been removed and the pulmonary parenchyma can be better visualized. It may also be useful in determining whether disease is bilateral or unilateral, although careful auscultation and percussion of the chest should determine this. The majority of cats and dogs show bilateral effusions; occasionally, a patient has unilateral disease, which may be secondary to a more localized process or the ability to wall off a particular area of the pleural space (Figure 12.6). Cats and dogs have both been reported to have an anatomically complete mediastinum but, because of the frequency of bilateral thoracic effusions, it seems unlikely that the mediastinum is intact in most cases. There may be individual anatomical variability in the completeness of the mediastinum in both species.

Ultrasonography: Thoracic ultrasonography can identify abscesses or masses in the pulmonary parenchyma or mediastinum, and can be used to help locate fluid for thoracocentesis, particularly if the fluid is pocketed.

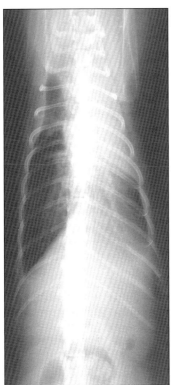

12.6 Unilateral pyothorax in a cat, shown on a ventrodorsal radiograph.

Thoracocentesis

Thoracocentesis (see above and Operative Technique 12.1) is indicated as soon as a strong suspicion of pleural effusion is present. If the fluid is caused by a septic process, it is often thick, opaque and foul-smelling and may be flocculant. Samples should be evaluated using biochemistry, cytology, cell counts and culture (see the *BSAVA Manual of Canine and Feline Clinical Pathology*).

Cytology should look for the presence of neutrophils, which are often degenerate and show signs of toxic change. Bacteria, both intracellular and extracellular, are usually present (Figure 12.7). However, the absence of bacteria does not exclude pyothorax from the differential list, especially if the patient has already been treated with antibiotics. Whenever an inflammatory exudate is present, the fluid should be submitted for aerobic and anaerobic culture and sensitivity testing. Sulphur granules, which are actually macroaggregates of bacteria, may also be seen in the effusion with *Actinomyces* and *Nocardia* infections. If the pyothorax has been chronic, increasing numbers of macrophages and plasma cells may be seen in the fluid.

A complete blood count often shows a marked leucocytosis, with or without an increased number of band neutrophils and toxic change. In severe cases, a leucopenia and degenerative left shift may be found. Anaemia may be present if the pyothorax is chronic.

Biochemical results may be normal or may show changes consistent with sepsis, including hypoalbuminaemia, hypoglycaemia and increased alanine aminotransferase and total bilirubin: the last two are consistent with cholestasis. Changes consistent with dehydration and haemoconcentration are seen in some patients.

Retrovirus testing is indicated for cats diagnosed with pyothorax; although not thought to be an underlying cause, positive retroviral status may certainly complicate treatment and increase the risk of recurrence.

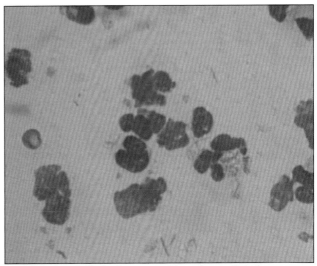

12.7 Pleural effusion from a cat with pyothorax. Note the degenerative neutrophils, and intra- and extracellular bacteria.

Emergency treatment

Stabilization of the patient with pyothorax presenting in respiratory distress should include oxygen supplementation, minimal handling and stress, thoracocentesis and intravenous catheter placement. Fluid therapy, including shock boluses, may be indicated depending on the patient's cardiovascular status at the time of presentation.

Broad-spectrum antibiotics should be administered intravenously as soon as possible, especially if the patient presents in septic shock.

Medical management

Antimicrobials: Broad-spectrum antimicrobials active against Gram-positive, Gram-negative and anaerobic bacteria are administered until culture and sensitivity results are available. A broad-spectrum approach is appropriate because of the frequency with which dogs and cats are infected with a mixed population of bacteria. Antibiotics are administered intravenously whilst the patient is critical, but can be administered by the oral route once the patient has been stabilized and culture and sensitivity results are available. Appropriate antibiotic therapy should be continued for 1–2 months following discharge from the hospital.

Fluid therapy: This should be continued at maintenance rates or higher, depending on the amount of pleural effusion that is produced. Keeping the patient adequately hydrated is essential in maintaining the effusion at a consistency that can be easily aspirated via thoracocentesis or thoracostomy tubes. These patients often become hypoalbuminaemic and may benefit from appropriate colloidal support.

Drainage: Drainage of pleural effusion is one of the mainstays of therapy for patients with pyothorax. This can be accomplished by intermittent thoracocentesis or by placement of thoracostomy tubes, with intermittent aspiration or continuous drainage (see above). Thoracostomy tubes are preferred because they allow more complete drainage of the thoracic cavity and are usually less stressful than the restraint required for multiple thoracocentesis procedures. Thoracostomy tubes are best placed with the patient under general anaesthesia, so initial stabilization with fluid therapy and pleural drainage by thoracocentesis should occur before anaesthetizing what can be very critical patients. Bilateral thoracostomy tubes are indicated unless the patient only has a unilateral effusion, although success has been reported with unilateral drainage in dogs (Johnson and Martin, 2007).

Lavage: Lavage of the thoracic cavity has been recommended by many authors. Warm physiological saline or other balanced electrolyte solutions can be used at 20 ml/kg, instilled over 10–15 minutes, q6–24h. Addition of antibiotics or other medications, including chymotrypsin, streptokinase and heparin, has been recommended in various reports. Antibiotic therapy is most useful when administered intravenously. A recent retrospective study found that there was increased survival in dogs treated medically if they received pleural lavage with 0.9% saline or lactated Ringer's solution at 10–20 ml/kg, and also increased survival if they received pleural lavage with heparin (10 IU/ml) compared with lavage without heparin (Boothe *et al.*, 2010). However, this was a retrospective study with a number of limitations, so it is difficult to make recommendations based on this report alone. A prospective randomized study is needed to determine the true value of these therapies. Lavage can be performed at the time of placement of the chest tube if the pleural effusion is too thick to aspirate easily through the tube. Risks of continuing to lavage the chest tube during hospitalization include placing a large volume of fluid into the chest without the ability to retrieve it and the potential introduction of a nosocomial infection resistant to the antimicrobials that the patient is already receiving.

Cats: In cats, medical treatment including thoracostomy tubes, intravenous fluids and intravenous antibiotic therapy is usually successful. If a cat is not responding to medical therapy, or if an obvious surgical lesion such as an abscessed lung lobe or foreign body is identified, surgical intervention is indicated. Failure of medical management can be defined as the inability to aspirate effusion through properly placed and functional thoracostomy tubes or failure of the effusion to resolve over a reasonable period of time (usually a week).

Surgical treatment

In one study, dogs were shown to have improved outcomes with surgical intervention for the treatment of pyothorax, and surgery should be considered sooner in this species than in cats, without first waiting for a response to medical therapy (Rooney and Monnet, 2002). However, further recent studies have shown excellent outcomes in dogs without surgical intervention (Johnson and Martin, 2007) or failed to support the finding that surgical treatment is superior to medical management (Boothe *et al.*, 2010).

Surgical treatment requires a complete exploratory thoracotomy. The goal is to identify and remove any necrotic tissue or foreign material, as well as to allow complete lavage of the thoracic cavity. Samples for aerobic and anaerobic culture are obtained at surgery. Options for surgical therapy include thoracoscopy (see below), median sternotomy and, occasionally, lateral thoracotomy (see Operative Technique 11.1). Advantages of thoracotomy include full exploration of the thoracic cavity and removal of all exudate from the pleural space with lavage. Disadvantages include the increased cost and length of stay in the hospital, the pain associated with the thoracotomy and the risks associated with general anaesthesia.

Median sternotomy (see Chapter 11) allows a full evaluation of the right and left hemithoraces. The lungs, pericardium, trachea, mediastinum, pleural surfaces and lymph nodes can all be evaluated for signs of abscessation, bleeding, inflammation or leakage of air. Adhesions of fibrous tissue may need to be broken down to allow complete evaluation, especially when looking for a possible foreign body. Any necrotic, abscessed or severely inflamed tissue should be resected, including lung lobes, lymph nodes, mediastinum and pericardium. A lateral thoracotomy is only indicated if the inflammatory process is limited to one hemithorax. Occasionally, the origin of a unilateral pyothorax can be isolated to a single abscessed lung lobe or foreign body, in which case a lateral thoracotomy may be preferred (Figure 12.8). When the cause of the pyothorax cannot be identified or localized to one side of the chest, a median sternotomy is the approach of choice. Even with surgical exploration of the thoracic cavity, the underlying cause of the pyothorax is often not identified. Thoracostomy tubes, either unilateral or bilateral as indicated, should be placed at the time of the surgery.

Thoracoscopy is a minimally invasive surgical procedure that can be used to explore the thoracic cavity. This technique has been recommended for assistance in treatment of pyothorax in humans and has resulted in shorter hospital stays when compared with thoracostomy tube drainage alone, thoracostomy tube drainage with fibrinolytics, and thoracotomy. The role of thoracoscopy has not been clearly defined for veterinary patients, but as the technique becomes more commonly used similar treatment benefits may be identified.

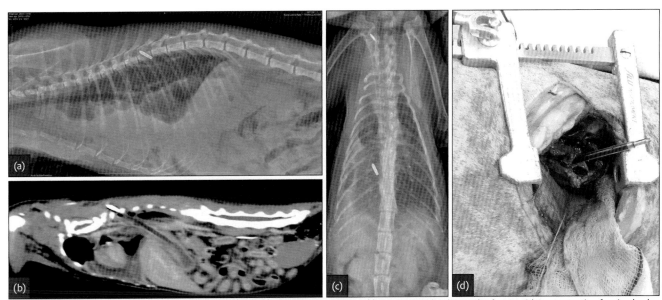

12.8 Lateral (a) radiograph and (b) sagittal computed tomographic image and (c) dorsoventral radiograph of a cat with a penetrating foreign body in the distal oesophagus removed via a right 10th intercostal thoracotomy. (d) The preoperative imaging was critical in determining the tract of the foreign body and therefore whether a lateral thoracotomy approach would be preferable to a median sternotomy.

Postoperative care: Animals with pyothorax require intensive care and monitoring, especially for the first 24–48 hours after surgery. Septic shock and systemic inflammatory response syndrome may develop. Fluid therapy in the postoperative phase is very important and often consists of crystalloids, colloids and blood products. Vasopressors may be needed to treat refractory hypotension once volume expansion has been accomplished. Respiratory, acid–base and electrolyte abnormalities should be evaluated and treated as needed. These patients are at high risk for the development of disseminated intravascular coagulation and need to have their coagulation parameters monitored closely. Daily evaluation of the complete blood count and cytology of the pleural effusion are necessary.

Prognosis

A poor prognosis and frequent recurrence have been reported in both cats and dogs. Many patients may be euthanased on the basis of these reports and because of owners' financial constraints, thereby perpetuating the poor prognosis. In cats and dogs that receive aggressive medical and surgical therapy, as deemed appropriate, survival is >50%, with a recurrence rate of <10%. Many of the patients with pyothorax that do not survive either die naturally or are euthanased within the first 24 hours of presentation; the survival rate increases significantly for patients that are alive 24 hours after admission (Rooney and Monnet, 2002; Waddell *et al.*, 2002).

Chylothorax

Chylothorax is an accumulation of lymphatic fluid leaking from the TDS into the pleural space. Thoracic duct fluid has three main sources: lymph from the intestines; lymph of hepatic origin; and lymph from the hindquarters. The term 'chyle' refers to lymphatic fluid drained from the intestines. It is the high fat content of intestinal lymph that gives chylous fluid its milky appearance. This fat is mainly in the form of chylomicrons, which are aggregates of triglycerides, phospholipids, lipoproteins and cholesterol, formed in the intestinal epithelial cells from dietary

fats that have been digested and absorbed. Once formed, the chylomicrons are secreted into intestinal lymphatics that drain into the cisterna chyli and thence into the TDS. Thoracic duct lymph also contains fluid and proteins similar in type and concentration to those of plasma. A large amount of fluid and protein leaks out of normal capillary beds continuously, and the TDS provides a major pathway for the return of fluid and protein from the interstitial space to the circulation. The proteins, including albumin and various globulins, are important in maintaining normal colloidal osmotic pressure and immune function, and in the transport of protein-bound hormones and drugs. Thoracic duct lymph also contains electrolytes and trace minerals. The main cellular component of lymph is the small lymphocyte.

Thoracic duct system

In both dogs and cats the anatomy of the 'thoracic duct' is quite variable, both in location and in the number of ducts present. The thoracic duct is probably more appropriately referred to as the 'thoracic duct system' (TDS).

Dogs: In dogs the TDS generally begins its course on the right side of the mediastinum dorsal to the aorta. In a study of 20 dogs, only one dog had a single vessel in the caudal mediastinum; five had two collateral vessels and 14 had three or more vessels (Kagen and Breznock, 1979). Most of the collateral vessels were in close relation. However, in some dogs, portions of the vessel system crossed the midline in widely distinct areas (over three vertebral spaces), creating a situation where there were lymphatic vessels on both the left and the right sides of the caudal mediastinum at the same time. In many dogs, the TDS crosses the midline from right to left between the levels of the fifth and 11th thoracic vertebrae. In others, the TDS remains right-sided and enters veins or lymph nodes in the right hemithorax. Many normal dogs develop a single lymphatic vessel in the cranial mediastinum that ends at the junction of the jugular and brachiocephalic veins with the cranial vena cava. Other dogs have multiple lymphatic vessels, which send some terminal branches to mediastinal lymph nodes.

Cats: In the normal cat, the TDS consists of a single duct on the left side of the caudal mediastinum. In the middle of the mediastinum there are multiple ducts in a vast majority of cats. In the cranial mediastinum, the duct is on the left side of the oesophagus in 90% of cases and terminates at the jugulosubclavian angle, the left external jugular vein or the brachiocephalic vein. These variations in anatomy have important implications for the surgical approach when considering thoracic duct ligation.

Aetiology

Chylothorax remains an enigmatic disease in many dogs and cats because of the difficulty in identifying a specific cause and in defining an effective treatment. Previously, many cases of chylothorax were presumed to be traumatic in origin, with chylous fluid thought to leak from a ruptured TDS. However, many cases had no history of major trauma, and experimentally the TDS in normal dogs heals rapidly after deliberate transection. Congenital cases have been described but these are also rare.

In the majority of dogs and cats, chylothorax is associated with dilatation of the TDS (lymphangiectasia) and leakage. Experimentally, ligating the cranial vena cava close to the right atrium can produce TDS lymphangiectasia, so conditions that increase pressure in the cranial vena cava have the potential to cause chylothorax. TDS lymphangiiectasia and leakage can also occur secondary to physical obstruction caused by neoplasia. Hence, chylothorax has been associated with:

- Congenital heart disease (e.g. tetralogy of Fallot, tricuspid dysplasia, cor triatriatum dexter)
- Heart base tumours
- Cardiomyopathies
- Mediastinal lymphosarcoma or thymoma
- Foreign body or fungal granulomas
- Heartworm disease
- Cranial vena caval thrombosis.

Chylothorax can also occur associated with more generalized lymphatic abnormalities such as intestinal lymphangiectasia and lymphangioleiomyomatosis.

The role of the pericardium in the aetiology of chylothorax has also received attention. Theoretically, restriction of the right atrium and ventricle by restrictive or effusive pericardial diseases could increase the pressure in the cranial vena cava and contribute to chylothorax. Whilst there are many dogs with significant pericardial effusions that have no associated chylothorax, pericardectomy is reported as an effective treatment for chylothorax in some cases.

The 'cause and effect' association between lung lobe torsion and chylothorax remains unclear. Some authors list lung lobe torsion as a potential cause of chylothorax. Whilst torsion of the right middle lung lobe could be argued to cause obstruction of, or increased pressure in, the TDS, it is equally possible that a chylous effusion may 'float' and mobilize the right middle lung lobe, facilitating torsion. Regardless of these arguments, it is important to realize that these two conditions can occur simultaneously.

In many instances, a search for diseases underlying chylothorax yields no definitive answer. The condition in these animals is thus classified as 'idiopathic'. Some of these cases may eventually reveal an identifiable underlying cause, such as microscopic neoplasia obstructing the TDS, which is undetectable without a surgical or post-mortem biopsy. In spite of these frustrations, the investigation for underlying causes is important when considering both an animal's prognosis and treatment. Identification of an underlying cause, such as heart disease or cranial mediastinal lymphoma, suggests a treatment plan that may resolve the chylothorax without the need for surgery. In idiopathic cases, the clinician is left to treat the consequences of the disease (i.e. the chylous pleural effusion) rather than its root cause.

Clinical signs

Chylothorax can affect any breed of dog or cat. However, Afghan Hounds and Shiba Inu dogs, and Oriental breeds of cat, such as Himalayan and Siamese, may be predisposed. Presentation to a veterinary surgeon (veterinarian) is usually precipitated by either dyspnoea, associated with the chylous pleural effusion, or persistent coughing. Coughing may be due to the pleural effusion or caused by a disease process underlying the chylothorax, such as cardiomyopathy or thoracic neoplasia. Other clinical signs can include anorexia, lethargy and weight loss. There is a great variability in the duration of clinical signs recognized by owners.

Physical examination

Findings usually include an increased respiratory rate and variably muffled lung and heart sounds. Poor body condition may reflect debilitation associated with the loss of fats and proteins into the pleural space.

Diagnostic imaging

Radiography: Thoracic radiographs should be taken unless positioning the animal causes worsening respiratory difficulty. In this instance, thoracocentesis (see Operative Technique 12.1) is performed before radiography, as both a diagnostic and a therapeutic measure. Thoracic radiographs should be taken in any animal with chronic coughing not responding to symptomatic treatment, as this can be the only clinical sign associated with chylothorax in some instances. Opposite lateral radiographs of the thorax allow better evaluation of the right and left lung fields. DV positioning is less stressful for the animal than VD. Radiographs will often show only non-specific signs of pleural effusion, such as rounding of the lung margins, interlobar fissure lines and separation of the lungs from the thoracic wall. Conditions underlying chylothorax may be visible on thoracic radiographs, depending on the severity of the pleural effusion. Caudal displacement of the cardiac silhouette and widening of the cranial mediastinum may indicate a cranial mediastinal mass. Enlargement of the cardiac silhouette may indicate pericardial effusion or cardiac disease. Marked consolidation of one lung lobe with a prominent, aberrantly located air bronchogram may indicate lung lobe torsion. Lung lobes that have a persistent shrunken, rounded appearance, even after removal of pleural effusion, may be affected by fibrosing pleuritis (Figure 12.9). Scarring and contraction of the lungs' visceral pleura appears to occur in response to chronic pleural effusion.

Ultrasonography: This is useful for evaluating the heart and mediastinum for diseases that might cause chylothorax. In many instances, identified masses can be biopsied or aspirated with ultrasound guidance, providing material for a definitive diagnosis. Ultrasonography can also be used to evaluate the hilus of a suspected lung lobe torsion and the cranial vena cava for evidence of thrombosis.

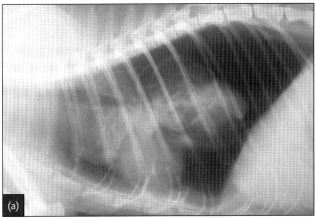

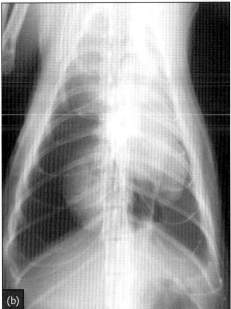

12.9 (a) Lateral and (b) dorsoventral radiographs of a cat with chronic chylothorax. Note the small rounded radiodense lung lobes visible on each view. This appearance is due to chronic fibrosis of the visceral pleura secondary to chylothorax.

Computed tomography: CT scans have been used to evaluate the thorax for underlying causes of chylothorax and to delineate the anatomy of the TDS to aid in surgical planning.

Thoracocentesis

Thoracocentesis (see Operative Technique 12.1) is performed to relieve respiratory distress and to obtain fluid for analysis. Chylous effusions are generally either white or pink. Redder effusions should raise concern for lung lobe torsion. Fluid from thoracocentesis is put in an EDTA tube. A fluid analysis (including cell count) is performed and fluid triglyceride levels are determined. The specific gravity of chylous effusions can range from 1.022 to 1.027 in dogs and from 1.019 to 1.050 in cats. Total protein concentrations can range from 0.25 to 0.62 g/l in dogs and from 0.26 to 0.1 g/l in cats. The total nucleated cell count is usually <10,000/ml in both species.

Chylothorax is diagnosed by evaluation of pleural fluid triglyceride levels. In true chylothorax, the concentration of pleural fluid triglycerides is higher than that of serum triglycerides. This difference is usually marked (10-fold difference or greater) unless the affected animal is anorexic, in which case pleural triglyceride levels can drop towards serum levels. Pleural fluid triglyceride concentrations >1 g/l are also considered diagnostic for chylothorax.

Medical management

Supportive care for animals with chylothorax involves correction of dehydration and electrolyte imbalances. Nutritional support should be considered in anorexic, severely malnourished animals and can be provided by a naso-oesophageal, oesophageal or gastric feeding tube. Enteral nutritional support will invariably increase the thoracic duct lymph flow and this may, in turn, necessitate more frequent thoracocentesis or even chest tube placement.

Treatment should be aimed at any identifiable disease causing chylothorax. Successful management of underlying disease may lead to resolution of the chylothorax, although this may take several months and intermittent thoracocentesis may be required. Experimentally, no diets tested reduced the volume of chyle transported in the TDS, although a homemade diet of boiled tuna and rice resulted in a lower thoracic duct fat content than either low- or high-fat commercial diets. Benzopyrone drugs have been used in humans to treat limb lymphoedema secondary to trauma or radical lymph node removal as part of breast cancer treatment. Benzopyrones have been given to animals with chylothorax in the hope of increasing chyle resorption from the pleural space. Whilst the chylous pleural effusion has resolved in some treated animals, it is not clear whether this is as a result of the benzopyrone treatment or represents spontaneous resolution of the disease. Benzopyrones have been administered to animals at doses ranging from 50 to 100 mg/kg q8h.

Surgical treatment

Surgery is indicated to:

- Obtain biopsy samples to confirm underlying disease
- Remove non-lymphomatous mediastinal masses or lung lobe torsions
- Treat cases that are idiopathic and have not responded to conservative therapy.

Anecdotally, many surgeons feel that fibrosing pleuritis is a contraindication to surgical treatment of chylothorax, especially in cats, so preoperative radiographs should be carefully evaluated for signs of this condition. Until recently, none of the surgical techniques described below had success rates better than 50–60% in dogs, and poorer success rates in cats. Many techniques (omentalization, pericardectomy, pleuroperitoneal shunting, thoracic duct embolization or 'combination' surgeries) are either described in published reports with few clinical cases, or have not had clinical case series published in peer-reviewed journals. It is, therefore, impossible to give indications for one technique over another in individual cases. Thoracic duct ligation and pericardectomy were reported to resolve idiopathic chylothorax in 10/10 dogs and 8/10 cats (Fossum *et al.*, 2004). In another study, thoracic duct ligation and cisterna chyli ablation was more successful than thoracic duct ligation and pericardectomy in resolving chylothorax in dogs (McAnulty, 2011).

Thoracic duct ligation: This has been the mainstay of the surgical treatment of chylothorax for many years. After thoracic duct ligation, many new lymphatic-to-venous anastomoses form in the abdominal cavity to transport lymph to the venous system, bypassing the TDS. Successful thoracic duct ligation resolves the chylothorax completely; however, in 50% of dogs and in 50–80% of cats, either chylothorax or a serosanguineous pleural effusion persists after surgery.

This procedure is technically demanding and should only be attempted by veterinary surgeons with thoracic surgical experience. Specialized equipment (monitoring equipment including Doppler or direct arterial blood pressure measurement, pulse oximeter or blood gas machine, end-tidal CO_2 monitor, chest retractors) is required.

The patient is fasted for 12 hours before surgery. Anaesthesia is induced and the animal prepared for aseptic surgery. Strategies for minimizing postoperative pain include preoperative placement of a fentanyl patch, 'high' epidural anaesthesia using morphine (0.1 mg/kg) and intercostal nerve blocks using bupivacaine (1.5 mg/kg). As discussed above, the TDS is generally found on the right side of the caudal mediastinum in dogs and on the left side of the caudal mediastinum in cats. Thus, the entire right or left lateral thorax and abdomen (depending on species) is clipped and prepared for surgery.

In dogs, a right eighth or ninth intercostal space thoracotomy is performed. The TDS lies between the aorta and the azygous vein. Visualization of the TDS is often difficult, even if corn oil or cream has been fed immediately preoperatively; sympathetic nerves in the caudal mediastinum can be confused with lymphatic vessels. Identification of the TDS is facilitated by exposing an abdominal lymph node through a flank incision. A single paracostal incision has also been described, allowing access to the abdomen for lymph node injection and the thorax, through the diaphragm, for thoracic duct ligation (Staiger et al., 2011). Usually, the easiest lymph node to locate is associated with the ileocolic junction. Once identified, a small volume (0.5–1 ml) of methylene blue is injected into the node. The TDS will turn blue shortly after this injection is made. At this point, some surgeons cannulate an abdominal lymphatic vessel with a 20–24 G over-the-needle catheter and perform a contrast lymphangiogram by injecting 1 ml/kg of water-soluble contrast agent diluted with 0.5 ml/kg of sterile saline into the lymphatic system. Although this allows identification of the number and location of lymphatic branches in the caudal mediastinum, it requires intraoperative fluoroscopic or radiographic capabilities.

The TDS is dissected and ligated using silk or Prolene sutures. At this point a contrast lymphangiogram may be repeated to help ensure ligation of all TDS branches. A thoracostomy tube is placed, and the thoracic and abdominal incisions are closed in the routine manner (see Chapter 11).

An 'en bloc' method for thoracic duct ligation without the use of lymphangiography has been reported in dogs and cats (Bussadori et al., 2011). The thoracotomy approach is similar to that described above. A separate flank incision was not performed as mesenteric lymphangiography was not used in the series of cases reported. All structures dorsal to the aorta and ventral to the thoracic vertebral bodies were dissected and ligated en bloc, sparing the sympathetic trunk. A subphrenic pericardectomy and omentalization were also performed. The results of this procedure in a limited number of dogs and cats were similar to those described for other techniques.

The thoracic duct can also be dissected thoracoscopically (Mayhew et al., 2012). This technique has the advantages of being minimally invasive and allowing a minimally invasive pericardectomy and/or cisterna chyli ablation to be performed in conjunction with thoracic duct ligation. It requires two thoracoscopes and associated towers. The surgeon and anaesthetist need to be experienced in thoracoscopic surgery and potentially one-lung ventilation.

Omentalization, pericardectomy and cisterna chyli ablation: Placing omentum into the thoracic cavity, removing the pericardium and cisterna chyli ablation are procedures that were initially used when thoracic duct ligation failed to resolve chylothorax. These procedures are now being used as 'primary' surgical treatments for chylothorax, generally combined with thoracic duct ligation. The omentum is thought either to act as a physiological drain, when placed in the thoracic cavity to treat chylothorax, or to assist in sealing a leaking TDS. The physiological drain theory is difficult to support logically, because the omental lymphatics drain back into the TDS. As mentioned above, primary pericardial disease or pericardial thickening in response to chronic chylous effusion is thought potentially to elevate caval pressure and contribute to chylothorax in some animals. Anecdotally, biopsy of a thickened pericardium removed to treat persistent chylothorax revealed microscopic carcinoma. Ablation of the cisterna chyli is thought to stimulate the formation of intra-abdominal lymphatic-ovenous anastomoses, bypassing the TDS.

Various combinations of thoracic duct ligation, pericardectomy, cysterna chyli ablation and omentalization are now performed. The approach for thoracic duct ligation is generally too caudal to allow a safe pericardectomy, so an additional fifth intercostal space thoracotomy is required for pericardectomy, unless the procedure can be performed thorascopically through the initial intercostal thoracotomy. The cisterna chyli ablation can often be performed through the abdominal approach used to access a mesenteric lymph node or lymphatic vessel for injection of methylene blue or contrast. The omentum can be identified and mobilized through the flank abdominal incision and passed into the thoracotomy via a small hole in the diaphragm.

Pleuroport placement: A pleuroport is a stainless steel subcutaneous access port that can be accessed percutaneously using a Huber needle that is connected to a silastic catheter placed in the pleural space. These devices allow the pleural space to be drained safely without the risk of lung injury associated with repeated needle thoracocentesis. They are, therefore, useful in situations where repeated thoracic drainage is anticipated (i.e. failure or inability to control fluid production). The patient is anaesthetized and the lateral thorax clipped. A small incision is made through the skin and lateral thoracic musculature. A small window is made between the ribs to allow the fenestrated end of the silastic tube to be fed into the pleural space. The other end is connected to the subcutaneous access port, which is sutured to the thoracic musculature in a subcutaneous pocket.

Pleuroperitoneal shunting: This has been used to treat chylothorax when thoracic duct ligation has failed. In this technique, a commercially available shunt catheter is implanted and the owner pumps pleural fluid into the peritoneal cavity.

The patient is anaesthetized and placed in lateral recumbency. The lateral thorax and abdomen are clipped and prepared for aseptic surgery. The pleuroperitoneal shunt is placed into a bowl of heparinized saline and primed by repeatedly compressing the pump chamber. Vertical skin incisions are made over the seventh or eighth rib and the 12th rib. The incisions are continued under the external abdominal oblique muscle and a tunnel is dissected between the two incisions at this level. The shunt is pulled through from the first incision to the second, taking care that the afferent tubing is positioned towards the thorax and the efferent tubing towards the abdomen. The pump chamber is positioned over the ninth rib. The afferent tubing is placed in the pleural space through a hole created at the seventh or eighth intercostal space, using haemostats. The efferent tubing is inserted into the abdomen behind the last rib. Purse-string sutures are placed around both afferent and efferent limbs. The cranial skin incision is enlarged as necessary to allow the pump backing to be sutured to intercostal muscles. Muscle, subcutaneous tissue and skin are closed routinely.

Postoperatively, the pump chamber is pumped 100–200 times every 4–6 hours initially; this is varied in the subsequent weeks to provide control of the clinical signs associated with the pleural effusion. Potential complications include dislodgement and flipping of the pump chamber, and obstruction of the pump chamber with fibrin.

Prognosis

In spite of the encouraging results of surgical treatment reported recently, the prognosis for dogs and cats with chylothorax must remain guarded. It is vital to identify an underlying cause and treat this condition whenever possible. Animals with chylothorax secondary to a potentially treatable condition (e.g. mediastinal lymphoma) have a better prognosis than those with, for example, diffuse carcinoma invading the TDS lymphatics. In truly idiopathic cases treated by thoracic duct ligation and pericardectomy, chylothorax resolved in 10/10 dogs and 8/10 cats (Fossum et al., 2004).

References and further reading

Birchard SJ, Smeak DD and Fossum TW (1988) Results of thoracic duct ligation in 15 dogs with chylothorax. *Journal of the American Veterinary Medical Association* **193**, 68–71

Boothe HW, Howe LM, Boothe DM *et al.* (2010) Evaluation of outcomes in dogs treated for pyothorax: 46 cases (1983–2001). *Journal of the American Veterinary Association* **236**, 657–663

Bussadori R, Provera A, Martano M *et al.* (2011) Pleural omentalization with en bloc ligation of the thoracic duct and pericardectomy for idiopathic chylothorax in nine dogs and four cats. *The Veterinary Journal* **188**, 234–236

Davies C and Forrester SD (1996) Pleural effusions in cats: 82 cases (1987 to 1995). *Journal of Small Animal Practice* **37**, 217–224

Demetriou JL, Foale RD, Ladlow J *et al.* (2002) Canine and feline pyothorax: a retrospective study of 50 cases in the UK and Ireland. *Journal of Small Animal Practice* **43**, 388–394

Dempsey SM and Ewing PJ (2011) A review of the pathophysiology, classification, and analysis of canine and feline cavitary effusions. *Journal of the American Animal Hospital Association* **47**, 1–11

Dewhurst E (2016) Body cavity effusions. In: *BSAVA Manual of Canine and Feline Clinical Pathology, 3rd edn*, ed. E Villiers and J Ristic, pp. 435–451. BSAVA Publications, Gloucester

Fossum TW and Birchard SJ (1986) Lymphangiographic evaluation of experimentally induced chylothorax after ligation of the cranial vena cava in dogs. *American Journal of Veterinary Research* **47**, 967–971

Fossum TW, Evering WN, Miller MW *et al.* (1992) Severe bilateral fibrosing pleuritis associated with chronic chylothorax in five cats and two dogs. *Journal of the American Veterinary Medical Association* **201**, 317–324

Fossum TW, Jacobs RM and Birchard SJ (1986) Evaluation of cholesterol and triglyceride concentrations in differentiating chylous and nonchylous pleural effusions in dogs and cats. *Journal of the American Veterinary Medical Association* **188**, 49–51

Fossum TW, Mertens MM, Miller MW *et al.* (2004) Thoracic duct ligation and pericardectomy for treatment of idiopathic chylothorax. *Journal of Veterinary Internal Medicine* **18**, 307–310

Hackett T (1999) Endocrine and metabolic emergencies. In: *BSAVA Manual of Canine and Feline Emergency and Critical Care*, ed. L King and R Hammond, pp. 187–189. BSAVA Publications, Gloucester

Hodges CC, Fossum TW and Evering W (1993) Evaluation of thoracic duct healing after experimental laceration and transection. *Veterinary Surgery* **22**, 431–435

Holt D and Wilson J (2012) Preoperative stabilization. In: *BSAVA Manual of Canine and Feline Surgical Principles*, ed. S Baines, V Lipscomb and T Hutchinson, pp.88–103. BSAVA Publications, Gloucester

Johnson MS and Martin MWS (2007) Successful medical treatment of 15 dogs with pyothorax. *Journal of Small Animal Practice* **48**, 12–16

Kagen KG and Breznock EM (1979) Variations in the canine thoracic duct system and the effects of surgical occlusion demonstrated by rapid aqueous lymphography using an intestinal lymphatic trunk. *American Journal of Veterinary Research* **40**, 948–958

Kovak JR, Ludwig LL, Bergman PJ, Baer KE and Noone KE (2002) Use of thoracoscopy to determine the aetiology of pleural effusions in dogs and cats: 18 cases (1998–2001). *Journal of the American Veterinary Medical Association* **221**, 990–994

Lappin MR (1998) Polysystemic viral diseases. In: *Small Animal Internal Medicine, 2nd edn*, ed. R Nelson and G Couto, pp.1290–1294. Mosby, St Louis

Lisciandro GR, Lagutchik MS, Mann KA *et al.* (2008) Evaluation of a thoracic focused assessment with sonography for trauma (TFAST) protocol to detect pneumothorax and concurrent thoracic injury in 145 traumatized dogs. *Journal of Veterinary Emergency and Critical Care* **18**, 258–269

Mayhew PD, Culp WTN, Mayhew KN *et al.* (2012) Minimally invasive treatment of idiopathic chylothorax in dogs by thoracoscopic thoracic duct ligation and subphrenic pericardectomy: six cases (2007–2010). *Journal of the American Veterinary Medical Association* **241**, 904–909

McAnulty JF (2011) Prospective comparison of cisterna chyli ablation to pericardectomy for treatment of spontaneously occurring idiopathic chylothorax in the dog. *Veterinary Surgery* **40**, 926–934

Mellanby RJ, Villiers E and Herrtage ME (2002) Canine pleural and mediastinal effusions: a retrospective study of 81 cases. *Journal of Small Animal Practice* **43**, 447–451

Neath PJ, Brockman DJ and King LG (2000) Lung lobe torsion in dogs: 22 cases (1981–1999). *Journal of the American Veterinary Medical Association* **217**, 1041–1044

Papsouliotis K and Dewhurst E (2005) Body cavity effusions. In: *BSAVA Manual of Canine and Feline Clinical Pathology, 2nd edn*, ed. E Villiers and L Blackwood, pp. 340–354. BSAVA Publications, Gloucester

Radlinsky MG (2012) Thoracic cavity. In: *Veterinary Surgery Small Animal*, ed. K Tobias and S Johnston, pp. 1787–1812. Elsevier Saunders, St Louis

Reetz JA, Caceres AV, Suran JN *et al.* (2013) Sensitivity, positive predictive value, and interobserver variability of computed tomography in the diagnosis of bullae associated with spontaneous pneumothorax in dogs: 19 cases (2003–2012). *Journal of the American Veterinary Medical Association* **243**, 244–251

Reichle JK and Wisner ER (2000) Non-cardiac thoracic ultrasound in 75 feline and canine patients. *Veterinary Radiology and Ultrasound* **41**, 154–162

Rooney MB and Monnet E (2002) Medical and surgical treatment of pyothorax in dogs: 26 cases (1991–2001). *Journal of the American Veterinary Medical Association* **221**, 86–92

Scott JA and Macintire DK (2003a) Canine pyothorax: pleural anatomy and pathophysiology. *Compendium on Continuing Education for the Practicing Veterinarian* **25**, 172–178

Scott JA and Macintire DK (2003b) Canine pyothorax: clinical presentation, diagnosis, and treatment. *Compendium on Continuing Education for the Practicing Veterinarian* **25**, 180–193

Smeak DD, Birchard SJ, McLoughlin MA *et al.* (2001) Treatment of chronic pleural effusion with pleuroperitoneal (Denver) shunts: 14 dogs (1985–1999). *Journal of the American Veterinary Medical Association* **219**, 1590–1597

Staiger BA, Stanley BJ and McAnulty JF (2011) Single paracostal approach to thoracic duct and cisterna chyli: experimental study and case series. *Veterinary Surgery* **40**, 786–794

Steyn PF and Wittum TE (1993) Radiographic, epidemiologic and clinical aspects of simultaneous pleural and peritoneal effusions in dogs and cats: 48 cases (1982–1991). *Journal of the American Veterinary Medical Association* **202**, 307–312

Valtolina C and Adamantos S (2009) Evaluation of small-bore wire-guided chest drains for management of pleural space disease. *Journal of Small Animal Practice* **50**, 290–297

Waddell LS, Brady CA and Drobatz KJ (2002) Risk factors, prognostic indicators, and outcome of pyothorax in cats: 80 cases (1986–1999). *Journal of the American Veterinary Medical Association* **221**, 819–824

Walker AL, Jang SS and Hirsch DC (2000) Bacteria associated with pyothorax of dogs and cats: 98 cases (1989–1998). *Journal of the American Veterinary Medical Association* **216**, 359–364

OPERATIVE TECHNIQUE 12.1

Needle thoracocentesis

PATIENT PREPARATION AND POSITIONING

A generous area around the site for needle insertion is clipped and surgically prepared. Local anaesthetic may be infiltrated under the skin at the site of needle insertion if desired. Sternal recumbency is usually the easiest position for the animal and the most efficient for drainage. Alternatively, a sitting position or lateral recumbency may be used. Thoracocentesis is usually performed on conscious animals. Sedation, or occasionally general anaesthesia, may be required in fractious animals.

ASSISTANT

One person is required to restrain the patient. It is useful, but not essential, to have another person available to perform drainage of the pleural space with the syringe, allowing the surgeon to concentrate solely on needle placement.

ADDITIONAL INSTRUMENTS

Butterfly needle or over-the-needle catheter (18–22 G); extension tubing; three-way tap; syringe (10–50 ml). A needle size that is appropriate for the size of animal is selected, e.g. 20–22 G for cats and small dogs; 18–20 G for medium to large dogs. A measuring bowl is helpful if a large amount of fluid is present.

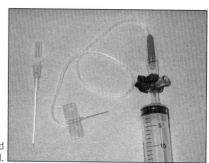

Thoracocentesis equipment. If an over-the-needle catheter is used instead of a butterfly cannula, a separate extension tube is also required.

SURGICAL TECHNIQUE

Approach

The seventh or eighth intercostal space is recommended unless radiography or ultrasonography indicates otherwise. If fluid and air are present within the pleural cavity the needle is inserted approximately half way up the chest wall. If only fluid is present, it is more efficient to insert the needle in the ventral third of the thorax, whereas the dorsal third is appropriate if just air is present. To avoid the intercostal vessels and nerve, which lie on the caudal aspect of each rib, the needle is introduced close to the cranial rib border.

Surgical manipulations

1. Advance the needle slowly in a slightly ventral direction (approximately 45 degrees to the body wall), with the bevel of the needle facing the lung (to reduce the risk of iatrogenic lung laceration).

2. Once the needle is felt to penetrate the pleura, apply gentle suction using the preattached syringe and extension tubing. The extension tubing allows the needle in the patient to move independently from the syringe, reducing the risk of lung laceration and minimizing the risk of the needle becoming dislodged from its desired position.
   If an over-the-needle catheter is used, withdraw the stylet once the pleural cavity is entered, followed by prompt attachment of the extension tubing and syringe. Redirection of the catheter after the stylet has been removed tends to result in kinking and obstruction of the catheter.

3. Drainage of both sides of the thorax is recommended to ensure complete evacuation of the pleural space.

WARNING

A negative finding does not rule out a pleural effusion

PRACTICAL TIP

Fluid in the pleural cavity may be present in 'pockets' and it is worth trying both sides and different sites if the expected amount of fluid is not forthcoming. If available, ultrasonography may help to identify specific areas of fluid accumulation and guide needle placement

POSTOPERATIVE CARE

Radiography should be performed after thoracocentesis to document change and confirm absence of iatrogenic injury.

OPERATIVE TECHNIQUE 12.2

Small-bore wire-guided chest drain placement in a closed chest

PATIENT PREPARATION AND POSITIONING

It is ideal if the animal tolerates pre-oxygenation, clipping and surgical preparation of the chest prior to sedation. A large area of the right or left lateral chest, including the entire rib cage, is clipped and surgically prepared. The animal is usually in sternal recumbency but can be in lateral recumbency if this is tolerated without respiratory compromise. A 2% lidocaine (0.2 ml/kg) local anaesthetic block is infused into the site of skin incision.

> **WARNING**
>
> Never attempt to place a chest drain in an animal with severe respiratory compromise. Stabilization with oxygen, thoracocentesis and cage rest is indicated first

ASSISTANT

One person is required to monitor and restrain the patient.

ADDITIONAL INSTRUMENTS

Multifenestrated 14 G chest drain catheter kit (Chest Tube – Guidewire inserted; MILA International), three-way tap, two bungs; 20–50 ml syringe.

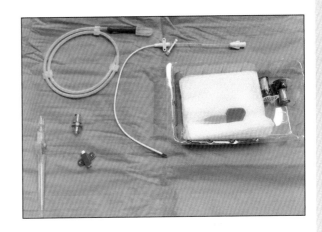

SURGICAL TECHNIQUE

1. The 14 G introducer catheter and stylette is tunnelled subcutaneously in a cranioventral direction for several rib spaces and inserted into the pleural cavity at the seventh or eighth intercostal space towards the cranial edge of the rib to minimize risk of injury to the caudally situated neurovascular bundle. Make sure the introducer catheter and stylette is fully advanced into the thorax.

2. Remove the stylette and immediately introduce a J-wire through the catheter in a cranioventral direction for 10–20 cm or until resistance is met.

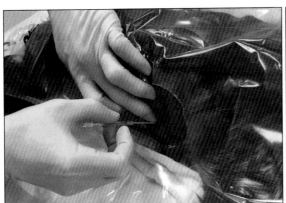
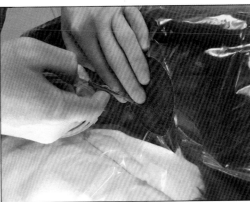

→ **OPERATIVE TECHNIQUE 12.2 CONTINUED**

3 Remove the introducer catheter, leaving the J-wire in place. Keep hold of the J-wire at all times to prevent inadvertent wire slippage out of the chest.

4 Advance the 14 G chest tube into the chest over the guidewire, keeping a firm hold of the wire at all times and making a small skin incision with a blade just large enough to allow advancement of the chest drain over the wire and into the chest.

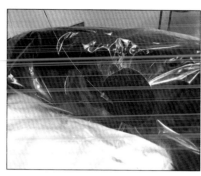 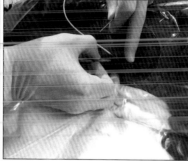 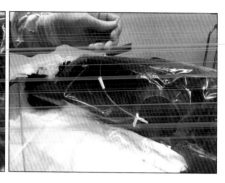

5 Remove the wire and drain any pleural air or fluid with a syringe.

6 Secure the chest drain to the skin using the suture holes in the chest tube.

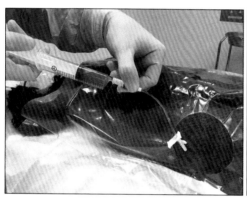 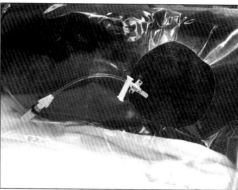

7 If the drain cannot be fully inserted (small patients) the tube can be secured using additional suture wing adaptors in the kit.

8 It is recommended that the tube is flushed with saline several times a day to decrease the risk of tube blockage.

POSTOPERATIVE CARE

- A dressing is placed over the site of chest drain insertion and held in place by a chest bandage.
- The dressing and bandage must be changed and all the connections checked at least once daily.
- The animal must wear an Elizabethan collar to prevent interference with the drain.
- Animals with chest drains should have constant, ideally continuous, supervision: to ensure security of the tube connections; to observe for changes in respiratory rate and effort; and to prevent interference with the drain.

OPERATIVE TECHNIQUE 12.3

Chest drain placement in an open chest

PATIENT PREPARATION AND POSITIONING

The patient is anaesthetized and positioned in lateral recumbency for an intercostal thoracotomy (see also Chapter 11), or dorsal recumbency for a median sternotomy.

ASSISTANT

One person is required to monitor the anaesthetic. A surgical assistant is optional.

ADDITIONAL INSTRUMENTS

Silicone chest drain (16–30 Fr); chest drain connector, three-way tap, two bungs, gate clamp; 20–50 ml syringe. A chest drain is selected that is approximately the width of the mainstem bronchus (16 Fr for cats and tiny dogs; 18–24 Fr for small to medium dogs; 26–30 Fr for large to giant dogs). The length of chest drain that will just place the tip of the drain at the level of the second rib is estimated.

SURGICAL TECHNIQUE

Approach

A small skin incision is made with a blade at approximately the 10th intercostal space, about two-thirds of the way up the chest wall.

Surgical manipulations

1 Insert a large pair of forceps under the skin and advance them in a cranioventral direction to approximately the eighth intercostal space. Introduce the forceps into the chest with a controlled push, while intrathoracic structures are protected by the other hand inside the chest.

2 Open the tips of the forceps and grasp the end of the chest drain.

3 Retract the chest drain and forceps together through the chest wall and skin incision.

4 Arrange the drain so that its tip lies at approximately the level of the second rib and all of the side holes reside within the chest.

5 Close the thoracotomy incision before the chest is drained.

6 Preplace a gate clamp on the chest drain and attach the drain to a connector, three-way tap and syringe.

7 After the syringe drainage, place two bungs on the three-way tap and secure the drain to the chest wall by means of a Chinese fingertrap suture.

POSTOPERATIVE CARE

- A dressing is placed over the site of chest drain insertion and held in place by a chest bandage.
- The dressing and bandage must be changed and all the connections checked at least once daily.
- The animal must wear an Elizabethan collar to prevent interference with the drain.
- Animals with chest drains should have constant, ideally continuous, supervision: to ensure security of the tube connections; to observe for changes in respiratory rate and effort; and to prevent interference with the drain.

Chapter 13

Surgery of the intrathoracic trachea and mainstem bronchi

Carolyn Burton and Eric Monnet

Surgical diseases of the intrathoracic trachea are uncommon in both dogs and cats. This low prevalence of surgical disease, coupled with the anatomical location of this part of the trachea, means that surgical intervention, when required, is best performed by a trained surgical specialist. Step-by-step technical detail of surgically managed conditions of these structures is therefore outside the scope of this manual. However, the authors hope that the following descriptions will improve the recognition and diagnosis of several conditions of the intrathoracic trachea and enhance understanding of the treatment options available at specialist centres.

For general guidelines on tracheal anatomy and surgical principles, please refer to Chapter 8.

Intrathoracic tracheal and bronchial trauma

As the trachea is protected by the thoracic wall, trauma to the thoracic trachea is uncommon in dogs and cats. Unlike the cervical trachea, penetrating or lacerating wounds are very rare. Perhaps the most common form of intrathoracic tracheal trauma is rupture of the trachea. Even these injuries are relatively rare, but over recent years they have become better recognized and more frequently diagnosed. Tracheal ruptures fall into two main categories:

- Tracheal avulsion injury following blunt trauma to the neck or thorax
- Iatrogenic tracheal rupture as a result of overinflation of an endotracheal tube cuff.

Both of these forms of tracheal injury are more common in the cat than in the dog.

Intrathoracic tracheal avulsion injury

There are many reports of feline tracheal avulsion injury in the veterinary literature. Such publications have improved the frequency of recognition of this condition and this has led to much more frequent diagnosis.

Aetiology

The condition is thought to be the result of a blunt traumatic incident to the neck or thorax that involves hyperextension of the neck. Most affected cats have been involved in road

traffic accidents, although falling from a height is known to have caused the same injury in some. The traumatic incident stretches the trachea and leads to a partial circumferential tear, or complete avulsion, of the intrathoracic trachea at a predictable site between 1 and 4 cm cranial to the tracheal bifurcation. Following avulsion, an airway lumen is maintained by the intact peritracheal adventitial tissue or by thickening of mediastinal tissue, creating a 'pseudotrachea' or 'pseudoairway' that allows continued respiration. The ends of the avulsed trachea gradually become stenotic as granulation tissue develops in an attempt to repair the damage. Clinical signs may, therefore, take days to weeks to develop.

Clinical signs

Cats with tracheal avulsion injuries present in two distinct groups:

- Those showing acute-onset dyspnoea immediately after the episode of trauma
- Those showing worsening dyspnoea days or weeks after the incident.

Cats that are presented acutely post trauma have radiographic signs of pneumomediastinum and discontinuity of the tracheal walls (see below), along with other evidence of traumatic disease. Such animals must undergo full evaluation and stabilization prior to definitive treatment of the tracheal injury. Cats presented days to weeks after trauma, with dyspnoea, rarely have persisting concurrent injuries. It is important to realize that screening thoracic radiographs taken at the time of the initial trauma can alert the clinician to the possibility of this injury, although it is possible for thoracic radiographs to appear remarkably normal in some cases. Prompt radiographic diagnosis allows treatment to be planned and undertaken before the severe dyspnoea associated with attempted healing develops. This considerably reduces the risk to these patients.

Diagnosis

Thoracic radiography is the most useful tool for diagnosing acute and chronic tracheal avulsion. In acute post-trauma patients, pneumomediastinum, pneumothorax and discontinuity of the trachea can usually be appreciated (Figure 13.1). In addition, other radiographic signs of trauma (fractured ribs, pulmonary alveolar infiltrate, long bone fracture) may be present. In most chronically affected

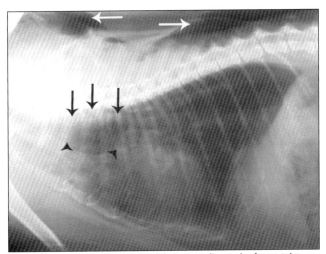

13.1 Tracheal avulsion: lateral thoracic radiograph of a cat taken on the day that it was hit by a car. The separated ends of the trachea are seen (arrowheads) along with a pseudotracheal membrane (black arrows) and evidence of leakage of air: subcutaneous emphysema (white arrows), pneumomediastinum and mild pneumothorax.

animals, plain lateral thoracic radiographs show a well defined spherical dilatation of the trachea at the level of the tracheal avulsion, with stenotic ends to the separated trachea (Figure 13.2). This avulsion is usually sited at the level of the second, third or fourth thoracic vertebra.

Tracheoscopy can be used to confirm the diagnosis, if necessary, and allows direct visualization of either circumferential tracheal ring disruption or tracheal stenosis. In animals with longstanding disease where the scarred ends of the trachea are cicatrized, stenosis will prevent the passage of the endoscope onwards into the pseudotrachea and particularly into the distal tracheal segment. Tracheoscopy is not without risk in these patients.

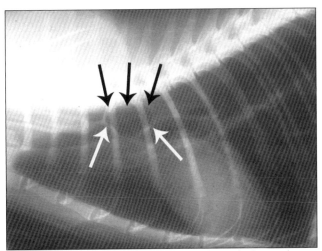

13.2 Tracheal avulsion: lateral thoracic radiograph of a cat taken 3 weeks after it was hit by a car. The stenotic ends of the separated trachea can be seen (white arrows) and the pseudotracheal membrane is obvious (black arrows).

Surgical correction

Surgical correction requires a right third or fourth intercostal space thoracotomy or, occasionally, a cranial sternotomy, allowing access to the pseudotrachea. The pseudotrachea has a typical appearance (Figure 13.3).

The pseudotrachea is opened and a sterile endotracheal tube passed into the distal tracheal segment via

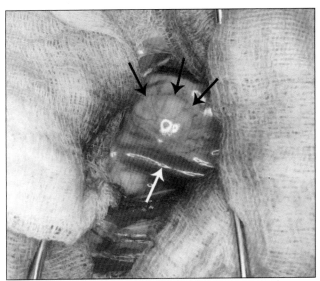

13.3 Tracheal avulsion: view of the bulging pseudotracheal membrane (black arrows) through a right third intercostal thoracotomy. The cranial vena cava is seen ventral to the trachea (white arrow).

the thoracotomy, allowing maintenance of the airway during the tracheal anastomosis (Figure 13.4a). Identification of the opening into the distal tracheal segment is not always easy, particularly in chronic cases, where it can be extremely small. There is often a considerable gap between the proximal and distal tracheal segments due to retraction as a result of the avulsion. Identification of the transected proximal segment can be improved with advancement of the orotracheal tube. Any damaged tracheal rings are then resected. Tracheal anastomosis is carried out, preplacing all sutures prior to tying (Figure 13.4b). Ventilation is resumed via a long orotracheal tube, which is advanced past the anastomotic site into the distal tracheal segment.

The surgical and anaesthetic management during correction of intrathoracic tracheal avulsion injuries is technically demanding, and referral is advised. However, with specialist input the success rate and long-term prognosis are extremely good following surgical correction.

PRACTICAL TIP

Tracheal stenosis can make positive pressure ventilation difficult in these cats. Prior to opening the thorax, these patients may do better if left to breathe spontaneously. Forceful positive pressure ventilation can lead to rupture of the pseudotracheal membrane and life-threatening tension pneumothorax. Once the thoracic cavity is open, spontaneous breathing efforts will be fruitless; the surgeon must therefore be prepared to secure an airway rapidly if positive pressure ventilation also proves ineffective. To prevent contamination of the operating theatre environment with anaesthetic gases total intravenous anaesthesia (TIVA) is recommended

Left principal bronchus avulsion/rupture

A similar injury to intrathoracic tracheal avulsion has also been reported, involving the left principal bronchus in two cats (White and Oakley, 2000). The aetiology in these cases was also thought to be traumatic; the clinical signs were tachypnoea and increased respiratory effort.

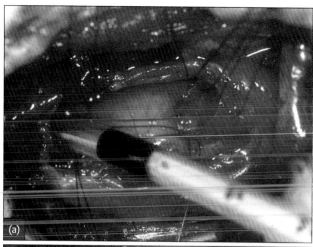

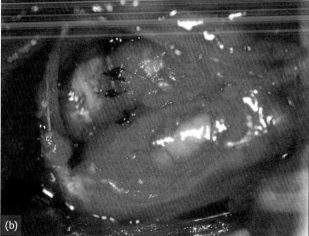

13.4 (a) The tracheal avulsion is exposed through a right lateral thoracotomy and a sterile endotracheal tube is used to secure the airway whilst the sutures are preplaced through the ends of the trachea. (b) Preplaced sutures are tied following removal of the endotracheal tube.

Diagnosis was achieved with thoracic radiography, bronchoscopy and computed tomography (CT). Radiographic findings included a spherical enlargement of the base of the left mainstem bronchus, pneumomediastinum, pneumothorax, pleural effusion and retraction of all lung lobes in the left hemithorax. Bronchoscopy confirmed almost complete stenosis of the left principal bronchus. In both cases successful surgical correction was achieved via a right fifth intercostal thoracotomy, resection of the damaged/stenosed segment and anastomosis of the bronchus.

Iatrogenic tracheal rupture
Aetiology

Tracheal injuries resulting from overinflation of an endotracheal tube cuff are more commonly seen within the cervical trachea than in the intrathoracic trachea. Such injuries are more common in cats, although it is possible to cause similar injuries in dogs (see Chapter 8).

The injury typically occurs as a result of the use of a cuffed endotracheal tube. Seventy percent of cats sustaining this injury are undergoing anaesthesia for a dental procedure. There is a tendency to overinflate the cuff during dental procedures to minimize the chance of aspiration of fluid into the patient's airway. In addition, animals are repositioned frequently; if this is done without disconnecting the anaesthetic delivery tube, shear forces develop that further damage the trachea. Tracheal rupture has also been caused during intubation as a result of using a stylet. The type of endotracheal tube cuff used in these procedures appears to have little influence on whether a rupture is caused, with both high pressure-low volume and low pressure-high volume cuffs reported as causing a problem. The most common site of injury is the dorsal wall of the trachea at the junction between the ends of the tracheal rings and the tracheal membrane. In some animals the tracheal injury results in 360-degree pressure necrosis of the tracheal wall, secondary either to cuff contact or to pressure from the tip of the endotracheal tube.

Clinical signs and management

Most cats are presented either immediately or within 1–6 days of injury because of subcutaneous emphysema. Other reported clinical signs include dyspnoea, gagging, regurgitation, pyrexia and cough. The diagnosis is often presumptive, with a history of a recent anaesthetic episode and subsequent development of subcutaneous emphysema.

Cervical and thoracic radiography can be helpful; subcutaneous emphysema, discontinuity or irregularity of the tracheal gas shadow, pneumomediastinum and pneumothorax are commonly identified abnormalities. If further confirmation of the diagnosis is required, tracheoscopy can be helpful; however, the tracheal mucosa and lumen can appear remarkably normal on tracheoscopy despite the presence of a large tear.

Careful examination of the tracheal mucosa, particularly around any areas of mild inflammation, is necessary to identify a defect.

Cats with mild to moderate clinical signs that resolve with cage rest can be successfully managed conservatively with rest, oxygen therapy and sedatives if required. Patients need to be carefully monitored, and serial re-evaluations of respiratory status and the amount of subcutaneous emphysema are necessary during this time. The subcutaneous emphysema can take some time to resolve, usually within 2 weeks, but up to 6 weeks has been reported. Cats with severe dyspnoea or worsening clinical signs during conservative management require surgical repair. This may be achieved via a right lateral third or fourth intercostal space thoracotomy or ventral midline cervical approach combined with a median sternotomy, depending on the position and extent of the rupture (Figure 13.5). Most ruptures occur at the junction of the tracheal cartilage and dorsal tracheal membrane, and gentle rotation of the trachea using stay sutures improves visualization of the rupture site. Once again, careful anaesthetic management is required and TIVA may be necessary if secure endotracheal intubation distal to the tear is not possible. The prognosis for these cats following resolution of clinical signs with conservative management or surgery is good.

It is important to note that, to the authors' knowledge, there are no reports of tracheal rupture associated with the use of non-cuffed endotracheal tubes. Prevention of aspiration of fluids can be achieved by using a non-cuffed tube together with packing of the pharyngeal area with a surgical swab. If cuffed endotracheal tubes are used they should be inflated carefully with the minimum volume of air needed to achieve a seal, the anaesthetic circuit should be disconnected each time the patient is moved, and the cuff deflated prior to extubation.

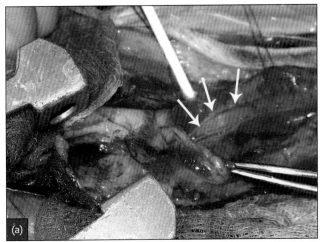

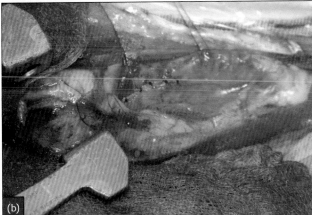

13.5 Cervical and intrathoracic tracheal tear caused by overinflation of an endotracheal tube cuff. (a) The tear is exposed via a ventral neck and sternotomy approach. The endotracheal tube can be seen through the tracheal defect (arrowed). (b) Closure of the defect with simple interrupted sutures of fine polydioxanone.

Intrathoracic tracheal laceration or penetration

Aetiology

Intrathoracic tracheal lacerations may be seen following severe dog bites or following ballistic injury (e.g. gunshot, arrow). In most instances the intrathoracic tracheal trauma following a bite wound is thought to occur when the trachea is crushed between the collapsing thoracic walls. This crush injury can be worsened by penetration of the trachea by a fractured rib or tooth in the case of a bite wound. A rather more obscure traumatic aetiology has been reported in a kitten that developed bronchial rupture following routine venepuncture (Godfrey, 1997).

Clinical signs and management

Intrathoracic tracheal injury is suspected in animals with focal or extensive subcutaneous emphysema and pneumomediastinum, and where no other source of leakage can be identified. Such patients could have either intrathoracic tracheal leakage or ruptured 'marginal alveoli'. Because marginal alveolar ruptures respond to conservative management, and because the presence of peritracheal tissue allows spontaneous healing of small defects to take place without surgical intervention, stable patients with these clinical and radiographic signs are rarely investigated further. The exact nature of the injury and the cause of air leakage often remain uncharacterized.

The distal portion of the trachea and the mainstem bronchi are less supported by peritracheal adventitial tissue, and in this region minor lacerations can produce extensive pneumomediastinum and pneumothorax. Again, the majority of these lacerations are self-limiting.

Severe pneumothorax should be controlled with thoracocentesis or thoracic drain placement until the tracheal laceration seals (see Chapter 12). In the rare instances where pneumomediastinum and pneumothorax are uncontrollable, or persist after 3–4 days of conservative treatment, further investigations (tracheobronchoscopy) and exploratory thoracotomy, followed by identification, debridement and surgical closure of the laceration, are indicated.

Non-traumatic tracheal and bronchial conditions

Tracheal and bronchial foreign bodies

Tracheal foreign bodies are seen more commonly in cats, whereas bronchial foreign bodies are more common in outdoor/hunting dogs. Extremely large foreign bodies that become wedged within the intrathoracic trachea can be inhaled by cats, which is surprising given the sensitivity of the feline larynx.

Clinical signs

Typically, these animals have a sudden onset of moist cough, respiratory noise and varying degrees of dyspnoea. However, many animals show remarkably few clinical signs despite the presence of relatively large foreign bodies.

Diagnosis

Many foreign bodies are radiodense or are visible as a soft tissue opacity within the tracheal lumen, for example stones, teeth, bone fragments, tree bark, pine cone fragments and coal. These are readily identified with plain lateral thoracic radiographs (Figure 13.6a). Non-radiodense foreign bodies, such as blades of grass, insects, pieces of plastic and feathers, are usually visible with endoscopy. In some cases the foreign body may not be directly visible but the exudate surrounding it is easily identifiable. Endoscopically guided suction, combined with gentle flushing with saline, often dislodges the exudate and allows the foreign body to be seen.

Treatment

Radiodense foreign bodies are most easily removed with forceps under fluoroscopic guidance (Figure 13.6b) or by using rigid or flexible tracheoscopy. In cases where the shape and smooth surface of the foreign body prevents successful grasping, fluoroscopic-guided placement of an over-the-wire balloon catheter caudal to the foreign body, followed by inflation and gradual retraction, has been successful. Many non-radiodense materials can be similarly grasped with forceps under direct visualization with endoscopy. Care is needed when manipulating the foreign body through the rima glottidis to prevent trauma and the development of laryngeal oedema. Care must also be taken to avoid pushing a tracheal foreign body into the carina and causing complete, life-threatening airway obstruction. Fragmentation of the foreign body

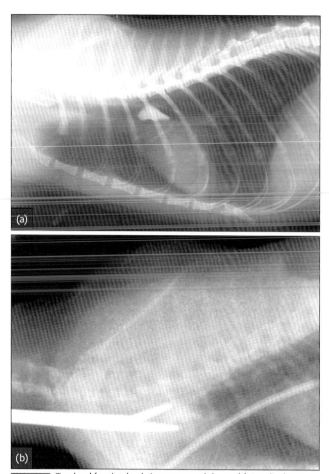

The mass is usually large and the disease process advanced at the time of diagnosis: at least 50% of the tracheal lumen must be obstructed for clinical signs to be recognized.

Clinical signs

Dogs and cats with tracheal tumours are usually presented with worsening dyspnoea, a progressive cough and exercise intolerance.

Diagnosis

Radiography (Figure 13.7a), CT (Figure 13.7b) and bronchoscopy can all be used to visualize a mass. Bronchoscopy is useful for identification and biopsy and even for debulking the tumour to improve clinical signs in the short term. In some cases surgery is performed without a histological diagnosis and is considered an excisional biopsy.

Treatment

For the majority of tracheal tumours surgical resection is recommended for definitive diagnosis, treatment and/or palliation of clinical signs. Surgical resection of tumours affecting the intrathoracic trachea is extremely challenging from both surgical and anaesthetic perspectives (Figure 13.8). Such surgery should only be attempted by trained anaesthesia and surgical personnel. Unfortunately, survival

13.6 Tracheal foreign body in a young adult cat. (a) A radiodense foreign body (pebble) is lodged at the tracheal bifurcation. (b) Removal of the foreign body was easily achieved by gentle use of grasping forceps under fluoroscopic guidance. The forceps may be placed through the larynx either via the endotracheal tube or under direct laryngoscopic visualization.

during removal can also occur, particularly with plant matter. Where these removal methods fail, which tends to be more common if the foreign body is within a bronchus, a more invasive approach with a thoracotomy and removal via a tracheotomy or bronchotomy is needed. Foreign bodies wedged further into the smaller airways, or those that have caused significant lung pathology, may require a lung lobectomy for removal and resolution of the problem. In general, successful removal of foreign bodies has a good long-term outcome.

Neoplasia of the trachea

Although tracheal neoplasms are rare in both the dog and the cat, many different tumour types have been seen, including lymphoma (the most common tracheal tumour in cats), plasmacytoma, chondrosarcoma, adenocarcinoma, mast cell tumour, squamous cell carcinoma, basal cell carcinoma and neuroendocrine tumour. Benign neoplasms such as leiomyoma and osteochondroma have also been reported. Not all tracheal masses are neoplastic, with more exotic parasitic lesions causing tracheal granulomas and obstruction being reported outside the UK, and even more unusually, a haematoma involving the dorsal tracheal membrane has been reported to cause an obstructive mass after a dog bite. Inflammatory masses and polyps of the feline trachea are less common than neoplastic masses, and the underlying aetiology for these is currently not clear.

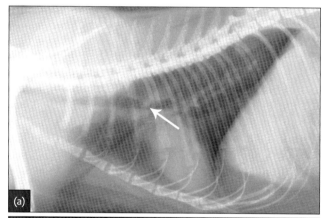

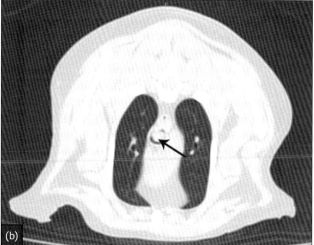

13.7 Intrathoracic tracheal apocrine gland carcinoma in a 9-year-old Domestic Shorthaired cat. (a) A lateral thoracic radiograph shows a soft tissue density within the tracheal lumen between ribs 4 and 5 (arrowed). (b) A computed tomographic image of the same case showing a mass lesion arising from the left dorsolateral aspect of the caudal tracheal wall and causing almost complete occlusion of the tracheal lumen (arrowed).

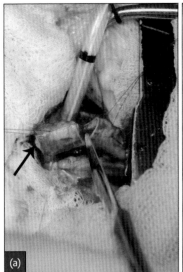 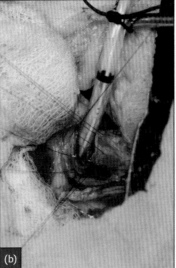 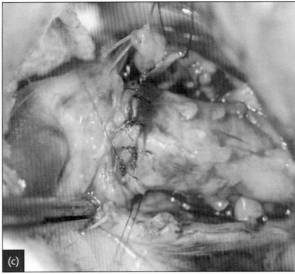

13.8 Intraoperative views of the tracheal apocrine gland carcinoma shown in Figure 13.7 seen through a right fifth intercostal thoracotomy following transection of the azygos vein. (a) The distal trachea has been sectioned and a sterile endotracheal tube placed in the carina to maintain the cat's airway. The tracheal mass can be seen inside the cut end of the trachea (arrowed). The proximal tracheal incision is being made to allow the section of trachea containing the mass to be removed. (b) Sutures of fine polypropylene are placed in each end of the sectioned trachea, with the sterile endotracheal tube still positioned in the carina, to align the cut ends of the trachea. (c) The preplaced sutures of fine polypropylene are tied to complete the end-to-end anastomosis of the trachea.

rates are often low owing to the advanced stage of disease when first seen. Intralumenal stenting may be a good palliative option for recurrent tumours or in selected elderly patients. Primary intratracheal lymphosarcoma is the exception in not requiring surgical management; it can be successfully treated/palliated with chemotherapy. Inflammatory masses can often be managed successfully with corticosteroid treatment and the prognosis is often better for these than is the case with neoplasia.

References and further reading

Burton CA (2003) Surgical diseases of the trachea in the dog and cat. *In Practice* **25**, 514–527

Godfrey DR (1997) Bronchial rupture and fatal tension pneumothorax following routine venipuncture in a kitten. *Journal of the American Animal Hospital Association* **33**, 260–263

Goodnight ME, Scansen BA, Kidder AC *et al.* (2010) Use of a unique method for removal of a foreign body from the trachea of a cat. *Journal of the American Animal Hospital Association* **237**, 689–694

Jakubiak MJ, Siedlecki CT, Zenger E *et al.* (2005) Laryngeal, laryngotracheal and tracheal masses in cats: 27 cases (1998–2003). *Journal of the American Animal Hospital Association* **41**, 310–316

Lowe JE, Bridgman AH and Sabistan DC Jr (1982) The role of bronchioplastic procedures in the surgical management of benign and malignant pulmonary lesions. *Journal of Thoracic and Cardiovascular Surgery* **83**, 227–234

Mitchell SL, McCarthy R, Rudloff E *et al.* (2000) Tracheal rupture associated with intubation in cats: 20 cases (1996–1998). *Journal of the American Veterinary Medical Association* **216**, 1592–1595

Schmierer PA, Schwarz A, Bass DA *et al.* (2014) Novel avulsion pattern of the left principal bronchus with involvement of the carina and caudal thoracic trachea in a cat. *Journal of Feline Medicine and Surgery* **16**, 695–698

Tivers MS and Hotston Moore A (2006) Tracheal foreign bodies in the cat and the use of fluoroscopy for removal: 12 cases. *Journal of Small Animal Practice* **47**, 155–159

Wendell N (2002) Diseases of the trachea and bronchi. In: *Textbook of Small Animal Surgery, 3rd edn*, ed. D. Slatter, pp. 858–880. WB Saunders, Philadelphia

White RN and Oakley MR (2001) Left principal bronchus rupture in a cat. *Journal of Small Animal Practice* **42**, 495–498

White RN and Burton CA (2000) Surgical management of intrathoracic tracheal avulsion in cats: long-term results in nine consecutive cases. *Veterinary Surgery* **29**, 430–435

Chapter 14

Surgery of the lung

Nicholas J. Trout, David A. Puerto and Philipp D. Mayhew

Anatomy and physiology

The lungs, which lie protected within the laterally compressed thoracic skeleton, are divided into distinct lobes by fissures, allowing them to accommodate the movements of the thoracic wall and diaphragm. On the left side, the lungs are divided into a cranial lobe, with a cranial and caudal part, and a caudal lobe. The left pulmonary artery lies cranial to the left bronchus; the left pulmonary vein lies ventral to the left bronchus. The larger right lungs are divided into cranial, middle, caudal and accessory lobes. The right pulmonary artery is located dorsal and slightly caudal to the right bronchus; the right pulmonary vein lies ventral to the right bronchus.

Lung is absent from a small area between the heart and body wall at the ventral aspect of the fourth intercostal space called the 'cardiac notch'. A layer of mesothelial connective tissue covers both the lungs and the lining of the thorax, forming the visceral and parietal pleura, respectively. These pleura come together at the caudal lung lobes to make the pulmonary ligament; this ligament is severed to facilitate caudal lung lobectomy.

The lungs serve to exchange gases between inspired air and pulmonary arterial blood, a process that occurs by simple diffusion at the level of capillaries and alveoli. In a resting state the process of inspiration is provided mainly by diaphragmatic contraction, with expiration occurring passively from the elastic recoil of the lungs. In more active states, inspiratory muscle groups are called upon to pull the ribs cranially, thereby increasing intrathoracic volume, and expiratory muscle groups can be recruited to force expiration actively. The lungs are 'coupled' to the thoracic wall by a small amount of pleural fluid, such that changes in thoracic volume result in changes in lung volume.

Careful maintenance of alveolar ventilation is essential during thoracic surgery. Thoracotomy disrupts the coupling of the lungs to the thoracic wall, allowing the lungs to separate from the wall and collapse. During anaesthesia, manual or mechanical ventilation is essential to maintain adequate oxygenation and ventilation, necessitating increased equipment and/or technical support to undertake thoracic surgical procedures. Inappropriate rates of ventilation can result in gaseous and metabolic abnormalities, and ventilation must be coordinated with the operating surgeon to prevent injury to the lungs during surgery. Inappropriate pressure of ventilation can result in barotrauma to the lungs. Positive-pressure ventilation can also result in decreased venous return and cardiac output when the chest is a closed cavity. For these reasons thoracic surgery should only be undertaken by more experienced practitioners.

Diagnostic approach

The canine and feline respiratory patient must first be assessed by physical examination and stabilized prior to any major diagnostics (see Chapters 1 and 2).

Imaging

Thoracic radiography is indicated for most respiratory patients (for emergency situations, see Chapter 2). Radiographs may reveal airway disease (e.g. foreign body, neoplasia, asthma, collapsing trachea), primary lung disease (e.g. pneumonia, lung lobe torsion, lung tumour), secondary lung disease (e.g. heart failure) or pleural space disease (e.g. space-occupying mass, effusion, pneumothorax). The initial radiographic evaluation will determine what additional diagnostics are appropriate for the patient.

Transthoracic ultrasonography can provide valuable information about thoracic structures. It can be used to detect effusions and evaluate lung tissue where there is consolidation or a mass lesion. Using ultrasound guidance, accurate sampling of small pleural effusions and lung lesions adjacent to the thoracic wall can be obtained via fine-needle aspiration or needle biopsy. In one study, diagnostic samples were obtained in 51 of 56 patients (Reichle and Wisner, 2000).

> **WARNING**
>
> A 31% incidence of pneumothorax has been reported following transthoracic needle biopsy of the lung (Teske et al., 1991)

> **PRACTICAL TIP**
>
> Radiographs should be taken after lung aspiration or biopsy to determine whether pneumothorax has occurred. In patients with unilateral air leakage, it may be beneficial to lay the patient in lateral recumbency with the affected side down (Zidulka, 1987)

Advanced imaging, such as computed tomography (CT) or magnetic resonance imaging (MRI), has increased sensitivity for detecting pulmonary changes and metastatic disease (i.e. lymph node involvement), and may be useful for surgical planning.

Lavage

Transtracheal wash (TTW), endotracheal wash (EW) and bronchoalveolar lavage (BAL) can be useful diagnostic tools in cases of pneumonia, parasitic disease, inflammatory disease and lung tumours. TTW is minimally invasive and easily performed on a conscious or lightly sedated patient; EW and BAL require general anaesthesia. EW requires intubation with a sterile endotracheal tube, or use of a laryngeal mask airway and careful insertion of a bronchoscope. BAL uses bronchoscopy to facilitate sampling of specific lung lobe bronchi. Samples should be evaluated for cytology, and both aerobic and anaerobic cultures performed. Anaerobic cultures were positive in 18/104 cultures in a recent study (Johnson *et al.*, 2013). Details of these techniques are given in the *BSAVA Manual of Canine and Feline Clinical Pathology*.

> **PRACTICAL TIP**
>
> Preoxygenation prior to performing TTW or EW is helpful to prevent hypoxia during the procedure

Thoracotomy

Exploratory thoracotomy can be a diagnostic and/or therapeutic tool. If the underlying disease process can be localized to one side, a lateral thoracotomy is indicated. If exploration of the entire thoracic cavity is necessary, then a median sternotomy should be performed (for surgical approaches, see Chapter 11). In cases of primary pulmonary neoplasia, thoracotomy with lung lobectomy is both therapeutic and diagnostic. See Operative Technique 14.1 for details of the technique for lung lobectomy. Lung biopsy may also be performed via a 'keyhole' (mini-thoracotomy) approach, and this has proven useful in the management of interstitial lung diseases (Norris *et al.*, 2002). The keyhole biopsy technique is best for diffuse lung disease or peripheral lung lesions because access to the hilus is difficult through a limited incision.

Thoracoscopy or video-assisted thoracoscopic surgery (VATS)

An alternative to open thoracotomy, VATS is a minimally invasive technique that offers the advantages of decreased postoperative pain and shorter recovery time. Disadvantages include the need for specialized equipment and a steep learning curve (Garcia *et al.*, 1998). Lung biopsy using VATS allows sampling of any lung lobe tip in cases of diffuse disease but requires careful port placement to target a specific lung lesion. VATS lung lobectomy (Lansdowne *et al.*, 2005; Mayhew *et al.*, 2013) and VATS-assisted lung lobectomies (Laksito *et al.*, 2010; Wormser *et al.*, 2014) have been described in dogs.

VATS lung biopsy

For lung biopsy, dorsal or lateral recumbency can be used. Using dorsal recumbency, a more complete examination of both hemithoraces is possible. In dorsal recumbency, a subxiphoid camera port is usually established along with two further instrument ports placed on the right or left sides to give access to the periphery of one of the lung lobes. In lateral recumbency it is important to place the ports in a triangulating pattern around the anticipated lobe to be biopsied. A VATS lung biopsy specimen can be harvested by use of a loop ligature placed around the periphery of the lobe or by using an endoscopic stapling device (Figure 14.1).

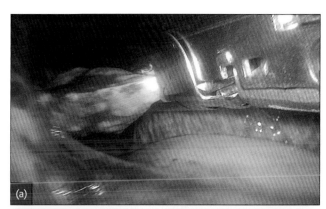
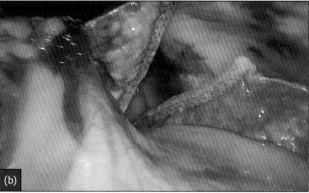

14.1 (a) An endoscopic stapler is seen in place across a section of lung lobe. (b) After discharge of the staple cartridge the triple rows of staples can be seen on either side of the resection site.

VATS and VATS-assisted lung lobectomy

In general, the VATS-assisted technique may be used in cases where the thoracic mass is modestly sized and located somewhat peripherally within the lobe, and where it requires larger thoracic wall incisions to exteriorize the lobe in question safely. It may be more challenging to resect masses close to the pulmonary hilus with this technique. However, the VATS-assisted technique does not involve induction of one-lung ventilation (OLV), which is considered mandatory for VATS lung lobectomy. A VATS-only approach allows resection of larger masses closer to the hilus, although the easiest cases remain those that are modestly sized and peripheral (Lansdowne *et al.*, 2005). The VATS technique is generally performed for masses ≤3–4 cm in size in dogs <20 kg, masses ≤4–7 cm in diameter in dogs 20–30 kg and masses ≤8–9 cm in dogs >30 kg.

For VATS-assisted and VATS lung lobectomy, most patients will be positioned in the corresponding left or right lateral recumbency depending on mass location. Recommended portal placement sites for VATS lobectomy are shown in Figures 14.2 and 14.3.

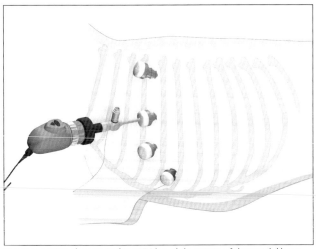

14.2 Port placement for VATS lung lobectomy of the caudal lung lobes. VATS = video-assisted thoracoscopic surgery.

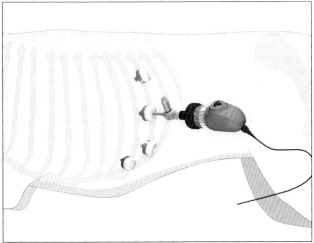

14.3 Port placement for VATS lung lobectomy of the cranial lung lobes. VATS = video-assisted thoracoscopic surgery.

VATS-assisted lung lobectomy – surgical technique

Once the lesion has been visualized from the telescope portal, an 'assist' incision is created one to two spaces caudodorsal (for cranial lobe lesions) or craniodorsal (for caudal lobe lesions) to the lesion. The length of this incision is generally made in proportion to the size of the lesion to be exteriorized, but in one report varied from 2 to 7 cm (Wormser *et al.*, 2014). It is helpful at this point to insert a commercially available wound retraction device (e.g. Alexis wound retractor, Applied Medical Inc., Rancho Santa Margarita, CA, USA) into the intercostal incision to facilitate lung lobe exteriorization without causing iatrogenic damage to the tissues. Once exteriorized, the lung lobe can be resected using either endoscopic staplers or traditional surgical stapling devices used for open thoracic surgery. The resulting thoracotomy incision is then closed in routine fashion.

VATS lung lobectomy – surgical technique

For VATS lung lobectomy, OLV is mandatory to enable sufficient visualization of the pulmonary hilus. OLV can be induced using a variety of modalities, including endobronchial blockers, double-lumen endobronchial tubes and selective intubation.

Initial placement of the telescope and blunt probe can assist the surgeon in visualization of the target lesion and in examination of any lymphadenopathy. If caudal lung lobes or accessory lobes are being resected, the pulmonary ligament must first be sectioned, which the authors prefer to do using a J-hook monopolar electrosurgical probe. An endoscopic stapler (e.g. EndoGIA, Covidien Inc., Mansfield, MA, USA) is mandatory for VATS lobectomy and will place three lines of staples on either side of the cut line, thus providing very secure closure of all airways and blood vessels within the lung tissue. Several cartridge lengths (30, 45 and 60 mm) and staple sizes (2.0, 2.5, 3.5 and 4.8 mm) are available. The 3.5 mm staple leg length is generally recommended for endoscopic lung stapling in dogs and appears to be very effective for a wide variety of patient sizes. Some stapler cartridges incorporate an 'articulating' tip, allowing the surgeon to angulate the direction of the staple line to suit their needs.

VATS tracheobronchial lymph node resection is possible and can be performed through a three-port approach (Steffey *et al.*, 2015).

Complications

Several important intra- and postoperative complications can be associated with VATS lung lobectomy. Haemorrhage from intercostal vessels has been reported, causing significant postoperative blood loss (Lansdowne *et al.*, 2005; Mayhew *et al.*, 2013). Haemorrhage or air leakage from the pulmonary hilus can also occur if the stapler does not function correctly or is incorrectly placed. Iatrogenic damage to surrounding structures (especially lung) can occur, and great care should be taken when passing instruments through thoracic cannulae. The most common reasons for conversion of a VATS lung lobectomy to an open approach are failure of OLV and haemorrhage (Lansdowne *et al.*, 2005; Mayhew *et al.*, 2013). Conversion to an open approach was necessary in 4/9 and 1/23 dogs operated on in two studies (Lansdowne *et al.*, 2005; Mayhew *et al.*, 2013). When resection of primary lung lobe tumours was compared between VATS and open approaches, there was no difference in the ability to obtain a clean margin of resection for these tumours with either approach (Mayhew *et al.*, 2013).

Postoperative considerations

Appropriate postoperative management of the thoracic surgery patient is essential for success (see also Chapter 1). Problems include: hypoventilation; haemorrhage; hypoxaemia; hypothermia; postoperative pain; acidosis; oliguria; shock; and death (Figure 14.4). Patients should be in a facility that is staffed with trained personnel 24 hours a day to allow close monitoring and optimal outcome.

Postoperative hypothermia is common and is treated by slowly warming the patient with warm blankets or forced hot air patient-warmers. Hypothermia exacerbates acidosis and hypotension and can potentiate oliguria. The surgery, postoperative haemorrhage, fluid losses, pain, anaesthetic drugs and hypothermia can lead to hypovolaemic shock. Intravenous fluids should be administered and urine output carefully monitored. Hypovolaemia and decreased urine output should be corrected early.

Hypoventilation results in respiratory acidosis and can worsen hypoxaemia. Hypoventilation may result from anaesthetic medications, postoperative pain, thoracic

Problem	Causes	Solutions
Hypothermia	Prolonged surgical time; open thorax; loss of thermoregulation due to anaesthesia	• Slow warming using water blankets or forced hot air warmers
Hypovolaemic shock	Fluid loss	• Intravenous fluid support; monitor urine output
	Pain	• Provide supplemental analgesia (note: opiates are respiratory depressants)
	Hypothermia	• Slow warming using water blankets or forced hot air warmers
	Acid–base disturbances (lactic acidosis from poor tissue perfusion)	• Fluid and colloid support to ensure good oxygen delivery to the tissues
Hypoventilation (blood pCO_2 ≥50 mmHg)	Anaesthetic protocols	• Partial reversal of opiate medication (if used) using butorphanol tartrate at 0.05 mg/kg
	Pain	• Provide supplemental analgesia (note: opiates are respiratory depressants) and local anaesthesia with intercostal blocks at surgery and interpleural bupivacaine postoperatively
	Pneumothorax	• Address pneumothorax • Provide oxygen therapy (maintain blood haemoglobin saturation ≥92–93%; pO_2 >80 mmHg)
	Thoracic bandage	• Loosen restrictive bandage
Hypoxaemia	Atelectasis	• Provide oxygen therapy (maintain blood haemoglobin saturation ≥92–93%; pO_2 >80 mmHg)
	Pleural space disease	• Aspirate thoracostomy tube and alternate recumbency of patient
Pain	Thoracic surgery; underlying disease	• Intercostal nerve blocks (1.5 mg/kg total dose bupivacaine) infiltrating the nerves at the thoracotomy and two rib spaces cranial and caudal to this incision • Interpleural bupivacaine (1.5 mg/kg total dose) infused via thoracostomy tube, incision-dependent, repeat q6–8h as needed • Regional anaesthesia with preservative-free morphine at 0.1 mg/kg given as high epidural or via epidural catheter • Systemic analgesics (e.g. morphine, oxymorphone, hydromorphone). Slow infusion of lidocaine into surgical wound using soaker/diffusion catheter at a rate of 1–2 mg/kg/h

14.4 Postoperative problems in the thoracic surgery patient.

bandages or pneumothorax. Hypoventilation is confirmed by an arterial blood pCO_2 ≥50 mmHg. If hypoventilation is suspected secondary to anaesthetic medications, a partial opiate reversal agent such as butorphanol tartrate can be used and benzodiazepines can be reversed with flumazenil. Hypoventilation secondary to pain should be addressed by providing supplemental analgesia, but caution should be used as many opiates are respiratory depressants at high doses. If a thoracic drain is in place it should be aspirated to rule out or address pneumothorax or accumulation of pleural effusion. Oxygen therapy should be provided during initial recovery as many patients are hypoxaemic secondary to the primary disease, acidosis or atelectasis. Oxygenation can be monitored with pulse oximetry and arterial blood gas analysis. The goal of the therapy is to maintain blood haemoglobin saturation ≥92–93% or pO_2 >80 mmHg, respectively.

In general, the patient will have had a thoracostomy tube placed intraoperatively for use in postoperative management (see also Chapter 12, or the *BSAVA Guide to Procedures in Small Animal Practice*). The thoracostomy tube is essential to monitor and manage complications such as pneumothorax or haemothorax. The thoracostomy tube should be aspirated every 2–6 hours until the fluid or air production is <2 ml/kg/day, at which time the tube may be removed. All connections should be secure and the tube should be handled aseptically to prevent iatrogenic pneumothorax and nosocomial infections. The tube should be covered with a light bandage to protect it, but care should be exercised so that the bandage does not interfere with ventilation. Possible postoperative haemorrhage should be monitored by periodic assessment of packed cell volume/total protein and blood pressure, and qualitative and quantitative assessment of thoracic drainage (Guillaumin and Adin, 2015).

Perioperative pain management is essential in the recovery of the thoracotomy patient. Intercostal nerve blocks may be performed intraoperatively with bupivacaine or ropivacaine at 1.5 mg/kg total dose, infiltrating the nerves of the intercostal incision and two rib spaces cranial and caudal to the incision. Long-acting liposome-encapsulated bupivacaine at a dose of 5.3 mg/kg can also be infiltrated into the tissues during closure. Regional anaesthesia and pain control with either a high epidural (single injection) or an epidural catheter for repeated injections can also be very useful. Preservative-free morphine is used at a dose of 0.1 mg/kg and may be administered every 12–24 hours via the epidural catheter. Alternatively, bupivacaine can be administered interpleurally (1.5 mg/kg total dose) via the thoracostomy tube. The patient should be placed in sternal or lateral recumbency with the incision down to deliver medication effectively to the surgical site. This method of local analgesia is useful for supplemental analgesia after surgery, as it can be repeated every 6–8 hours as needed. Another option is the use of wound/diffusion catheters (MILA International, Inc.), which are polyurethane catheters with micropores in the distal end. They can be placed in the thoracotomy incision at the time of closure, like a drain, but infused with local anaesthetic (2 mg/kg lidocaine and 1.5 mg/kg bupivacaine) (see *BSAVA Manual of Canine and Feline Anaesthesia and Analgesia*). Systemic analgesia, in the form of opiates such as morphine, oxymorphone or hydromorphone, can be used as necessary. It is generally safer to start with the lower doses and repeat dosing to titrate analgesia while trying to avoid excess respiratory depression.

Lung trauma

Causes of traumatic injuries to the lungs fall into two broad categories:

- Blunt, e.g. road traffic accident, kick, fall from a height
- Penetrating, e.g. gunshot, stick, knife, arrow, deep bite from a large dog on a small dog, secondary to displaced ends of fractured ribs.

These injuries can result in pneumothorax (see Chapter 12), haemothorax, pulmonary contusions, rib fractures, lung lacerations and diaphragmatic hernia (see Chapter 17). In all cases, life-threatening problems must be addressed initially. Once the patient is sufficiently stable, plain thoracic radiographs should be taken, preferably without the use of general anaesthesia, to assess for the presence of fractured ribs, lung contusions, oedema, or free air and fluid in the thorax.

If the patient has an open chest wound, the area should be clipped, prepared and dressed as quickly as possible to maintain the continuity of the thoracic wall. Objects that penetrate the thorax should be left *in situ*, where possible, to be removed via a lateral thoracotomy or median sternotomy once the patient is stable.

> **PRACTICAL TIP**
>
> Some projectiles may be seen on thoracic radiographs as an incidental finding. There is no perfect guideline regarding when to explore a penetrating chest wound. The risk for contamination and infection must be considered on a case-by-case basis

Occasionally, lung lacerations can occur when the chest is compressed laterally by trauma with the glottis closed; this may lead to a dramatic increase in intra-airway pressure and cause rupture of the conducting airways or alveoli of the lung. Another mechanism of injury is tearing of the trachea, mainstem bronchi or pulmonary parenchyma due to shearing forces generated by rapid acceleration or deceleration (e.g. road traffic accidents, 'high-rise syndrome').

The majority of animals that sustain thoracic trauma do not require surgical intervention. Pulmonary contusion and mild pneumothorax as a result of road traffic accidents are common and are frequently managed with supportive care. Most lung lacerations self-seal as a result of clot formation, elastic recoil and transpulmonary pressure. If the patient shows signs of respiratory distress (increased respiratory rate and effort) despite appropriate pain management, or the degree of pneumothorax is moderate or severe (based on plain thoracic radiographs), periodic thoracocentesis should be performed (see Chapter 12) in combination with serial thoracic radiographs to monitor resolution.

> **PRACTICAL TIP**
>
> The severity of pulmonary contusions may not be fully appreciated until 6–12 hours after lung trauma

If pneumothorax persists, worsens or fails to respond, a thoracostomy tube may be placed (see Chapter 12). If intermittent suction of a thoracostomy tube fails to empty the pleural space, continuous suction will be necessary. If the pneumothorax still fails to resolve (after 2–3 days with

a chest tube), exploratory thoracotomy is indicated. Other indications for exploratory thoracotomy include: rib fracture that impales lung tissue; penetrating wounds in which gross contamination of the thoracic cavity is suspected; the presence of penetrating objects within the thorax; or haemothorax producing >2 ml/kg/h for 3–4 hours.

Bite wounds over the thorax always require careful and thorough exploration once the patient is stable, particularly where a large dog has attacked and shaken a small dog (Figure 14.5) (see Chapter 11).

Puncture wounds that appear to be innocuous on the surface may be associated with large intercostal muscle tears and rib fractures. Deep palpation of the affected area of the thorax under anaesthesia can reveal large defects in the thoracic wall, beneath the skin. Plain radiographs may prove useful in locating the site of lung and thoracic trauma; otherwise, a median sternotomy may be necessary. Absence of pneumothorax on thoracic radiographs does not rule out significant thoracic pathology in bite wound cases.

When performing surgery for traumatic lung injury, air leaks should be located by filling the thorax with warm

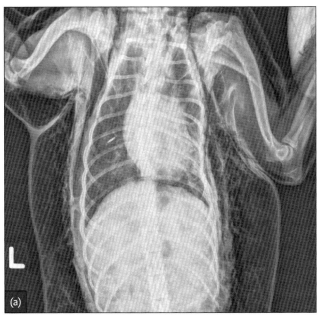

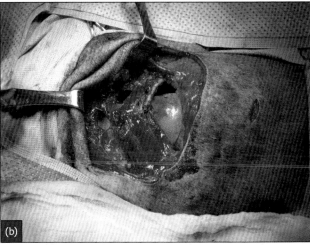

14.5 (a) Radiograph showing severe subcutaneous emphysema and multiple rib fractures in a 2-year-old Miniature Poodle that had sustained thoracic bite wounds. (b) At surgery, severe damage to ribs and thoracic wall musculature can be appreciated. The dog also sustained a traumatic impalement of a lung lobe caused by the sharp ends of one of the fractured ribs.

sterile saline, inflating the lungs and watching for air bubbles. Increasing airway pressure at the time of leak testing will improve detection rates. Superficial lung lacerations can be sealed using a simple continuous inverting mattress (Lembert) pattern (1.5 metric (4/0 USP) or 1 metric (5/0 USP) absorbable suture material). Deeper lacerations may require deep interrupted mattress sutures (2 metric (3/0 USP) or 1.5 metric (4/0 USP) absorbable suture material) to achieve haemostasis and pneumostasis, followed by a simple continuous pattern (1.5 metric (4/0 USP) or 1 metric (5/0 USP) absorbable suture material). Contused or oedematous lung tissue may be so friable that attempts to close the laceration can be difficult. In these cases partial or complete lung lobectomy should be considered if the injuries are confined to a single lung lobe (see below).

As much gross foreign material, such as grit or hair, should be removed from the wound and thoracic cavity as possible. A sample of pleural fluid should be retained for cytology and culture.

Fractured rib ends that protrude into the thorax can be cut short using a rongeur. They may also be reapposed using a K-wire inserted into the medullary cavity on the distal rib segment, and 'shuttled' into the proximal segment (Figure 14.6), or reapposed using cerclage wire or large-gauge (4 metric (1 USP) or 3.5 metric (0 USP)) absorbable suture material. The thorax must be thoroughly lavaged with several litres of sterile saline flush before testing for leaks.

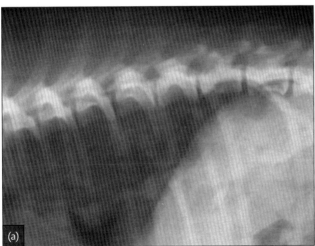

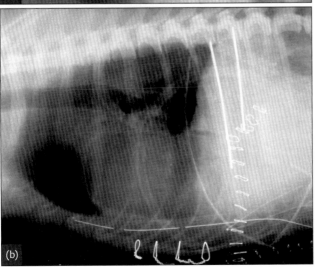

14.6 (a) Rib fractures (b) repaired using Kirschner wires.

Pulmonary abscess

Patients with pulmonary abscesses may present with a variety of clinical signs, including coughing, tachypnoea, haemoptysis, lethargy and fever. Radiography may be helpful; identification of a mass lesion with a gas–fluid interface in the lung is diagnostic of a pulmonary abscess. Such a radiographic appearance, however, is uncommon when radiographs are made in lateral recumbency and further diagnostic tests may be necessary. Medical testing should include a complete blood count, chemistry profile, urinalysis and thoracic radiography. One of the most useful aids to diagnosing pulmonary abscessation is transthoracic ultrasonography and aspiration of the lesion. CT imaging may also aid in the identification of a foreign body and accurate localization of the lesion.

If the lesion is solitary, the treatment of choice is thoracotomy with lung lobectomy. Once the affected lobe has been removed, it should be submitted for histopathology and culture and sensitivity testing, and appropriate antibiotic therapy should be instituted. One of the more common causes of pulmonary abscess formation is inhaled plant material (e.g. a grass awn). If there are multiple pulmonary abscesses, aggressive medical management may be indicated.

Pneumonia and bronchiectasis

Chronic lower respiratory tract infections can result in the accumulation of mucopurulent and purulent exudates or plugs that obstruct bronchi and bronchioles. Local inflammatory mediators cause loss of collagen and elastin in the bronchial walls, which dilate, causing further retention of infected secretions and creating a chronic disease. Clinical signs include recurrent fever, anorexia, debilitation and exercise intolerance. Brachycephalic dogs (Darcy *et al.*, 2016), spaniels and older dogs are over-represented (Hawkins *et al.*, 2003).

Pneumonia and bronchiectasis affect cranial and middle lung lobes most profoundly and are usually suspected on the basis of plain radiography. Most cases of chronic pneumonia should be managed medically, based on cytology and culture and sensitivity testing results following BAL. Affected dogs can survive for years. Complete or partial lobectomy has been described as a definitive diagnostic and therapeutic option where one or two isolated lobes are involved and the pneumonia has not responded to appropriate aggressive medical treatment. Pulmonary lobectomy in such circumstances resulted in a resolution of the pneumonia in 54% of animals treated

(Murphy *et al.*, 1997). Bacterial or fungal pneumonia was less likely to resolve when compared with foreign body pneumonia, and mortality increased when multiple lung lobes were involved.

Lung lobe torsion

Lung lobe torsion (LLT) occurs when a lung lobe rotates on its longitudinal axis, resulting in twisting of the bronchus and the pulmonary vessels at the hilus. LLT is a rare condition that has been reported in both dogs and cats and occurs most frequently in large, deep-chested dogs such as Afghan Hounds (the right middle and left cranial lung lobes have a higher incidence of torsion), although one atypical breed, the Pug, is apparently also predisposed (left cranial lung lobe more often affected). Reported clinical signs are non-specific and include dyspnoea, tachypnoea, lethargy, coughing, anorexia and weight loss. On physical examination, dull heart and lung sounds are the most common clinical abnormalities.

Pleural effusion is a common finding in dogs with LLT and has been reported to be chylous in nearly one-third of LLT cases (Neath *et al.*, 2000). Radiographic findings of abnormal bronchial position and blunting of the bronchial lumen are suggestive of LLT (Figure 14.7). Thoracic ultrasonography and thoracic CT may also be useful for diagnosis. CT characteristically shows an abruptly ending

bronchus with enlargement and emphysema of the affected lobe (Seiler *et al.*, 2008).

Thoracotomy with lobectomy of the affected lung lobe is the treatment of choice. The lung lobe should not be untwisted or repositioned prior to lobectomy, to prevent release of toxins or vasoactive substances into the systemic circulation. The prognosis for treatment of patients with LLT is fair to guarded. Although nearly all patients survive the initial surgery, there is a high complication rate, with only 55% of patients having non-complicated recovery (Neath *et al.*, 2000). The prognosis for Pugs is more favourable (Murphy and Brisson, 2006). There can be recurrence of LLT in some patients, or persistence of pleural effusion. The finding of a chylous effusion has been associated with a poor prognosis (Fossum *et al.*, 1985). Adjunctive procedures for treatment of the chylothorax may be necessary (see Chapter 12).

> **PRACTICAL TIP**
>
> Submit excised lung lobe for histopathology and perform culture and sensitivity testing of pleural fluid. Examine the thoracic cavity for any evidence of a primary disease process (e.g. neoplasia)

Spontaneous pneumothorax

Spontaneous pneumothorax is defined as a closed pneumothorax resulting from air leakage from the lung parenchyma, without any history of trauma. This is a rare condition in dogs and cats, although there appears to be a predilection in Huskies (Puerto *et al.*, 2002). The most common causes of spontaneous pneumothorax in dogs are pulmonary blebs (Figure 14.8) and bullous emphysema; other reported causes are neoplasia, pulmonary abscesses, bacterial pneumonia, heartworm and migration of plant foreign bodies. Seven cases of spontaneous pneumothorax have been reported in cats with small airway disease or asthma (Cooper *et al.*, 2003; White *et al.*, 2003).

In dogs, initial stabilization with thoracocentesis or thoracostomy tube placement may be necessary. Initial diagnostics include a complete blood count, chemistry profile, heartworm testing and thoracic radiography or CT. Early surgical exploration is recommended for dogs that do not have identifiable non-surgical disease or diffuse

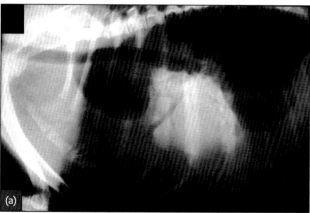

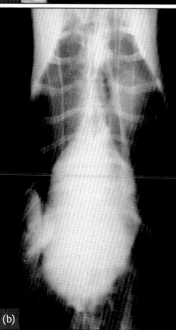

14.7 (a) Lateral and (b) ventrodorsal radiographs of an Afghan Hound with a right middle lung lobe torsion. Note the pleural effusion and prominent air bronchogram secondary to congestion of the affected lobe on the lateral view, and the appearance of the right middle lobe on the ventrodorsal view.

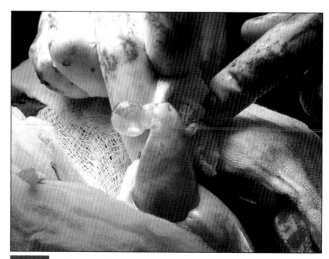

14.8 Pulmonary bleb in a 7-year-old Old English Sheepdog.

pulmonary disease. Radiography is good for detecting pneumothorax but has low sensitivity for detecting pulmonary bullae. CT is more sensitive than radiography for detection of bullae, but the positive predictive value is low and its clinical usefulness is poor as lesions may be missed or incorrectly diagnosed (Reetz *et al.*, 2013). Median sternotomy is the surgical approach of choice because it allows evaluation of all lung lobes, including the accessory lobe (see Chapter 11). Alternatively, a transdiaphragmatic thoracoscopic approach allows inspection of both hemithoraces. Immersion of the lung lobes in saline can help in localization of the affected lobe; once identified, a partial (Figure 14.9) or complete lobectomy is performed. Thoracoscopy with partial lung lobectomy has been reported for the surgical treatment of spontaneous pneumothorax (Brissot *et al.*, 2003).

Surgical treatment resulted in resolution of spontaneous pneumothorax with only a 3% recurrence rate in one study (Puerto *et al.*, 2002). Non-surgical treatment can be offered if surgical treatment is not feasible, but owners should be advised of higher recurrence and mortality rates. Blood-patch pleurodesis has also been reported for treating spontaneous pneumothorax and can be attempted following failure of conservative or surgical management (Oppenheimer *et al.*, 2014). Omentalization of all lung lobes is also a treatment option for dogs that have bullae in multiple lung lobes or where previous surgical management has failed.

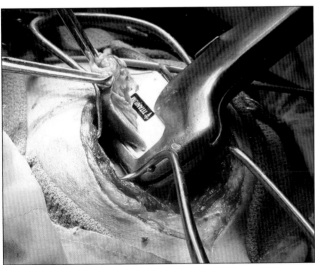

14.9 Ruptured bulla excised by using a thoracoabdominal stapler to perform partial lung lobectomy.

PRACTICAL TIP

Do not rely on radiographs for diagnosis of pulmonary bullae. Radiography is inconsistent and surgical findings often differ from what would be expected based on radiographs

Lung neoplasia

Primary pulmonary neoplasia is far less common than metastatic pulmonary neoplasia. Most primary lung tumours are malignant adenocarcinomas and metastasize early in the course of the disease. Affected cats and dogs are often relatively old (>10 years); affected dogs are more commonly of larger breeds (>10 kg). About one-quarter of all cats and dogs with primary lung neoplasia are free of clinical signs, with the remainder presenting with a non-productive cough of several weeks' to months' duration, anorexia, weight loss, lethargy, haemoptysis or spontaneous pneumothorax.

Diagnosis

The diagnosis is usually made on plain thoracic radiographs (Figure 14.10). Metastatic lung disease from other neoplasia tends to be small, circumscribed and located in the peripheral or middle portions of the lung. Primary lung tumours are usually solitary large masses. If there are metastases, there are usually additional smaller masses.

Evaluation of BAL fluid may also be useful in the early diagnosis of malignant primary or metastatic neoplasia (Danielski *et al.*, 2007). CT should also be considered for staging of patients with pulmonary neoplasia because it has a high sensitivity for detecting tracheobronchial lymphadenopathy (Paoloni *et al.*, 2006).

Hypertrophic osteopathy, involving soft tissue swelling and palisading periosteal proliferation of the bones of the extremities (Figure 14.11), is uncommon but can result in limb pain and lameness. Pulmonary metastatectomy produces early and sustained alleviation of the clinical signs of hypertrophic osteopathy (Liptak *et al.*, 2004). Metastasis of primary lung tumours to one or more digits is quite common in cats.

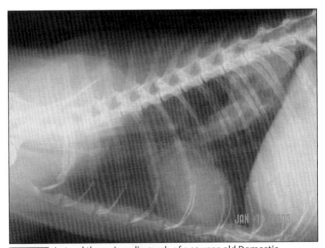

14.10 Lateral thoracic radiograph of a 14-year-old Domestic Longhaired cat with a primary lung tumour.

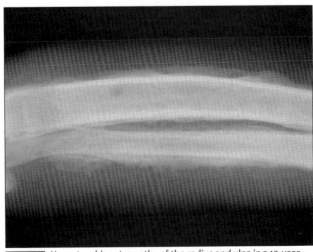

14.11 Hypertrophic osteopathy of the radius and ulna in a 10-year-old mixed-breed dog with a primary lung tumour.

Thorough physical examination for other primary sites of neoplasia should be combined with haematology, serum chemistry profile and urinalysis. Cytological evaluation of pleural fluid obtained via ultrasound- or CT-guided fine-needle aspiration can be helpful to provide more information prior to surgery.

Surgical treatment

Partial or complete lobectomy is indicated if there is a solitary lesion or multiple lesions within a single lobe. A partial lung lobectomy can be performed if the lesion involves the distal two-thirds of the affected lung lobe; otherwise, a complete lung lobectomy is necessary. These procedures (described in Operative Technique 14.1) require the use of a mechanical ventilator or an assistant dedicated to providing manual ventilation. Use of pulse oximetry, capnography and blood pressure monitoring equipment to monitor the patient is recommended. If using perioperative antibiotics, these should be given intravenously at the time of anaesthetic induction.

Use of mechanical stapling devices to perform partial or complete lung lobectomies provides a rapid and reliable alternative to hand suturing (Figure 14.12). Thoraco-abdominal (TA) staplers come in a variety of sizes to create staggered staple lines of 30 mm (TA30), 55 mm (TA55) and 90 mm (TA90). For the TA55 and TA90 there are two sizes of staple available: 3.5 mm (blue cartridge) and 4.8 mm (green cartridge). For partial or complete lung lobectomy, the authors prefer to use the blue 3.5 mm cartridge (compressing to 1.5 mm) or the white 30V3, which provides three staggered rows of 3 mm staples (compressing to about 1 mm) for additional security ('V' stands for vascular). The green 4.8 mm cartridge is for thick tissue and the staples compress to a size of about 2 mm, which is inadequate compression in the lung and will result in significant haemorrhage. Staplers can add to the cost of the procedure but this may be offset by decreased anaesthetic time and reduced risk for a critical patient.

Thoracoscopic lung lobectomy may also be performed in select cases as described earlier in this chapter.

WARNING

Mechanical staplers are relatively simple to use but some experience is necessary to select the appropriate size of device and to manipulate this equipment within the tight confines of the thorax

Testing for leaks can be performed by filling the thorax with sterile saline, inflating the lungs to a pressure of 25–30 cmH$_2$O and looking for bubbles. Small leaks may seal spontaneously, but application of small titanium clips (Surgiclips, Covidien Inc.) can prove useful to ensure a surgical seal. Excised tissue should be submitted for histopathological evaluation. It is important to examine the hilar lymph nodes, especially in cases of suspected neoplasia. Wedge biopsy or lymph node extirpation should be performed where possible. A thoracostomy tube should be placed and the pleural space emptied at the end of the surgery.

Prognosis

Survival times for dogs and cats are dependent on the grade and/or differentiation of the tumour. In one study (McNeil et al., 1997), dogs with well differentiated tumours had a median survival time (MST) of 790 days, whereas dogs with poorly differentiated tumours had an MST of 251 days. A more dramatic difference was found in cats with primary lung tumours: cats with moderately differentiated tumours had an MST of 698 days, which was significantly longer than that for cats with poorly differentiated tumours (MST = 75 days) (Hahn and McEntee, 1998). Solitary lung tumours in dogs carry a poor prognosis unless local lymph nodes are clean and metastatic disease is absent (Polton et al., 2008). For further details regarding primary lung neoplasia and adjunctive treatment options, see the BSAVA Manual of Canine and Feline Oncology.

14.12 Complete lung lobectomy (right middle lung lobe) using thoracoabdominal stapling equipment.

References and further reading

Bexfield N and Lee K (2014) BSAVA Guide to Procedures in Small Animal Practice, 2nd edn. BSAVA Publications, Gloucester

Brissot HN, Dupre GP, Bouvy BM and Paquet L (2003) Thoracoscopic treatment of bullous emphysema in 3 dogs. Veterinary Surgery 32, 524–529

Cooper ES, Syring RS and King LG (2003) Pneumothorax in cats with a clinical diagnosis of feline asthma: 5 cases (1990–2000). Journal of Veterinary Emergency and Critical Care 13, 95–101

Danielski A, Diaz Otero MA and Quintavall F (2007) The bronchoalveolar lavage (BAL) in metastatic lung cancer investigation in dogs and cats: a retrospect. Annali della Facolta ta di Medicina Veterinaria 22, 2791–2804

Darcy H, ter Haar G and Humm K (2016) Retrospective analysis of aspiration pneumonia in brachycephalic dogs (incidence, presentation and prognosis) at a university teaching hospital: preliminary results. *Journal of Small Animal Practice* **57**, 52–53

Dobson JM and Lascelles BDX (2003) *BSAVA Manual of Canine and Feline Oncology, 2nd edn.* BSAVA Publications, Gloucester

Duke-Novakovski T, de Vries M and Seymour C (2016) *BSAVA Manual of Canine and Feline Anaesthesia and Analgesia, 3rd edn.* BSAVA Publications, Gloucester

Fossum TW, Birchard SJ and Jacobs RM(1985) Chylothorax in 34 dogs. *Journal of the American Veterinary Medical Association* **188**, 1315–1318

Garcia F, Prandi D, Pena T, French J and Trasserra O (1998) Examination of the thoracic cavity and lung lobectomy by means of thoracoscopy in dogs. *Canadian Veterinary Journal* **39**, 285–291

Guillaumin J and Adin CA (2015) Postthoracotomy management. In: *Small Animal Critical Care Management*, ed. D Silverstein and K Hopper, pp. 703–707. Elsevier, St Louis

Hahn KA and McEntee MF (1998) Prognosis in cats after removal of primary lung tumor: 21 cases (1979–1994). *Veterinary Surgery* **27**, 307–311

Hawkins EC, Basseches J, Berry CR, Stebbins ME and Ferris KK (2003) Demographic, clinical, and radiographic features of bronchiectasis in dogs: 316 cases (1988–2000). *Journal of the American Veterinary Medical Association* **223**, 1628–1635

Johnson LR, Queen EV, Vernau W, Sykes JE and Byrne BA (2013) Microbiologic and cytologic assessment of bronchoalveolar lavage fluid from dogs with lower respiratory tract infection: 105 cases (2001–2011). *Journal of Veterinary Internal Medicine* **27**, 259–267

Laksito MA, Chambers BA and Yates GD (2010) Thoracoscopic-assisted lung lobectomy in the dog: report of two cases. *Australian Veterinary Journal* **88**, 263–267

Lansdowne JL, Monnet E, Twedt DC and Dernell WS (2005) Thoracoscopic lung lobectomy for treatment of lung tumors in dogs. *Veterinary Surgery* **34**, 530–535

Liptak JM, Monnet E, Dernell WS and Withrow SJ (2004) Pulmonary metastatectomy in the management of four dogs with hypertrophic osteopathy. *Veterinary and Comparative Oncology* **2**, 1–12

Mayhew PD, Hunt BG, Steffey MA *et al.* (2013) Evaluation of short-term outcome after lung lobectomy for resection of primary lung tumors via video-assisted thoracoscopic surgery or open thoracotomy in medium- to large-breed dogs. *Journal of the American Veterinary Medical Association* **243**, 681–688

McNeil EA, Ogilvie GK, Powers BE *et al.* (1997) Evaluation of prognostic factors for dogs with primary lung tumors: 67 cases (1985–1992). *Journal of the American Veterinary Medical Association* **211**, 1422–1427

Murphy KA and Brisson BA (2006) Evaluation of lung lobe torsion in Pugs: 7 cases (1991–2004). *Journal of the American Veterinary Medical Association* **228**, 86–90

Murphy ST, Mathews KG, Ellison GW and Bellah JR (1997) Pulmonary lobectomy in the management of pneumonia in dogs: 59 cases (1972–1994). *Journal of the American Veterinary Medical Association* **210**, 235–239

Neath PJ, Brockman DJ and King LG (2000) Lung lobe torsion in dogs: 22 cases (1981–1999). *Journal of the American Veterinary Medical Association* **217**, 1041–1044

Norris CR, Griffey SM and Walsh P (2002) Use of keyhole lung biopsy for diagnosis of interstitial lung diseases in dogs and cats: 13 cases (1998–2001). *Journal of the American Veterinary Medical Association* **221**, 1453–1459

Oppenheimer N, Klainbart S *et al.* (2014) Retrospective evaluation of the use of autologous blood-patch treatment for persistent pneumothorax in 8 dogs (2009–2012). *Journal of Veterinary Emergency and Critical Care* **24**, 215–220

Paoloni MC, Adams WM, Dubielzig RR *et al.* (2006) Comparison of results of computed tomography with histopathologic findings in tracheobronchial lymph nodes in dogs with primary lung tumors: 14 cases (1999–2002). *Journal of the American Veterinary Medicine Association* **228**, 1718–1722

Polton GA, Brearley MJ, Powell SM and Burton CA (2008) Impact of primary tumour stage on survival in dogs with solitary lung tumours. *Journal of Small Animal Practice* **49**, 66–71

Puerto DA, Brockman DJ, Lindquist C and Drobatz K (2002) Surgical and nonsurgical management of and selected risk factors for spontaneous pneumothorax in dogs: 64 cases (1986–1999). *Journal of the American Veterinary Medical Association* **220**, 1670–1674

Reetz JA, Caceres AV, Suran JN *et al.* (2013) Sensitivity, positive predictive value, and interobserver variability of computed tomography in the diagnosis of bullae associated with spontaneous pneumothorax in dogs: 19 cases (2003–2012). *Journal of the American Veterinary Medical Association* **243**, 244–251

Reichle JK and Wisner ER (2000) Non-cardiac thoracic ultrasound in 75 feline and canine patients. *Journal of Veterinary Radiology and Ultrasound* **41**, 154–162

Seiler G, Schwarz T, Vignoli M and Rodriguez D (2008). Computed tomography features of lung lobe torsion. *Veterinary Radiology and Ultrasound* **49**, 504–508

Steffey MA, Daniel L, Mayhew PD *et al.* (2015) Video-assisted thoracoscopic extirpation of the tracheobronchial lymph nodes in dogs. *Veterinary Surgery* **44**, 50–58

Teske E, Stokhof AA, van den Ingh TSGAM *et al.* (1991) Transthoracic needle aspiration biopsy of the lung in dogs with pulmonic disease. *Journal of the American Animal Hospital Association* **27**, 289–294

Villiers E and Ristic J (2016) *BSAVA Manual of Canine and Feline Clinical Pathology, 3rd edn.* BSAVA Publications, Gloucester

White HL, Rozanski EA, Tidwell AS, Chan DL and Rush JE (2003) Spontaneous pneumothorax in two cats with small airway disease. *Journal of the American Veterinary Medical Association* **222**, 1573–1575

Wormser C, Singhal S, Holt DE and Runge JJ (2014) Thoracoscopic-assisted pulmonary surgery for partial and complete lung lobectomy in dogs and cats: 11 cases (2008–2013). *Journal of the American Veterinary Medical Association* **243**, 1036–1041

Zidulka A (1987) Position may reduce or stop pneumothorax formation in dogs receiving mechanical ventilation. *Clinical and Investigative Medicine* **10**, 290–294

OPERATIVE TECHNIQUE 14.1

Partial or complete lung lobectomy

PATIENT POSITIONING

Right or left lateral recumbency, depending on the side of the lesion. Placing a rolled towel under the opposite side widens the near-side intercostal space and can simplify the surgical approach.

ASSISTANT

Useful for retraction.

ADDITIONAL INSTRUMENTS

Electrocautery; Finochietto rib retractor (appropriate size for patient); laparotomy pads (counted); sterile saline flush and sterile bowl; trochar chest tube (appropriate size for patient); lung lobe retractors; sterile cotton-tipped applicators; right-angled forceps; DeBakey forceps; Satinsky forceps; crushing forceps; long-handled Metzenbaum scissors.

SURGICAL TECHNIQUE

Approach

As for lateral thoracotomy (see Chapter 11). The affected lung lobe should be located. Unaffected lung lobes may inflate and obscure the surgical field. These lobes should be gently packed cranially or caudally within the thorax using moistened laparotomy pads, to allow isolation of the affected lobe. Careful resection of pleural attachments can further mobilize the lobe and simplify its removal.

Surgical manipulations

Partial lobectomy

1 Apply crushing forceps at the level of resection.

2 Place a continuous overlapping suture pattern (2 metric (3/0 USP) or 1.5 metric (4/0 USP) absorbable suture material) and tie it 0.5 cm proximal to the forceps to provide haemostasis/pneumostasis.

3 Transect the lung between the forceps.

4 Oversew the viable distal lung tissue in a simple continuous pattern (1.5 metric (4/0 USP) or 1 metric (5/0 USP) absorbable suture material).

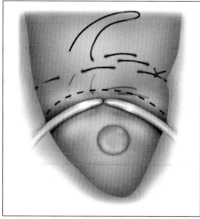 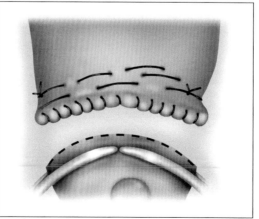

Partial lung lobectomy for removal of an apical lesion (dark circle). A haemostatic/pneumostatic overlapping continuous suture pattern is placed 5 mm proximal to the forceps. The lobe is incised along the dotted line and oversewn using a simple continuous pattern.

→ **OPERATIVE TECHNIQUE 14.1 CONTINUED**

Complete lobectomy

1 Triple-ligate the pulmonary arterial supply and transfix with 3 metric (2/0 USP) or 2 metric (3/0 USP) non-absorbable suture material.

2 Transect the pulmonary artery between the two distal sutures.

3 Carefully dissect the venous supply and ligate in a similar fashion.

4 Dissect the bronchus free and transect it between two pairs of crushing forceps.

PRACTICAL TIP
Sterile cotton-tipped applicators can be useful for gently teasing and bluntly isolating the artery, vein and bronchus

5 Remove the affected lobe.

6 Preplace a series of interrupted horizontal mattress sutures (3 metric (2/0 USP) or 2 metric (3/0 USP) non-absorbable suture material) in the bronchus before placing sutures to seal the bronchus.

7 Oversew the distal tissue using a simple continuous pattern (1.5 metric (4/0 USP) or 2 metric (3/0 USP) absorbable suture material).

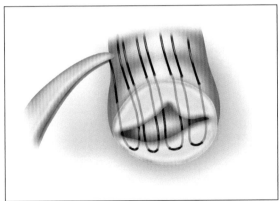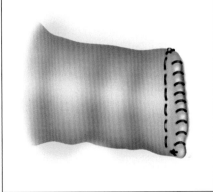

Preplacement of interrupted horizontal mattress sutures in the bronchus. The mattress sutures are then tied and the end of the bronchus is oversewn using a simple continuous pattern.

Closure

See Chapter 11.

Chapter 15

Surgery of the heart, pericardium and great vessels

Daniel J. Brockman

Introduction

There are a wide variety of acquired and congenital conditions that affect the heart, pericardium or great vessels for which there are either proven or potential surgical treatments. The operations required to effect these therapies are divided into two broad categories: extracardiac and intracardiac. The most common conditions that require extracardiac dissection to execute the surgical treatment are patent ductus arteriosus (PDA), vascular ring anomalies (VRA) and diseases that require partial pericardectomy for either palliation or definitive treatment. More occasionally, animals with neoplasms such as right atrial haemangiosarcoma, and those with some rare congenital heart conditions, such as tetralogy of Fallot, can be managed successfully using extracardiac manipulations.

As is the case in humans, intracardiac surgery that needs prolonged 'open heart' time requires cardiopulmonary bypass (CPB) to be done safely. Although CPB is in widespread use in human medicine, it is only available at a few specialist veterinary centres around the world. Intracardiac surgical therapy can be performed successfully under conditions of temporary vascular occlusion (typically total venous inflow occlusion (TVIO)), providing the intracardiac manipulations required are not complicated and can be completed within the 5–8-minute window that TVIO can provide. Such conditions include some types of valvular pulmonic stenosis, double-chambered right ventricle and cor triatriatum dexter. Even though these conditions can be managed successfully without cardiopulmonary bypass, in humans these operations are done more safely, more accurately and, therefore, with more consistent results, under conditions of CPB. It is anticipated that, in centres that offer these techniques for animals, this will also be the case for open heart surgery under CPB in dogs. Such techniques are beyond the scope of this manual.

This chapter will focus on conditions and techniques that would be appropriate and reasonable for a skilled practitioner to attempt. It is safe for the reader to assume, however, that all of these procedures could be quite reasonably designated 'specialist', from either a diagnostic perspective, a therapeutic perspective, or both, and as such would always benefit from the attention of a specialist team. That said, owners may decide not to pursue specialist treatment for a variety of reasons and so the only option, if therapy is to be pursued, will be to attempt such surgery in a practice setting. Of course, there is a learning curve with all surgical procedures, but a detailed understanding of the anatomy and pathoanatomy of VRA, PDA, and the pericardium and associated structures should allow most practised surgeons to attempt these procedures. Again, this may be justified if the alternative is euthanasia.

Optimizing safety when dissecting near the heart and great vessels

Although this chapter is not going to describe intracardiac surgical techniques, there are two surgical manoeuvres that are useful when dissection around the heart and great vessels is undertaken. These techniques will allow short-term cessation of blood flow through the heart so that vascular forceps can be placed accurately, should bleeding occur from a major vessel. Bleeding from a ruptured PDA or the right auricular appendage can be profuse and rapidly fatal, so these 'safety' manoeuvres should be prepared before any dissection around these structures is done, and deployed when needed. The two techniques are TVIO and total cardiac outflow occlusion (TCOO). In addition to these surgical manoeuvres, it is important that the anaesthesia and surgery team are appropriately prepared, blood products are available and the patient has sufficient intravenous access sites to allow rapid infusion of blood, should it become necessary. In the author's practice, pre-operative, intraoperative and postoperative checklists have been created for all surgical procedures, in an attempt to minimize the risk of errors. They have also adopted a 'time out' culture where the surgery, anaesthesia and nursing teams confirm the patient identification, procedure to be performed, anticipated concerns and equipment availability, immediately prior to commencing surgery, to reduce errors and focus the team.

Total venous inflow occlusion

TVIO is achieved by placing Rummel snares around the cranial and caudal vena cavae and the azygos vein. These vessels are easily identified from a right lateral approach or a ventral sternotomy but require a little more dissection from a left-sided approach. Typically, these tourniquets are placed and kept loose until they are needed. In healthy dogs, uneventful resuscitation should be possible after up to 8 minutes of TVIO. In dogs with diseased hearts, the permissible time for complete occlusion may be reduced. The objective, in the scenarios presented in this chapter, is to perform TVIO for as short a period of time as is necessary to achieve haemostasis using vascular clamps. Once the vascular clamps are in place, TVIO is concluded and blood circulation restored. The author's tip for using Rummel snares is to make the tubing that creates the snare long enough to be 'out of the way' once the snare is clamped (Figure 15.1).

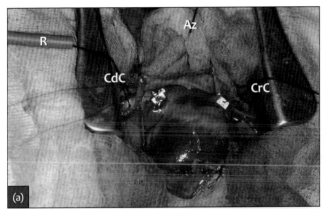

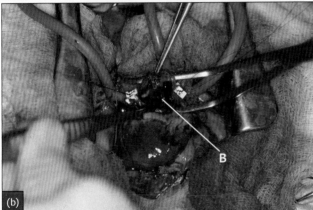

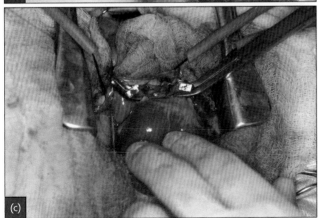

15.1 (a) In this dog with cor triatriatum dexter, thick (3.5 metric (o USP)) silk has been placed around the cranial vena cava (CrC), azygos vein (Az) and caudal vena cava (CdC) via a right fifth intercostal approach. Each silk suture passes through a length of rubber tubing (R) to make a Rummel snare in preparation for total venous inflow occlusion. Pericardial basket sutures keep the lung out of the surgical field. (b) The snares are tightened and held in place by clamps on the silk suture as it exits the rubber tubing (out of photograph), to arrest venous inflow and allow intracardiac manipulations. The fibromuscular band dividing the right atrium, which is to be resected, can be seen (B). (c) Once the atrium is sealed by the vascular (Satinsky) clamp, the snares are released and the circulation of blood resumes. The atrial incision is closed 'inside' the clamp.

Total cardiac outflow occlusion

TCOO is usually achieved by placing a straight vascular clamp from the left side of the chest, across the main pulmonary artery and the aortic root simultaneously. This manoeuvre is achieved by opening the pericardium directly ventral to the left phrenic nerve such that one jaw of the vascular clamp passes across the base of the heart via the transverse pericardial sinus and the more cranial jaw of the vascular clamp passes cranial to the pulmonary artery and aorta so that closing the jaws occludes them at the same time. This manoeuvre, in combination with traction on the aortic noose (see the section on PDA), should stop blood flow from a torn ductus, for example, sufficient to allow the placement of haemostatic vascular forceps. Again, occlusion time should be kept as short as is possible (Figure 15.2).

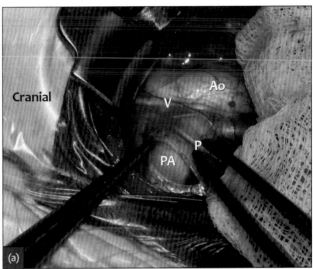

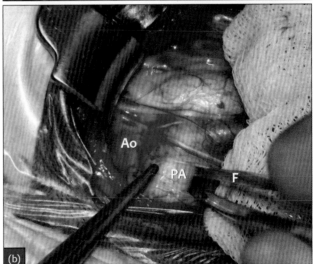

15.2 (a) The view of the heart and pericardium via a left fourth intercostal thoracotomy in a 1.4 kg dog with patent ductus arteriosus. An incision has been made in the pericardium ventral to the phrenic nerve (P), revealing the pulmonary artery trunk (PA). The vagus nerve (V) and aorta (Ao) are also visible. (b) The closed Potts forceps (F) are passing across the transverse pericardial sinus (TPS), isolating the aortic and pulmonary artery roots, which lie cranially. If bleeding occurs during dissection, a straight vascular clamp with the caudal jaw passing across the TPS and the cranial jaw cranial to the aorta allows total cardiac outflow occlusion to be achieved. Along with traction on the aorta, this manoeuvre should allow time to place a haemostatic vascular clamp across the bleeding ductus.

Pericardial diseases

The pericardium is continuous with the mediastinum and consists of a dense fibrous pericardial sac, which is covered by mesothelium on its pleural and parietal surfaces. The pericardial sac normally contains a small volume of fluid that lubricates the surfaces of the parietal serous pericardium and the visceral serous pericardium (epicardium). Because of the dense fibrous tissue in the pericardium, it is relatively inelastic, although it can become 'stretched' over time, as is seen in dogs with chronic pericardial effusion. As mentioned above, a tube of epicardium traverses the base of the heart caudal to the aorta and the pulmonary artery, the transverse pericardial sinus, which creates a direct communication between the two sides of the pericardial sac. This feature can assist placement of a TCOO clamp (see earlier).

Clinical features of pericardial disease

Cardiac tamponade is the term used to describe the detrimental effect of increased intrapericardial pressure on heart chamber filling and, therefore, on ventricular ejection. Such an increase in intrapericardial pressure can result from an abnormal volume of pericardial fluid or secondary to fibrous 'restrictive' pericardial disease. Permanent relief from tamponade is typically a key goal of pericardial surgery. Clinically, animals in tamponade will be presented because of signs associated with right-sided heart failure such as exercise intolerance and ascites. Physical examination can reveal tachycardia, muffled heart sounds, a consistent variation in peripheral arterial pulse quality associated with the different phases of respiration (pulsus paradoxus), jugular distension with pulsation, hepatomegaly and free peritoneal fluid. Although a transient increase in pericardial fluid can accompany many disease processes (viral infections, trauma, anticoagulant intoxication), most commonly tamponade is caused by the effusion associated with heart-base tumours, idiopathic pericardial disease and, occasionally, bacterial infective pericarditis. In addition, haemorrhage from a bleeding tumour (e.g. right atrial haemangiosarcoma), or from a 'tear' in the left atrial wall secondary to degenerative mitral valve disease, can cause either a gradual or an acute increase in intrapericardial pressure, resulting in tamponade. The diagnosis can be confirmed most rapidly using cardiac ultrasonography. Once the patient is stable, a thorough investigation should be undertaken in an attempt to identify an underlying cause for the effusion along with any concurrent disease processes.

Patient stabilization

Short-term relief of cardiac tamponade secondary to increased pericardial fluid volume can be achieved by pericardiocentesis. This technique involves draining the pericardium using a needle or catheter, via a right lateral thoracic approach (fifth intercostal space). Ultrasound guidance is ideal, and local anaesthetic infiltration of the skin and full aseptic technique should be used in all but the most urgent circumstances. Intermediate-term relief of tamponade can be achieved using a Seldinger technique to place a short-term indwelling catheter or to facilitate balloon dilation of the pericardial 'hole' to allow prolonged drainage. Typically, needle holes and balloon holes seal over time. (See the BSAVA Guide to Procedures in Small Animal Practice.)

Pericardial surgery

The indications for pericardial surgery include incision, to allow access to the heart for surgical manipulation, and excision (subtotal pericardectomy) to treat a range of conditions including neoplastic and idiopathic pericardial effusions, bacterial pericarditis and chylothorax. Subtotal pericardectomy, the removal of as much pericardium as is reasonably achievable, can be done via a left or right thoracotomy, via median sternotomy or thoracoscopically. Selecting the correct patient for pericardial surgery and matching that patient with the correct technique is the first step to minimizing both disease-related and technical complications. For example, dogs suspected to be suffering from bacterial infective pericarditis are probably best treated by open thoracic exploration and pericardectomy, to maximize the ability of the surgeon to identify any underlying cause (e.g. foreign body) and optimize the debridement of infected and diseased tissue whilst minimizing the risk of iatrogenic phrenic nerve injury. Alternatively, a dog with suspected right atrial haemangiosarcoma may be best approached via a right fifth intercostal thoracotomy to facilitate complete assessment of the right atrium. Finally, an aged dog with a presumptive chemodectoma at the heart base causing pericardial effusion may be palliated sufficiently by the minimally invasive creation of a pericardial window, whereas the same procedure may be inferior for the treatment of idiopathic pericardial effusion. Because of the difficulty in achieving a definitive diagnosis, it is recommended that any pericardium removed is submitted for microscopic examination, along with pleural biopsy material and sternal lymph node biopsy specimens.

Open subtotal pericardectomy

This is best performed via a left or right fifth intercostal thoracotomy or median sternotomy. Release of pericardial fluid can cause significant haemodynamic improvement and should be done as soon as possible once the chest cavity is open, and the anaesthetist should be made aware when this is happening. Usually, it is possible to elevate the phrenic nerve gently from the pericardium and protect this structure using a silicone vessel loop or Penrose drain, at least on the side of the thoracotomy, thus allowing the pericardial resection to be carried out close to the dorsal pericardial reflection. Once the phrenic nerve has been elevated, the pericardium is incised parallel to the heart base and the incision is continued towards the heart apex to form a T-shaped incision. Stay sutures in the pericardial edges will help with these manipulations, and the incision in the often quite vascular pericardium can be made using electrosurgery or a harmonic instrument to aid haemostasis, providing the myocardium and phrenic nerve are well protected. The incision around the base of the heart is continued either above or below the level of the phrenic nerve, depending on whether it has been mobilized, on the contralateral side of the heart.

These manipulations may require temporary displacement of the heart and can cause a significant temporary reduction in venous return and systemic blood pressure. The anaesthetist should also be made aware when the heart is being manipulated in such a way and it may be necessary to perform this part of the resection in 'stages' if severe hypotension develops. Completing the pericardial incision from 'inside' the pericardium will prevent the surgeon inadvertently wandering into the mediastinal adipose tissue (which can be voluminous) and damaging other structures therein. Once the heart base incision is complete, the sternopericardial ligament must be cut, preferably using electrosurgery, and the pericardium can be removed (Figure 15.3). The site of pericardial excision must be carefully evaluated, especially the mediastinal reflections, as small bleeding vessels that require attention can be hidden within mediastinal fat. The thorax should be flushed with sterile saline and a thoracostomy tube placed.

Thoracoscopic pericardial window and subtotal pericardectomy

The thoracoscopic creation of a pericardial window is, perhaps, most appropriate for palliation in older dogs with slow-growing tumours of the aortic body (chemodectoma) that have developed tamponade. In addition, subtotal (subphrenic) pericardectomy can be performed on dogs with presumed idiopathic pericardial effusions. The techniques can be performed from a lateral or ventral approach, although the author has only performed this from a ventral approach with the camera in a subxiphoid position and two ports for surgical manipulation, one on either side of the thorax in the sixth or seventh intercostal position.

Complications

Potential complications associated with subtotal pericardectomy include: haemorrhage; cardiac herniation (through a restrictive pericardial window); phrenic nerve injury; and recurrence of either pericardial or pleural effusion.

Postoperative care

The thoracostomy tube is maintained until the thorax is completely evacuated and until the volume of fluid production has fallen to an acceptable level. Routine post-thoracotomy care is recommended (see Chapters 1 and 11).

Patent ductus arteriosus

The ductus arteriosus, which joins the descending aorta to the left main pulmonary artery, is required in the developing fetus to allow blood ejected by the right ventricle to avoid the highly resistant pulmonary vasculature and gain access to the systemic circulation (right to left shunt) in order for the fetus to receive oxygen from the placenta. Normally, the ductus should close in the first few days of extrauterine life, in response to changes in blood oxygen content and reduced resistance to blood flow associated with lung ventilation. If this closure mechanism fails, the ductus remains patent (PDA) and, providing the pulmonary vasculature has developed normally, blood flow through the ductus typically reverses (i.e. becomes left to right), creating a relative overload of the pulmonary vasculature, left atrium and left ventricle. This overload can ultimately lead to fatal left heart failure, if left untreated.

James Buchanan (Buchanan, 1978, 2001) described the anatomy of the ductus arteriosus in a series of animals with naturally occurring PDA. His description of the overall

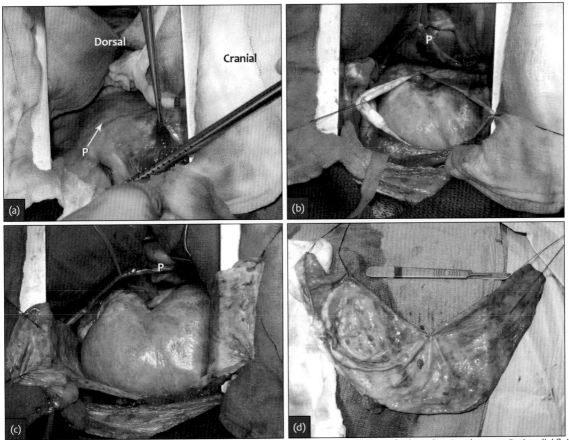

15.3 (a) The view from a right fifth intercostal thoracotomy in a dog undergoing 'open' subtotal pericardectomy. Pericardial fluid is seen gushing from a small incision in the pericardium made almost immediately on entry to the thorax to relieve any tamponade. The phrenic nerve (P) can also be seen. (b) The phrenic nerve (P) has been dissected free of the pericardium and is gently held dorsally using a silicone vessel loop. Silk stay sutures are holding the pericardium open after a vertical incision has been made from the base to the apex of the pericardial sac. (c) Elevation of the phrenic nerve allows the T-shaped incision to be made close to the dorsal pericardial reflection. If the left phrenic nerve can be isolated in a similar way, the incision in the pericardium is continued at this level all the way around the base of the heart. (d) Once removed, the pericardium is inspected and a sample of tissue submitted for microbiological analysis with the remainder submitted for histopathological analysis. It is good practice to submit pleural biopsy specimens and sternal lymph node samples from dogs with presumed idiopathic disease.

shape of the different forms of PDA, and his analysis of the histology of the ductus wall, which suggested that the eccentric distribution of muscular and elastic fibres therein were the cause of failure of the normal closure mechanism, have proved to be definitive studies. These studies also demonstrated that certain regions of the ductus and the section of the aortic wall through which the ductus courses (called the 'ductus aneurysm') were very thin in comparison with the normal aorta. This finding could explain, in part, the fragility of the ductus/aorta occasionally experienced during dissection in some animals. In addition, certain anatomical types of ductus (very short and wide) may be even more challenging to dissect free. These cases, it is suggested, would be better suited to clamping, division and oversewing of the cut ends of the ductus (Buchanan, 1967).

Clinical features

Animals with left to right shunting of blood frequently have a palpable 'thrill' associated with a 'machinery' murmur most easily heard at the left fourth intercostal space and radiating cranially. This murmur is often identified during routine pre-vaccination examination. Affected animals will typically develop congestive left heart failure within the first 12 months of life. Dogs with 'balanced flow' across the PDA and dogs with right to left shunting PDA will have minimal to no audible murmur and such animals may be presented with a combination of exercise intolerance and apparent lumbar pain, and will frequently sit down following modest exercise. Affected dogs will often have differential cyanosis (i.e. pink mucus membranes cranially with contemporaneous blue mucus membranes in the caudal body), reflecting the admixture of deoxygenated blood with the left ventricular output 'downstream' to the site where the brachycephalic trunk and left subclavian arteries leave the aorta.

Diagnosis of heart enlargement and the presence of pulmonary oedema can be made radiographically, so radiographs should be obtained of any dog with such a murmur and pulmonary 'crackles'. Abnormal heart chamber enlargement and the flow through a ductus can be confirmed using ultrasonography.

Patient stabilization

If pulmonary oedema is present, loop diuretics (furosemide) should be administered for a short period (a couple of days) prior to anaesthesia for occlusion of the PDA. Animals with 'balanced flow' may benefit from pulmonary vasodilators, such as sildenafil, prior to surgical intervention.

PDA occlusion

Ductal occlusion is normally recommended for dogs and cats with left to right shunting PDA. Animals with 'balanced flow' through a PDA and, therefore, concomitant pulmonary hypertension, may also be considered candidates for PDA occlusion, but PDA occlusion is contraindicated in animals with established pulmonary hypertension (presumed persistent fetal pulmonary circulation) with permanent right to left shunting of blood. Although more complications are seen in older dogs with PDA and dogs with more severe left heart dilatation (causing severe mitral incompetence and/or atrial fibrillation), such complications are not usually of a 'technical' surgical nature and these animals usually still benefit haemodynamically from ductus occlusion (van Israël et al., 2003; Bureau et al., 2005).

Non-surgical occlusion of PDA with intravascular thrombogenic coils, the Amplatz™ ductal occluder or the specifically designed Amplatz™ canine ductal occluder, using interventional radiology techniques, has become the most common therapy used in referral practice. As non-surgical occlusion has evolved, refinements in occluder and delivery system design have meant that surgical ligation of PDA is only considered for either very small or very large animals, where non-surgical occlusion is not possible for technical reasons. As a consequence, even highly trained surgeons are not practised at the dissection required for successful surgical ligation of a PDA; in addition, surgery is only ever required for the most challenging patients. Although operative mortality rates of 0% have been reported by individuals highly experienced in cardiac surgery (Bureau et al., 2005), for most, lack of familiarity with the procedure means that the risk of a fatal 'technical' complication is considerable. However, if owners cannot afford referral for specialist treatment (surgery or minimally invasive occlusion) this operation can be successful in the hands of any practised surgeon familiar with intrathoracic surgery.

Several surgical techniques that allow the successful placement of circumferential ductal ligatures have been described in the peer-reviewed literature and surgical texts. Broadly, these are: predominantly extrapericardial dissection; predominantly intrapericardial dissection; and an indirect approach to encircling the ductus by dissection around the aorta cranial and caudal to the ductus (Jackson and Henderson, 1979). The author of this chapter has no personal experience with the last technique so it will not be mentioned further. It is important, however, to select a technique and to practise that technique almost exclusively, since familiarity will bring better results. Both Buchanan (1967) and Eyster (1985) advocated performing manoeuvres that would be useful in the event of ductal haemorrhage. Although rarely needed, these manoeuvres have formed a routine part of the author's preparation, in case intraoperative complications develop (see earlier comments on TCOO). As previously mentioned (see also Chapter 1), prior to commencing any surgical procedure, it is critical that any contingency plans are made (blood products, familiarization with anatomy, equipment availability and team preparation). In the author's team, the custom is to have 'time out' prior to initiating surgery to ensure that everyone in the operating room is aware of what is being done and is alert to any potential complications and also prepared to take mitigating actions. Only once the team is certain these are all 'in place' does the surgery begin.

Ductus dissection can be performed through the left fourth intercostal space in most animals. Occasionally, a fifth intercostal incision is preferable in cats and some dogs; the evaluation of the position of the ductus relative to the chest wall, based on preoperative radiographs, can assist in this decision. Once the chest is opened, the pericardium is opened immediately ventral to the phrenic nerve, to provide access to the transverse pericardial sinus, therefore facilitating the placement of a straight vascular clamp across the ascending aorta and main pulmonary artery trunk, to allow temporary TCOO in the event of haemorrhage (see Figure 15.2). The author prefers either extrapericardial dissection alone or combined extra- and intrapericardial dissection (in very small patients), so no further intrapericardial manipulations are done at this stage. The phrenic nerve and the vagus nerve are dissected free from the pericardium and retracted ventrally using stay sutures or a silicone vessel loop. The left recurrent laryngeal nerve is identified as it leaves the left vagus and travels caudal to the PDA so as to avoid inadvertent damage.

A right-angled dissection instrument (Mixter or Lahey bile duct forceps) is then used to dissect around the aorta caudal to the ductus but cranial to the first intercostal artery. Either moist umbilical tape or a 6.4 mm (¼ inch) Penrose drain, or a silicone vessel loop (depending on the size of the animal) is placed loosely around the aorta and secured with artery forceps. Using gentle traction on this aortic noose, the space caudal to the ductus between the aorta, ductus and pulmonary artery trunk can be opened and extended medially by gentle dissection under direct visualization (Figure 15.4ab). This dissection is done first because it provides access for the placement of straight ductus clamps, should haemorrhage develop during future dissection. Cranial to the ductus, the space between the aortic wall and the ductus can be opened by gentle dissection (Figure 15.4c). In very small animals this dissection does not always remain extrapericardial but in larger animals it should. The preparation caudal to the

ductus should help the surgeon gain a good understanding of the dimensions of the ductus and allow gentle passage of a dissection instrument (usually Mixter or Halsted mosquito forceps, as appropriate) either from cranial to caudal or caudal to cranial, at an appropriate level to complete the ductus dissection (Figure 15.4d). Once dissection is complete, the author prefers to pass two appropriately sized surgical silk sutures around the ductus, along with one fine (1 metric (5/0 USP)) polypropylene suture (Figure 15.4e). The silk suture on the aortic side is tied first, with the aim of arresting blood flow through the ductus and abolishing the machinery murmur. Next, the polypropylene suture is tied and finally the silk suture on the pulmonary artery side is tied (Figure 15.4f). Frequently, abolition of blood flow through the ductus is associated with an acute increase in diastolic blood pressure and, therefore, mean blood pressure; this increased 'afterload' is sensed by baroreceptors in the aortic wall, which in turn trigger a bradycardic response (Branham sign). This is typically short-lived and rarely requires treatment, although it can be temporarily disconcerting.

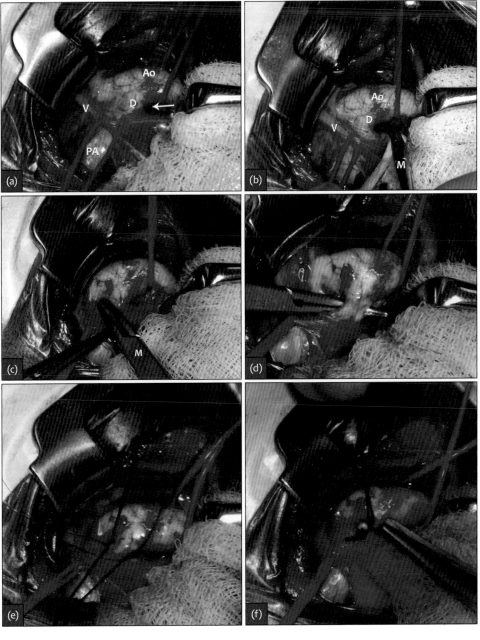

15.4 (a) The view of the heart and pericardium via a left fourth intercostal thoracotomy in a 1.4 kg dog with patent ductus arteriosus. With a vessel loop around the vagus nerve (V) and one around the aorta (Ao), the ductus arteriosus (D) is apparent. With gentle dorsal traction on the aorta, the dissection plane caudal to the ductus is made obvious (arrowed). PA = pulmonary artery trunk. (b) This dissection can be developed gently using a Mixter (M) or Halsted mosquito forceps, as appropriate. (c) The dissection plane between the cranial ductus and the aorta is identified by a 'crease' in the overlying mediastinum. This plane is gently developed using Mixter (M) or Halsted mosquito forceps, as appropriate. (d) The dissection around the ductus was completed using mosquito forceps in this small dog. (e, f) Two sutures of surgical silk and one fine polypropylene suture are passed around the ductus and tied.

Complications

Haemorrhage most commonly occurs during dissection of the craniomedial ductus, although the author has also experienced haemorrhage as the ligatures were being tied after apparently uneventful dissection. Care must be taken not to continue the dissection too 'deep' in relation to the ductus because the right pulmonary arterial branch is vulnerable in this position. Similarly, a 'shallow' dissection can lead the instrument directly into the medial ductus wall. Occasionally, when haemorrhage is minimal, a change in the direction of dissection (i.e. changing from cranial–caudal to caudal–cranial) will allow completion of the dissection. If haemorrhage is more brisk, the duct can be clamped. As previously mentioned, the author prefers straight (ductus) clamps placed in a caudal to cranial direction following elevation of the descending aorta using the noose that was placed previously. In over 25 years performing PDA surgery, the author has had to use TCOO only once but has clamped and oversewn the ductus in more than six animals, including one cat.

With ductus clamps in place and haemorrhage under control (see Figure 15.2), it is important to create enough room to transect the ductus and oversew the cut ends (hopefully incorporating the iatrogenic tear). This can be achieved either by carefully repositioning the clamps or by placing additional clamps alongside the initial haemostatic clamps, further away from the intended division site, to create enough room once the primary clamps are removed. The ductus ends can be closed using fine polypropylene suture material (1.5 metric (4/0 USP) to 0.7 metric (6/0 USP), depending on the size of the animal) either in two overlapping rows of simple continuous sutures or one continuous horizontal mattress suture oversewn by a simple continuous suture. Secure knots must be tied at each end and these knots should be augmented by expanded polytetrofluroethylene (ePTFE) pledgets in large dogs. Additional suture material should be ready prior to the removal of the vascular clamps. If haemorrhage is seen once the clamp is removed, the leak can be sutured either immediately or following replacement of the clamp. It is common to see a small amount of leakage adjacent to the suture, through suture needle holes, but application of a topical haemostatic agent (e.g. cellulose: Surgicel®, Ethicon) usually facilitates the formation of blood clots that stop this bleeding.

Once the duct is ligated, the stay sutures are removed and the pericardial incision repaired. The chest is closed in a routine way, over a thoracostomy tube.

Postoperative care

The thoracostomy tube is maintained until the thorax is completely evacuated, then it is removed. Routine post-thoracotomy care is recommended. Ideally, cessation of flow across the ductus should be demonstrated by cardiac ultrasonography prior to discharge from the hospital. Depending on the severity of left heart enlargement, a mitral murmur (secondary to mitral annular dilatation) may persist for some time, but reassessment 1–2 months later should demonstrate some reverse remodelling of the myocardium along with reduction in intensity, if not complete abolition, of the murmur.

Outcome of ductus ligation

In experienced hands, ligation of PDA is a very safe and successful procedure. For animals that survive the surgery, residual flow or 'recanalization' (defined as return of blood flow through a previously occluded ductus) is considered a technical complication that can be avoided. As previously mentioned, to reduce the risk of recanalization or limit its effect, the author commonly places a third ligature of polypropylene between the two traditional silk ligatures so that if the silk ligatures fail over time, the ductus will remain constrained by the polypropylene and will, therefore, be unable to 'reopen'. Alternatively, polypropylene could be used as the primary ligation suture. The use of polypropylene means that even if some flow returns as a result of silk ligature failure, or following atrophy of additional connective tissue inadvertently included in the original ligatures, the flow through the duct should be permanently limited to a haemodynamically insignificant volume.

Vascular ring anomalies

Vascular ring anomalies are secondary to abnormalities of embryogenesis of the great vessels that result in encirclement of the oesophagus and the trachea by abnormally positioned vascular structures. These conditions are rare. Different configurations have been described, including: persistent right aortic arch (PRAA); double aorta; aberrant left subclavian; aberrant right subclavian; and persistent right ductus/ligamentum with a left aortic arch. PRAA accounts for approximately 95% of all 'vascular ring' anatomical variants and often occurs along with an aberrant left subclavian artery. The encircled oesophagus has a focally narrowed lumen secondary to external vascular compression, which limits the size of particles of ingesta that can pass. Food accumulates in the oesophagus cranial to the constriction, creating dilatation and reducing effective peristalsis.

Clinical features

Affected animals are often presented because of regurgitation of food and an associated failure to thrive. The clinical signs are often most obvious once an affected animal is weaned from a liquid diet on to more solid foods. Frequent bouts of regurgitation will increase the risk of aspiration pneumonia in affected animals, which, despite their condition, usually remain bright with a ravenous appetite. Plain thoracic radiographs will often reveal a dilatated oesophagus containing particulate ingesta, cranial to the base of the heart. Good-quality dorsoventral thoracic radiographs may reveal an abrupt deviation in the caudal trachea as it is pushed to the left side of the thorax by the abnormal right aortic arch (Figure 15.5). The latter finding is pathognomonic for PRAA. A barium oesophagogram will confirm the presence of cranial thoracic megaoesophagus, identify the site of narrowing and provide information about the function of the caudal thoracic oesophagus, especially if fluoroscopy can be used (Figure 15.6). Thoracic radiographs will also help determine the presence or absence of pulmonary infiltrates, suggestive of aspiration pneumonia. Angiographic studies using fluoroscopy or computed tomographic angiography can be an invaluable aid to understanding the vascular configuration and planning surgical therapy, especially for non-PRAA vascular rings.

Stabilization

If an affected animal has aspiration pneumonia, antibiotic therapy based on culture and sensitivity testing of bronchoalveolar lavage samples should be initiated. If the

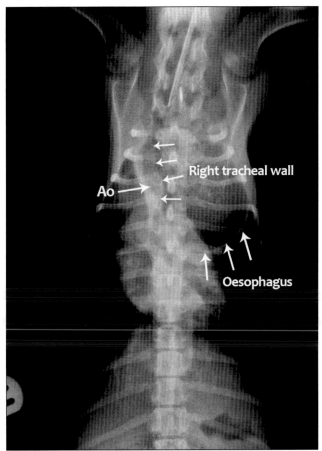

15.5 In a dog with persistent right aortic arch, the aortic root (Ao) can be seen to the right of the trachea, causing an abrupt deviation in the airway that can be seen on good-quality dorsoventral thoracic radiographs exposed (or digitally post-processed) to visualize the mediastinum. The deviated right tracheal wall and the oesophagus are delineated by arrows.

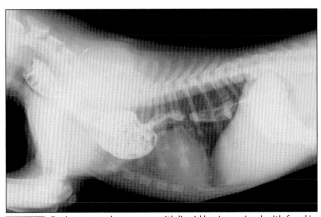

15.6 Barium oesophagogram with liquid barium mixed with food in a dog with persistent right aortic arch. The oesophagus cranial to the heart base is dilatated and there is a narrowing of the oesophagus at the base of the heart. Barium and food are also in the caudal oesophagus and the stomach. Fluoroscopy can help evaluate motility in the caudal oesophagus.

animal tolerates liquid feeding better than solid feeding, a return to a calorie-dense liquid diet fed from an elevated position may help the animal recover by increasing energy intake and decreasing the frequency of regurgitation episodes. The author has stopped short of surgical placement of a gastrostomy tube to provide enteral nutrition prior to surgical management of the vascular ring,

because the duration of anaesthesia required for tube placement is similar to that for division of the ligamentum. It is preferable to address the underlying cause as a means to improve swallowing function.

Surgical management of PRAA

Division of the ligamentum arteriosum in a dog with PRAA can be achieved via a left fourth intercostal thoracotomy incision (Figure 15.7a) or using thoracoscopic dissection during anaesthesia with one-lung ventilation. With PRAA, the trachea is often the most immediately identified structure dorsal to the heart base and to the left of the (right-sided) aorta. This surgical finding confirms the diagnosis of PRAA. Identification of the oesophagus can be facilitated by having an oesophageal tube in place. Typically, the ligamentum arteriosum, which completes the constrictive ring around the oesophagus and trachea, can be palpated either between the pulmonary artery and the aorta or, occasionally, between the pulmonary artery and an aberrant left subclavian artery (Figure 15.7b). The ligamentum is dissected free by blunt dissection using right-angled Mixter or Lahey forceps. Once encircled, the ligamentum is divided between ligatures and any residual fibrous tissue constricting the oesophagus is also divided. If an aberrant left subclavian is identified wrapping around, and constricting, the oesophagus in the cranial thorax, it can also be divided between secure (double) ligatures, to release the oesophagus further. A large-bore stomach tube is then gently guided along the oesophagus beyond the vascular ring to confirm that there is no further constriction (Figure 15.7c). The chest is closed in a routine manner over a thoracostomy tube. In severely emaciated animals, a surgical gastrostomy tube is placed upon completion of the thoracotomy, to aid enteral nutrition in the postoperative recovery period.

Postoperative care

Routine post-thoracotomy care is recommended (see Chapters 1 and 11). The thoracostomy tube is maintained until the thorax is completely evacuated, then it is removed. Because oesophageal dysfunction persists in the short term, and may persist in the longer term, feeding liquidized food from an elevated position and ensuring the animal remains upright for a period of several minutes (up to 20 minutes has been recommended) must be continued after surgery. Once it is clear that the animal can tolerate this food consistency and feeding method, the food consistency and feeding pattern may be changed. The process of trialling foods of different consistencies and different periods of time in an elevated position is continued over a period of weeks to months to work out the optimal regime for each animal.

Outcome of PRAA division

As previously mentioned, the majority of dogs that undergo division of PRAA will be substantially improved by surgery and many will become 'trouble-free' in terms of oesophageal function. Occasionally, animals will continue to require feeding of soft food from an elevated position followed by a period of 'front end' elevation after feeding to allow gravity to assist the persistently compromised oesophageal motility (Figure 15.8). If the owners are prepared to facilitate this lifestyle modification, these dogs can have an excellent quality of life too, although 'dietary indiscretion' will frequently be followed by a bout of regurgitation.

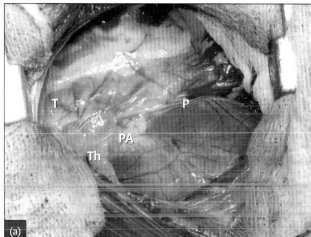

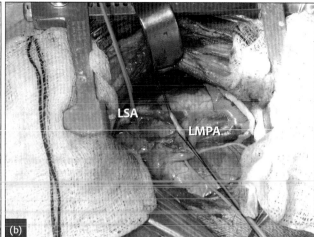

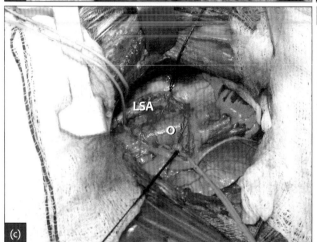

15.7 (a) A left fourth intercostal thoracotomy in a dog with persistent right aortic arch. The trachea (T) is visible in the cranial thorax, along with thymus (Th) ventrally. The aorta is not immediately visible but the pulmonary artery (PA) can be seen through the pericardium just ventral to the phrenic nerve (P). (b) In this dog, the ligamentum arteriosum joins the left main pulmonary artery (LMPA) to an aberrant left subclavian artery (LSA). (c) With silk ligatures tied around the ligamentum, it is divided and a large-bore stomach tube is passed through the narrowed oesophagus (O). Any restricting fibrous bands are sectioned. The course of the LSA should also be examined and if it causes narrowing of the oesophagus in the cranial thorax, it too can be divided between ligatures.

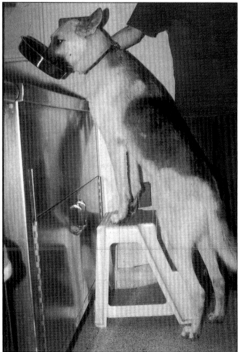

15.8 Although most dogs are significantly improved after surgery, some may need to be fed from an elevated position, and will need to remain in that position for several minutes in order to allow gravity to assist with the passage of food through the oesophagus, throughout their lives.

Other conditions/techniques

Although intracardiac treatment of pulmonic stenosis, cor triatriatum dexter and selected septal defects can be done without CPB, these are techniques that are beyond the scope of this chapter. Similarly, the modified Blalock–Taussig shunt to palliate dogs with tetralogy of Fallot, which is an entirely extracardiac procedure, is not covered in this text. There are, however, rare circumstances where additional techniques may be useful.

Right atrial mass

When managing a dog with haemorrhagic pericardial effusion of unknown aetiology, and if the right atrium/auricular appendage has not or cannot be interrogated echocardiographically, the author prefers to do open pericardectomy via a right lateral approach so that the right atrium can be inspected. The right atrium is a well known site for haemangiosarcoma and the primary tumour may be very small. Removing the pericardium will alleviate tamponade but if the tumour is actively bleeding it will have to be removed too. Theoretically, this is no different from removing a bleeding splenic mass, although technically there are some differences. The goals of resection of a bleeding right auricular mass are: to stabilize the animal by arresting active haemorrhage; to achieve a definitive diagnosis; and to reduce the total body tumour burden to improve the efficacy of follow-up anti-cancer drug therapy.

This resection can be achieved using a vascular stapling device or vascular clamps to facilitate hand-sewn atrial closure after resection of the atrial wall containing the tumour. Having Rommel tourniquets in place to perform TVIO prior to tumour resection is important in this instance. If a tangential (e.g. Satinsky) clamp is used, it is important to incorporate sufficient atrial wall to allow suturing of the atrium with the clamp still in place, after resection of the tumour (Figure 15.9a). This is relatively straightforward if the tumour is at the tip of the auricle but can be more difficult if the mass is in the central part of the atrial wall. If a stapling device is used, ideally the stapler should deploy an overlapping double or triple row of staples that close with a 1 mm gap. Depending on the size of the dog, 1 metric (5/0 USP) or 1.5 metric (4/0 USP) polypropylene sutures can be used in a continuous horizontal mattress suture pattern that is oversewn by a simple continuous pattern (Figure 15.9b). Initial postoperative management is as for any thoracotomy patient that has undergone blood loss. Ultimately, the management will depend on the histological diagnosis and owner preferences.

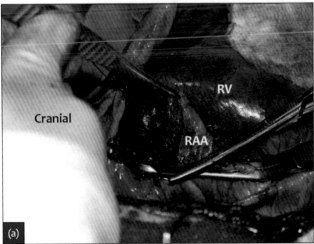

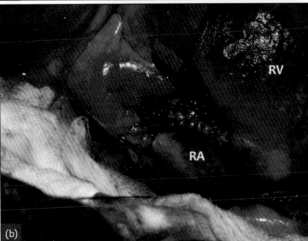

15.9 (a) Via a median sternotomy, a Satinsky clamp has been placed across the right atrial appendage (RAA) so that the tumour and its associated thrombus can be resected. The right ventricle (RV) is seen above the right atrium in this photograph. There is sufficient tissue left in the clamp to allow suturing to be done before the clamp is removed. (b) Appearance of the right atrium (RA) after removal of the Satinsky clamp. The atrial wall was closed using 1.5 metric (4/0 USP) polypropylene in a continuous horizontal mattress suture pattern that was oversewn with a simple interrupted pattern.

References and further reading

Aronsohn M (1985) Cardiac hemangiosarcoma in the dog: a review of 38 cases. *Journal of the American Veterinary Medical Association* **187**, 922–926

Aronson LR and Gregory CR (1995) Infectious pericardial effusion in five dogs. *Veterinary Surgery* **24**, 402–407

Bexfield N and Lee K (2014) *BSAVA Guide to Procedures in Small Animal Practice, 2nd edn.* BSAVA Publications, Gloucester

Birchard SJ (1990) Results of ligation of patent ductus arteriosus in dogs: 201 cases (1969–1988). *Journal of the American Veterinary Medical Association* **196**, 2011–2013

Buchanan JW (1967) Surgical treatment of congenital cardiovascular diseases. In: *Current Veterinary Therapy II*, ed. RW Kirk, pp. 87–103. WB Saunders, Philadelphia

Buchanan JW (1978) Morphology of the ductus arteriosus in fetal and neonatal dogs genetically predisposed to patent ductus arteriosus. *Birth Defects Original Article Series* **14**, 349–360

Buchanan JW (2001) Patent ductus arteriosus morphology, pathogenesis, types and treatment. *Journal of Veterinary Cardiology* **3**, 7–16

Buchanan JW (2004) Tracheal signs and associated vascular anomalies in dogs with persistent right aortic arch. *Journal of Veterinary Internal Medicine* **18**, 510–514

Buchanan JW (1968) Thoracic surgery in the dog and cat. 3. Patent ductus arteriosus and persistent right aortic arch surgery in dogs. *Journal of Small Animal Practice* **9**, 409–428

Bureau S, Monnet E and Orton EC (2005) Evaluation of survival rate and prognostic indicators for surgical treatment of left-to-right patent ductus arteriosus in dogs: 52 cases (1995–2003). *Journal of the American Veterinary Medical Association* **227**, 1794–1799

Case JB, Maxwell M, Aman A *et al.* (2013) Outcome evaluation of a thoracoscopic pericardial window procedure for subtotal pericardectomy via thoracotomy for the treatment of pericardial effusion in dogs. *Journal of the American Veterinary Medical Association* **242**, 493–498

Ehrhart N, Ehrhart EJ, Willis J *et al.* (2002) Analysis of factors affecting survival in dogs with aortic body tumors. *Veterinary Surgery* **31**, 44–48

Eyster GE, Eyster JT, Cords GB *et al.* (1976) Patent ductus arteriosus in the dog: characteristics of occurrence and results of surgery in 100 consecutive cases. *Journal of the American Veterinary Medical Association* **168**, 435–438

Eyster GE (1985) Basic cardiac procedures. In: *Textbook of Small Animal Surgery*, ed. D Slatter, pp. 893–918. W B Saunders, Philadelphia

Glaus TM, Martin M, Boller M *et al.* (2003) Catheter closure of patent ductus arteriosus in dogs: variation in ductal size requires different techniques. *Journal of Veterinary Cardiology* **5**, 7–12

Holt D, Heldmann E, Michel K and Buchanan JW (2000) Esophageal obstruction caused by a left aortic arch and an anomalous right patent ductus arteriosus in two German Shepherd littermates. *Veterinary Surgery* **29**, 264–270

Hunt GB, Simpson DJ, Beck JA *et al.* (2001) Intraoperative hemorrhage during patent ductus arteriosus ligation in dogs. *Veterinary Surgery* **30**, 58–63

Jackson J, Richter KP and Launer DP (1999) Thoracoscopic partial pericardectomy in 13 dogs. *Journal of Veterinary Internal Medicine* **13**, 529–533

Jackson WF and Henderson RA (1979) Ligature placement in closure of patent ductus arteriosus. *Journal of the American Animal Hospital Association* **15**, 55–58

Mayhew KN, Mayhew PD, Sorrell-Raschi L *et al.* (2009) Thoracoscopic subphrenic pericardectomy using double-lumen endobronchial intubation for alternating one-lung ventilation. *Veterinary Surgery* **38**, 961–966

Meijer M and Beijerink NJ (2012) Patent ductus arteriosus in the dog: a retrospective study of clinical presentation, diagnostics and comparison of interventional techniques in 102 dogs (2003–2011). *Tijdschrift Voor Diergeneeskunde* **137**, 376–383

Mellanby RJ and Herrtage ME (2005) Long-term survival of 23 dogs with pericardial effusions. *Veterinary Record* **156**, 568–571

Muldoon MM, Birchard SJ and Ellison GW (1997) Long-term results of surgical correction of persistent right aortic arch in dogs: 25 cases (1980–1995). *Journal of the American Veterinary Medical Association* **210**, 1761–1763

Olsen D, Harkin KR, Banwell MN *et al.* (2002) Postoperative rupture of an aortic aneurysmal dilation associated with a patent ductus arteriosus in a dog. *Veterinary Surgery* **31**, 259–265

Singh MK, Kittleson MD, Kass PH *et al.* (2012) Occlusion devices and approaches in canine patent ductus arteriosus: comparison of outcomes. *Journal of Veterinary Internal Medicine* **26**, 85–92, doi: 10.1111/j.1939-1676.2011.00859.x. Epub 2011 Dec 23

Stanley BJ, Luis-Fuentes V and Darke PG (2003) Comparison of the incidence of residual shunting between two surgical techniques used for ligation of patent ductus arteriosus in the dog. *Veterinary Surgery* **32**, 231–237

Vicari ED, Brown DC, Holt DE *et al.* (2001) Survival times of and prognostic indicators for dogs with heart base masses: 25 cases (1986–1999). *Journal of the American Veterinary Medical Association* **219**, 485–487

van Israël N, Dukes-McEwan J and French AT (2003) Long-term follow-up of dogs with patent ductus arteriosus. *Journal of Small Animal Practice* **44**, 480–490

Walsh PJ, Remedios AM, Ferguson JF *et al.* (1999) Thoracoscopic *versus* open partial pericardectomy in dogs: comparison of postoperative pain and morbidity. *Veterinary Surgery* **28**, 472–479

Weisse C, Soares N, Beal MW *et al.* (2005) Survival times in dogs with right atrial hemangiosarcoma treated by means of surgical resection with or without adjuvant chemotherapy: 23 cases (1986–2000). *Journal of the American Veterinary Medical Association* **226**, 575–579

Chapter 16

Surgery of the mediastinum

Daniel J. Brockman and Arthur K. House

Anatomy

The mediastinum is the potential space between the right and left pulmonary pleural sacs that, in the normal dog or cat, contains the:

- Heart
- Great vessels
- Trachea
- Oesophagus
- Lymph nodes
- Thymus.

Occasionally, ectopic thyroid and parathyroid tissue resides within the mediastinum. The thoracic spine forms the dorsal mediastinal border and the sternum forms the ventral border. The cranial and caudal borders are formed by the thoracic inlet and diaphragm, respectively. The lateral borders are formed by the mediastinal or parietal pleura, which separate one hemithorax from the other. Although the mediastinal pleura is not truly 'fenestrated' tissue its

delicate nature frequently allows extension of disease from one side of the chest to the other. In the cranial thorax, the mediastinum is just to the left of the midline; the mediastinal pleura joins the costal pleura to form the pleural cupula, which extends cranially beyond the first rib on each side. The cranial mediastinum (Figure 16.1) communicates with fascial planes of the neck. In the caudal thorax, the mediastinum is continuous with the pericardium and resides to the left of the midline to accommodate the accessory lung lobe. It attaches to the left side of the diaphragm, contacting the left thoracic wall near the ninth costochondral junction to form the sternopericardial ligament. Caudally, the mediastinum communicates with the retroperitoneal space through the aortic hiatus. The caudal vena cava resides in a reflection of the parietal pleura, the plica venae cavae, on the right side of the mediastinum (Figure 16.2). To assist radiographic interpretation, the mediastinum is divided into five regions: craniodorsal, cranioventral, middle, caudodorsal and caudoventral. Structures contained within each region are outlined in Figure 16.3.

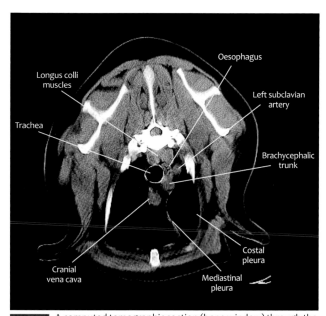

16.1 A computed tomographic section (bone window) through the cranial thorax of a dog, cranial to the heart. The mediastinum at this level contains the cranial vena cava, trachea, longus colli muscles, oesophagus and primary branches of the aorta such as the brachycephalic trunk, right subclavian artery and left subclavian artery. The thymus is not visible in this dog.

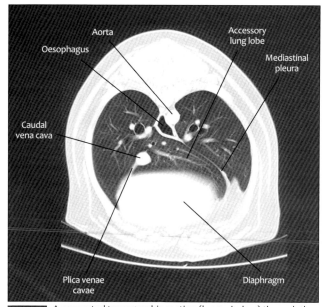

16.2 A computed tomographic section (lung window) through the caudal thorax of a dog, caudal to the heart. Note the vena cava residing in a reflection of the parietal pleura, which forms the plica venae cavae. The mediastinum attaches to the left side of the diaphragm near the ninth costochondral junction to accommodate the accessory lung lobe situated in the right hemithorax.

Organ	Region				
	Craniodorsal	Cranioventral	Middle	Caudodorsal	Caudoventral
Cranial vena cava	+				
Aortic arch	+				
Mediastinal lymph nodes	+				
Trachea	+		+	+	
Oesophagus	+		+	+	
Thoracic duct	+		+		
Brachycephalic trunk	+				
Left subclavian artery	+				
Thymus		+			
Sternal lymph nodes		+			
Mainstem bronchi			+		
Heart			+		
Right and left phrenic nerves	+		+	+	
Pulmonary arteries and veins			+		
Tracheobronchial lymph nodes			+		
Broncho-oesophageal arteries and veins			+		
Descending aorta			+	+	
Principal bronchi			+		
Right and left vagus nerves				+	
Azygos vein			+	+	
Caudal vena cava					+

16.3 Location of organs and structures within the five regions of the mediastinum. + = present.

(Adapted from Thrall (2002))

Clinical features of mediastinal disease

Diseases of the mediastinal structures may cause acute clinical signs such as regurgitation associated with an oesophageal foreign body (see Chapter 9) or dyspnoea associated with traumatic intrathoracic tracheal avulsion (see Chapter 13). Other neoplastic or inflammatory conditions of the mediastinum are associated with vague clinical signs such as pyrexia, weight loss, reduced appetite and malaise. Such disease processes may also affect the recurrent laryngeal nerves (causing laryngeal paralysis) the vagosympathetic trunk (causing Horner's syndrome) and may compress the oesophagus, trachea and major vessels resulting in regurgitation, coughing and dyspnoea and either cranial or caudal venous hypertension and oedema (cranial or caudal caval compression syndrome).

Because of the anatomy, diseases affecting the mediastinum may extend into the neck or abdomen (and *vice versa*), along the continuous fascial planes. Cervical oesophageal perforation can, therefore, lead to septic mediastinitis; conversely, intrathoracic tracheal injury may lead to cervical and subcutaneous emphysema. In cats, a large mass occupying the cranial mediastinum will often reduce the compressibility of the cranial rib cage. In addition, some mediastinal neoplasms are associated with paraneoplastic syndromes such as the hypercalcaemia occasionally associated with lymphoma, causing polyuria and polydipsia, and focal or generalized myasthenia gravis associated with mediastinal thymoma. A wide variety of non-specific clinical signs can, therefore, be associated with mediastinal disease.

Evaluation of the mediastinum

Physical examination of the mediastinum is limited to establishing the compressibility of the cranial thorax, and to thoracic auscultation. Abnormalities found using these physical examination techniques are not specific to mediastinal disease. Diagnostic imaging techniques including survey and contrast radiography, ultrasound examination and endoscopy are non-invasive steps that may be necessary to characterize mediastinal disease. Advanced imaging techniques such as computed tomography (CT) and magnetic resonance imaging (MRI) are being used increasingly to provide more specific information about the relationship of mediastinal neoplasia, in particular, to other structures contained within the mediastinum (Fujimoto *et al.*, 1992; Pirronti *et al.*, 2002). For tissue diagnosis or collection of samples for culture or biochemistry, more invasive techniques such as ultrasound-guided fine-needle aspiration or core tissue biopsy and surgical exploration are required.

Radiography

In the absence of disease the mediastinum is an unclear radiographic anatomical region that lacks contrasting tissue densities except for the air-filled trachea. The cranioventral region is more radiopaque because it is thicker.

The craniodorsal and caudodorsal regions of the mediastinum are best viewed using a combination of ventrodorsal (VD) and dorsoventral (DV) radiographic views (Brinkman *et al.*, 2006; Kirberger and Avner, 2006). Caudal mediastinal masses can be highlighted on DV views by the contrasting adjacent pulmonary parenchyma and magnification (Kirbeger and Avner, 2006). Similarly, a DV view can allow improved definition of the cranial mediastinum when compared with a VD view, owing to better inflation of the cranial pulmonary cupula. In the normal patient the mediastinum is no wider than twice the width of the thoracic spine, although in obese animals the craniodorsal region may become wider owing to the accumulation of fat. The middle region of the mediastinum is best viewed on a lateral view. In young dogs the thymus is viewed as a triangular structure in the cranioventral region of the mediastinum, often referred to as the thymic sail (Figure 16.4).

Four general radiographic observations are made in the presence of disease: mediastinal shift, pneumomediastinum, mediastinal fluid and mediastinal masses. Mediastinal shift occurs secondary to a unilateral increase or decrease in lung volume or secondary to the presence of an intrathoracic mass. Mediastinal shift generally does not indicate disease of the mediastinum but disease in the lungs, bronchi, thoracic wall or pleura. Pneumomediastinum is the accumulation of free gas within the mediastinum; this provides contrast and enhances the outer walls of mediastinal structures such as the trachea, oesophagus and great vessels. Pneumomediastinum is best observed on a lateral radiograph, as the width of the mediastinum is not significantly increased. The source of air may be the trachea, mainstem bronchi, marginal alveoli or oesophagus. Extension of gas from the cervical region caudally or from the retroperitoneum cranially into the mediastinum may occur. Pneumomediastinum occasionally progresses to a pneumothorax, especially in trauma cases or when large

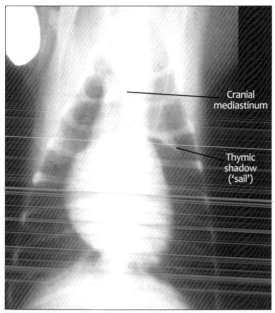

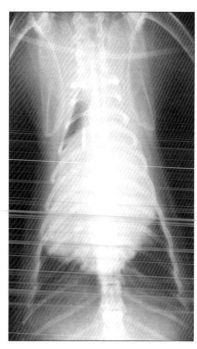

16.6 Ventrodorsal thoracic radiograph of the same cat as in Figure 16.5. Again, the mass effect of the neoplasm is resulting in distortion of adjacent structures. The heart and trachea have been displaced to the right with loss of the typical cardiac silhouette. A large soft tissue structure occupies the mid-thorax.

16.4 Ventrodorsal thoracic radiograph of a young dog. The thymus is clearly visible as a triangular structure in the cranial mid-thorax. Note the width of the cranial mediastinum in comparison with the caudal mediastinum on this view.

defects are present in the trachea or mainstem bronchi. As previously mentioned, concurrent subcutaneous emphysema may develop in such animals.

Mediastinal widening, viewed on VD or DV radiographic views, can be secondary to diffuse mediastinal disease such as mediastinitis or mediastinal fluid accumulation, or to focal mediastinal disease such as mediastinal neoplasia (Figures 16.5 and 16.6). In the latter, distortion of adjacent structures, especially the trachea, is frequently seen. Mediastinal fluid accumulation causes diffuse soft tissue opacity and may occur in conjunction with a mediastinal mass or secondary to inflammatory disease. Diffuse widening of the mediastinum is more typical of mediastinal fluid and inflammatory disease, whereas focal widening is more consistent with a neoplasm.

Ultrasonography

Ultrasonographic examination of the normal mediastinum is limited by the lack of a reliable acoustic window. In the presence of a pleural effusion or a cranial mediastinal mass, however, significant information can be acquired using thoracic ultrasound examination. The transducer may be positioned parasternally or alternatively at the cardiac

notch, using the heart as an acoustic window. Transoesophageal transducers can be used to acquire images of the heart base and major vessels within the mediastinum. In the investigation of cranial mediastinal masses, ultrasonography can provide useful information with regard to the architecture of the mass and its relationship with adjacent structures. Ultrasound-guided fine-needle aspiration or core biopsy techniques can be performed.

Advanced imaging

CT and MRI are the most powerful imaging modalities for estimating the location, volume and invasiveness of mediastinal neoplasms (Figure 16.7). However, difficulties in distinguishing a mass from collapsed lung may be experienced with both modalities. Radionuclide studies with either iodine-131 or technetium-99m have been used to identify ectopic or metastatic thyroid tissue in the mediastinum.

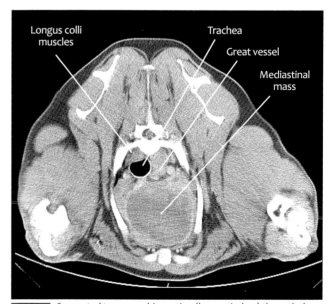

16.7 Computed tomographic section (bone window) through the cranial thorax of a dog, cranial to the heart. A large soft tissue mass occupies the majority of the cranial thorax. No invasion of adjacent structures such as the trachea or great vessel is observed.

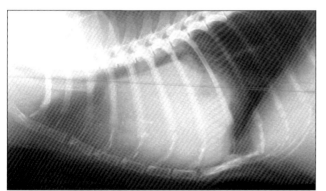

16.5 Lateral radiograph of a cat with a mediastinal thymoma. Owing to the mass effect of the neoplasm, dramatic elevation of the trachea and loss of the typical cardiac silhouette are observed. A soft tissue density occupies a large volume of the mid-thorax.

Pneumomediastinum

Conditions causing pneumomediastinum that require surgery are dealt with elsewhere in this book (see Chapters 9, 13 and 14). Pneumomediastinum can occur as a spontaneous event secondary to pulmonary pathology, severe dyspnoea and/or coughing, or following rupture of the oesophagus, trachea, mainstem bronchi or marginal alveoli. Road traffic accidents or bite wounds are the common traumatic insults, whereas mechanical ventilation, transtracheal aspiration, tracheostomy tube placement and endotracheal intubation are the typical iatrogenic events leading to pneumomediastinum (Brown and Holt 1995; Jordan et al., 2013). Pneumomediastinum may also result from migration of air within the cervical fascia, as observed following rupture of the cervical trachea. Pneumothorax, subcutaneous emphysema and pneumoperitoneum may all develop as a result of air leakage into the mediastinum. Whereas pneumothorax may develop secondary to pneumomediastinum, the converse is extremely unlikely. Although theoretically a rapidly forming pneumomediastinum could cause pressure on mediastinal vessels, reducing venous return to the heart, the flimsy nature of the canine and feline mediastinum means that pneumothorax develops prior to mediastinal tamponade. Consequently, emergency mediastinal decompression is rarely needed. Thoracocentesis may be necessary if mediastinal structures are leaking profusely (see Chapters 11 and 12).

Mediastinitis

Mediastinal inflammation may be either focal or diffuse. It develops as a primary disease process or secondary to perforation of the oesophagus or trachea, or extension of infectious or inflammatory processes in the deep cervical soft tissue, pericardium, pulmonary parenchyma or pleural space. Chronic granulomatous mediastinitis can develop secondary to infection with fungal organisms such as *Histoplasma*, *Blastomyces*, *Cryptococcus* or *Coccidioides* or bacterial organisms such as *Actinomyces*, *Nocardia* and *Corynebacterium* (Meadows et al., 1993).

Treatment requires management of the underlying disease process with surgical resection of diseased tissue and appropriate drainage of the mediastinum. Oesophageal perforation secondary to foreign body ingestion is one of the more common causes of mediastinitis. These cases may require aggressive surgical intervention and critical care. The management of oesophageal foreign bodies is discussed in Chapter 9.

Mediastinal haemorrhage

Haemorrhage within the mediastinum commonly results from trauma but may occur secondary to congenital or acquired coagulopathy, neoplastic erosion of vessels and occasionally from the thymus during involution. Blood vessels within the thymus undergo degenerative changes and become dilatated and fragile during thymic involution. Consequently, spontaneous thymic haemorrhage may be seen after relatively minor trauma such as stopping abruptly at the end of a lead. The haemorrhagic event normally occurs in dogs less than 2 years of age and may be fatal. German Shepherd Dogs and Cocker Spaniels appear to be over-represented.

Mediastinal neoplasia

Soft tissue masses within the mediastinum are rare, but when present they can usually be seen readily on plain thoracic radiographs (see Figures 16.5, 16.6 and 16.8). Primary and metastatic neoplastic lesions account for the majority of masses observed.

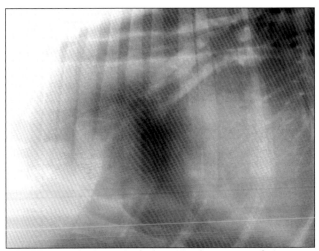

16.8 Lateral radiograph of a dog with a thymoma. A soft tissue mass can be observed in the cranial thorax. Given the small size of the mass no distortion of adjacent structures is observed. Despite the relatively innocuous appearance of this mass, invasion into the cranial vena cava was demonstrated at surgery (see Figure 16.9).

Differential diagnosis

Other mass lesions include: mediastinal lipoma; pleural, bronchial or thymic neoplasia; enlarged mediastinal lymph nodes; abscesses and granulomas; oesophageal foreign bodies; congenital diaphragmatic hernias; gastro-oesophageal intussusception; adenomatous ectopic thyroid or parathyroid tissue; vascular lesions (such as chemodectoma); and benign cysts arising from embryonic branchial pouch. Opacities that are occasionally confused with mediastinal masses include: fat in obese dogs; the thymus of young dogs; tumours of the pulmonary parenchyma, especially those affecting the accessory lung lobe; and occasionally diseases of the oesophagus and the oesophageal hiatus.

Clinical features

The clinical features of any mediastinal neoplasm depend on either invasion or compression of local structures. Compression of the oesophagus and trachea in the cranial mediastinum may result in coughing, dyspnoea, dysphagia and regurgitation. Occasionally, oedema of the head, neck and forelimbs is observed secondary to compression of the cranial vena cava (cranial vena cava syndrome). If the vagus nerves are infiltrated or compressed, changes such as altered phonation (dysphonia), inspiratory stridor and chronic cough, associated with laryngeal paralysis, may be present. Consequently, the diagnostic investigation of suspected laryngeal paralysis should include thoracic radiographs to rule out the presence of a mediastinal mass. Similarly, the sympathetic trunk may be damaged, leading to the development of Horner's syndrome. In conjunction with these potential clinical signs, pleural effusion, pneumothorax, chylothorax, chylopericardium and haemothorax have been observed with mediastinal lymphoma and invasive thymoma in dogs in particular.

As previously mentioned, paraneoplastic syndromes have been observed in association with thymic neoplasia in humans, dogs and cats, most notably acquired myasthenia gravis and megaoesophagus and less commonly hypercalcaemia and other immune-mediated diseases (Bellah *et al.*, 1983; Atwater *et al.*, 1994). A large percentage of human patients with myasthenia gravis have thymic abnormalities, either neoplastic or non-neoplastic (Robertson *et al.*, 1998; Mantegazza *et al.*, 2003). The incidence of acquired myasthenia gravis in dogs with thymoma is approximately 40% (Bellah *et al.*, 1983; Aronsohn, 1985; Atwater *et al.*, 1994).

Malignant mediastinal lymphadenopathy

Mediastinal lymphadenopathy affecting the sternal, cranial mediastinal or tracheobronchial lymphocentra is most commonly due either to multicentric neoplasia such as lymphoma, mastocytosis or malignant histiocytosis or to metastatic disease. All of the neoplastic causes are considered multicentric and, as such, surgical excision is of no therapeutic value once a diagnosis is confirmed. With the exception of lymphoma, they are poorly responsive to anticancer drug protocols (see the *BSAVA Manual of Canine and Feline Oncology*).

Thymic neoplasia

Thymoma and thymic carcinoma are the most commonly reported primary thymic tumours in dogs and cats. Of these, thymoma is the most common.

Clinical features

The clinical features of thymoma are vague and often mild until compression of the lungs and/or airways causes breathing difficulty. Occasionally, animals with this disease will present with signs referable to a paraneoplastic syndrome such as myasthenia gravis or hypercalcaemia.

Diagnosis

The diagnosis is often suspected on the basis of plain thoracic radiographs and may be confirmed by cytological examination of fine-needle aspirates. Cytological evaluation of fine-needle aspirate samples has been shown to correlate well with the definitive histological diagnosis (Reichle and Wisner, 2004; Pintore *et al.*, 2014). Thymoma and lymphoma may both contain large numbers of lymphocytes, making definitive diagnosis by examination of fine-needle aspirates alone challenging. Core biopsies or excisional biopsies are occasionally required to achieve a definitive diagnosis (Zitz *et al.*, 2008).

Biological behaviour

The biological behaviour of thymoma does not correlate well with the histological appearance of the neoplasm. Several histological subtypes of thymoma are described, epithelial, lymphocyte-rich and clear cell, among which lymphocyte-rich thymoma may have a better prognosis (Atwater *et al.*, 1994; Zitz *et al.*, 2008). Because the histological appearance of thymoma does not correlate well with the biological behaviour, thymomas are predominantly classified on the presence or absence of local invasion. Thymomas are, therefore, described as 'non-invasive' or 'invasive', on the basis of gross local tissue invasion. Local metastases are uncommon but can be seen in the lungs,

lymph nodes, diaphragm and pericardium. Distant metastasis is rare but has been reported to the kidneys, liver and spleen. Local invasion of the vascular system is also seen occasionally (Figure 16.9).

The prognosis is good for animals with non-invasive non-metastatic thymoma following complete excision (providing that paraneoplastic syndromes are not present), whereas the prognosis for animals with invasive or metastatic thymoma is poor. Theoretically, preoperative assessment of local disease should be critical to clinical decision-making. The degree of local tissue invasion is difficult to determine on the basis of plain thoracic radiography, so advanced imaging such as MRI and CT is often recommended to provide additional information about the local disease. Unfortunately, many animals are presented with extremely large mediastinal masses, which complicates differentiation between invasion and 'mass effect' (Fujimoto *et al.*, 1992; Pirronti *et al.*, 2002) (Figure 16.10); consequently, it may be impossible to differentiate invasive from non-invasive forms of thymoma on the basis of diagnostic imaging alone.

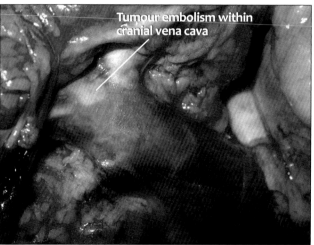

16.9 Intraoperative photograph of the case in Figure 16.8. A large neoplastic embolism can be seen within the cranial vena cava.

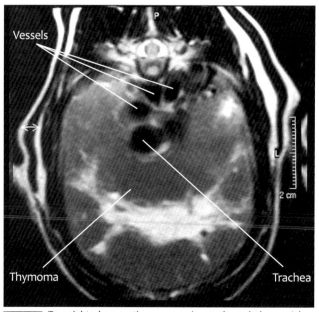

16.10 T2-weighted magnetic resonance image through the cranial thorax of a cat, cranial to the heart. The massive volume of the soft tissue mass makes differentiation of mass effect from invasiveness difficult. Note that blood vessels appear black because moving fluid is black on T2 images, compared with free fluid, which is white.

Treatment

Surgical excision is indicated in the management of thymoma, and exploration of the thorax is generally required to confirm or refute the suspicion of local invasion based on imaging. Although exploration can be performed via lateral thoracotomy, sternotomy is often preferable because of the size of the tumour. Non-invasive thymomas can be readily removed with blunt dissection (Figures 16.11 and 16.12). Preservation of structures such as the phrenic nerves and accurate haemostasis of larger vessels are essential. Attempted excision of invasive thymomas can be unrewarding owing to the invasion of vital structures; however, the slow-growing nature of these tumours means that incomplete excision may be palliative for some time. Cranial caval replacement with a jugular autograft has been described in dogs to achieve *en bloc* tumour excision when the cranial vena cava has been invaded. Cytoreductive surgery such as this may be palliative for a prolonged period of time. Postoperative monitoring by physical examination and thoracic radiography every 3–6 months is recommended, to detect tumour recurrence or development of myasthenia gravis and secondary megaoesophagus.

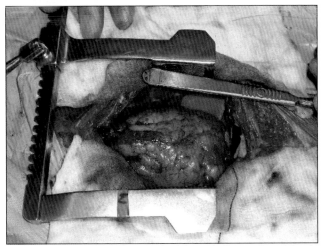

16.11 Intraoperative photograph of the cat in Figures 16.5, 16.6 and 16.10. A midline sternotomy has been performed to gain access to the thorax and tumour.

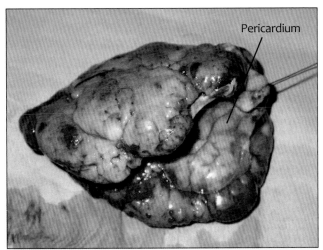

16.12 Gross anatomy of the thymoma removed from the cat in Figures 16.5, 16.6, 16.10 and 16.11. This thymoma was not invasive. Note how the mass has conformed to the shape of the surrounding thoracic wall and adjacent heart. The pericardium has been removed *en bloc* with the tumour.

Recurrence rates are not well documented, but based on the limited literature available, recurrence appears to occur in approximately 30% of dogs (Aronsohn 1985; Gores *et al.*, 1994). Cats seem to respond extremely well to surgical excision, with long-term remission. In a retrospective study of 10 cats, no recurrence was observed in a 6–36-month follow-up period (Gores *et al.*, 1994). A more recent study of thymoma in both dogs and cats documented a median survival time of 1825 days, with 1-year and 3-year survival rates being 89% and 74% in cats (Zitz *et al.*, 2008). A staging system is used in humans that is of prognostic value. In non-invasive forms, the rate of recurrent disease is approximately 2%, compared with 20% for invasive forms that are successfully excised at surgery (Monden *et al.*, 1984, 1985). In dogs, myasthenia gravis and megaoesophagus are the most important prognostic indicators. Dogs with non-invasive thymoma and no paraneoplastic megaoesophagus appear to have a good prognosis for survival, with median survival times of approximately 2 years (635–790 days) being reported (Zitz *et al.*, 2008; Robat *et al.*, 2013). Invasive thymoma and the presence of megaoesophagus carry a grave prognosis, with high postoperative morbidity and mortality in several studies (Bellah *et al.*, 1983; Atwater *et al.*, 1994; Scherrer *et al.*, 2008; Zitz *et al.*, 2008). A more recent study in dogs suggested that the presence of hypercalcaemia, myasthenia gravis or megaoesophagus did not influence survival, but pathological grade based on the Masaoka–Koga staging system did (Robat *et al.*, 2013).

In humans, resolution of myasthenia gravis following thymectomy occurs in approximately 30% of patients, with significant improvement in approximately 60–70% (Drachman, 1994). The response of acquired myasthenia gravis to thymectomy in dogs and cats is poorly described, with single reports of persistent or resolved disease following surgery (Gores *et al.*, 1994; Lainesse *et al.*, 1996). The development of myasthenia gravis following excision of thymoma has been observed in both humans and dogs. The pathogenesis of acquired myasthenia gravis in thymoma patients is not understood, but appears to involve immune dysfunction and the development of autoantibodies to acetylcholine receptors (Garlepp *et al.*, 1984; Paciello *et al.*, 2003). Other immune-mediated diseases that have been associated with thymoma in dogs and cats include polymyositis, granular cell proliferation and immune-mediated skin disease in the dog, and myositis, acute moist dermatitis, pemphigus foliaceus, superficial necrolytic dermatitis and hypogammaglobulinaemia in cats (Willard *et al.*, 1980; Carpenter and Holzworth, 1982; Day, 1997; Forster-Van Hijfte *et al.*, 1997; Smits and Reid, 2003). How these diseases respond to excision of the thymoma is unknown.

Non-thymic tumours are occasionally seen in association with thymoma in dogs, cats and humans. Up to 10% of human patients with thymoma may have additional non-thymic neoplasia, and seven of 22, five of 23 and 31 of 116 dogs with thymoma in three separate retrospective studies had additional neoplasms (Bellah *et al.*, 1983; Atwater *et al.*, 1994; Robat *et al.*, 2013). Lymphoma and primary lung tumours are the most commonly reported concomitant tumours in dogs and cats. A failure of thymus-dependent immune surveillance is thought to be responsible for the development of these concomitant tumours. This fact means that great care should be taken when evaluating animals with thymoma both before and during surgery.

Radiation therapy has been used as an adjunctive therapy prior to or post surgery or as a solitary protocol in both dogs and cats. In one study of 17 dogs and seven cats complete resolution of the tumour was rare, although partial responses were observed in 75% of cases, with greater than 50% reduction in tumour size and improvement in clinical signs (Smith *et al.*, 2001). Median survival times reported were 248 days in dogs and 720 days in cats. Fatal pneumonitis occurred in one animal, with minimal side effects reported in the other cases.

The value of chemotherapy has not been demonstrated in canine and feline patients with thymoma. Following surgical excision, chemotherapy is not required because metastasis is rare. Response to chemotherapy, typically protocols using cisplatin, has been observed in human patients with invasive thymoma.

References and further reading

Aronsohn M (1985) Canine thymoma. *Veterinary Clinics of North America: Small Animal Practice* **15**, 755–767

Atwater SW, Powers BE, Park RD *et al.* (1994) Thymoma in dogs: 23 cases (1980–1991). *Journal of the American Veterinary Medical Association* **205**, 1007–1013

Bellah JR, Stiff ME and Russell RG (1983) Thymoma in the dog: two case reports and review of 20 additional cases. *Journal of the American Veterinary Medical Association* **183**, 306–311

Brinkman EL, Biller D and Armbrust L (2006) The clinical usefulness of ventrodorsal *versus* dorsoventral thoracic radiograph in dogs. *Journal of the American Animal Hospital Association* **42**, 440–449

Brown DC and Holt D (1995) Subcutaneous emphysema, pneumothorax, pneumomediastinum, and pneumopericardium associated with positive-pressure ventilation in a cat. *Journal of the American Veterinary Medical Association* **206**, 997–999

Burgess R, Freeman L, Jennings R *et al.* (2011) An alternative pathway electrosurgical unit injury in a dog. *Veterinary Surgery* **40**, 509–514

Carpenter JL and Holzworth J (1982) Thymoma in 11 cats. *Journal of the American Veterinary Medical Association* **181**, 248–251

Day MJ (1997) Review of thymic pathology in 30 cats and 36 dogs. *Journal of Small Animal Practice* **38**, 393–403

Dobson J and Lascelles D (2011) *BSAVA Manual of Canine and Feline Oncology, 3rd edn.* BSAVA Publications, Gloucester

Drachman DB (1994) Myasthenia gravis. *New England Journal of Medicine* **330**, 1797–1810

Ettinger SJ and Feldman EC (2000) *Textbook of Veterinary Internal Medicine: Diseases of the Dog and Cat, 5th edn.* WB Saunders, Philadelphia

Forster-Van Hijfte MA, Curtis CF and White RN (1997) Resolution of exfoliative dermatitis and *Malassezia pachydermatis* overgrowth in a cat after surgical thymoma resection. *Journal of Small Animal Practice* **38**, 451–454

Fujimoto K, Nishimura H, Abe T *et al.* (1992) MR imaging of thymoma – comparison with CT, operative, and pathological findings. *Nippon Igaku Hoshasen Gakkai Zasshi* **52**, 1128–1138, in Japanese

Garlepp MJ, Kay PH, Farrow BR and Dawkins RL (1984) Autoimmunity in spontaneous myasthenia gravis in dogs. *Clinical Immunology and Immunopathology* **31**, 301–306

Gores BR, Berg J, Carpenter JL and Aronsohn MG (1994) Surgical treatment of thymoma in cats: 12 cases (1987–1992). *Journal of the American Veterinary Medical Association* **204**, 1782–1785

Jordan C, Halfacree Z and Tivers M (2013) Airway injury associated with cervical bite wounds in dogs and cats: 56 cases. *Veterinary and Comparative Orthopaedics and Traumatology* **26**, 89–93

Kirberger RM and Avner A (2006) The effect of positioning on the appearance of selected cranial thoracic structures in the dog. *Veterinary Radiology and Ultrasound* **47**, 61–68

Lainesse MF, Taylor SM, Myers SL, Haines D and Fowler JD (1996) Focal myasthenia gravis as a paraneoplastic syndrome of canine thymoma: improvement following thymectomy. *Journal of the American Animal Hospital Association* **32**, 111–117

Mantegazza R, Baggi F, Antozzi C *et al.* (2003) Myasthenia gravis (MG): epidemiological data and prognostic factors. *Annals of the New York Academy of Sciences* **998**, 413–423

Meadows RL, MacWilliams PS, Dzata G and Meinen J (1993) Chylothorax associated with cryptococcal mediastinal granuloma in a cat. *Veterinary Clinical Pathology* **22**, 109–116

Monden Y, Nakahara K, Iioka S *et al.* (1985) Recurrence of thymoma: clinicopathological features, therapy, and prognosis. *Annals of Thoracic Surgery* **39**, 165–169

Monden Y, Nakahara K, Kagotani K *et al.* (1984) Myasthenia gravis with thymoma: analysis of and postoperative prognosis for 65 patients with thymomatous myasthenia gravis. *Annals of Thoracic Surgery* **38**, 46–52

Morrison WB (1998) *Cancer in Dogs and Cats, Medical and Surgical Management.* Williams and Wilkins, Baltimore

Paciello O, Maiolino P, Navas L and Papparell S (2003) Acquired canine myasthenia gravis associated with thymoma: histological features and immunohistochemical localization of HLA type II and IgG. *Veterinary Research Communications* **27**, 715–718

Pintore L, Bertazzolo W, Bonfanti U *et al.* (2014) Cytological and histological correlation in diagnosing feline and canine mediastinal masses. *Journal of Small Animal Practice* **55**, 28–32

Pirronti T, Rinaldi P, Batocchi AP *et al.* (2002) Thymic lesions and myasthenia gravis. Diagnosis based on mediastinal imaging and pathological findings. *Acta Radiologica* **43**, 380–384

Reichle JK and Wisner ER (2004) Non-cardiac thoracic ultrasound in 75 feline and canine patients. *Veterinary Radiology and Ultrasound* **41**, 154–162

Robat CS, Cesario L, Gaeta R *et al.* (2013) Clinical features, treatment options and outcomes in dogs with thymoma: 116 cases (1999–2010). *Journal of the American Veterinary Medical Association* **243**, 1448–1454

Robertson NP, Deans J and Compston DA (1998) Myasthenia gravis: a population based epidemiological study in Cambridgeshire, England. *Journal of Neurology, Neurosurgery and Psychiatry* **65**, 492–496

Scherrer WE, Kyles AE, Samii VF *et al.* (2008) Computed tomographic assessment of vascular invasion and resectability of mediastinal masses in dogs and a cat. *New Zealand Veterinary Journal* **56**, 330–333

Slatter DH (2003) *Textbook of Small Animal Surgery, 3rd edn.* WB Saunders, Philadelphia

Smith AN, Wright JC, Brawner WR *et al.* (2001) Radiation therapy in the treatment of canine and feline thymomas: a retrospective study (1985–1999). *Journal of the American Animal Hospital Association* **37**, 489–496

Smits B and Reid MM (2003) Feline paraneoplastic syndrome associated with thymoma. *New Zealand Veterinary Journal* **51**, 244–247

Thrall DE (2002) *Textbook of Veterinary Diagnostic Radiology, 4th edn.* WB Saunders, Philadelphia

Willard MD, Tvedten H, Walshaw R and Aronson E (1980) Thymoma in a cat. *Journal of the American Veterinary Medical Association* **176**, 451–453

Withrow SJ and MacEwen EG (2001) *Small Animal Clinical Oncology, 3rd edn.* WB Saunders, Philadelphia

Zitz JC, Birchard SJ, Couto GC *et al.* (2008) Results of excision of thymoma in cats and dogs: 20 cases (1984–2005). *Journal of the American Veterinary Medical Association* **232**, 1186–1192

Chapter 17

Surgery of the diaphragm

Stephen Baines

Anatomy

General structure

The diaphragm is a musculotendinous sheet that separates the thoracic and abdominal viscera. It projects cranially into the thoracic cavity like a dome, giving it a convex thoracic surface and a concave abdominal surface. The mesothelial linings of these two cavities, the pleura and peritoneum, are separated from the diaphragmatic surface by the endothoracic and transversalis fascia, respectively.

Anatomical relationships

The mediastinum attaches to the diaphragm in the midline, dorsal to the oesophagus, but, ventral to the oesophagus, the mediastinum deviates to the left in a wide arc, across the surface of the costal muscles, returning to the midline just dorsal to the sternum. On the right side, a reflection of the mediastinum, the plica venae cavae, is attached to the diaphragm. This plica and the mediastinum form a recess between the heart cranially and the diaphragm caudally, which invests the accessory lung lobe. The oesophagus is attached to the diaphragm by a reflection of the diaphragmatic and endothoracic fascia that attaches around the entire circumference of the thoracic oesophagus. The stronger diaphragmatic fascial reflection is referred to as the phrenico-oesophageal ligament. On the abdominal surface, the diaphragm is attached to the liver by the triangular ligaments, and the coronary ligaments surround the caudal vena cava at the caval hiatus.

Detailed structure

The diaphragm is composed of a central tendon and a peripheral muscular part. The muscle fibres arise from the axial skeleton peripherally and radiate towards the central tendon.

The **central tendon** is relatively small and Y-shaped, formed by a ventral triangular body with narrow dorsal extensions on either side. The muscular part is formed by lumbar, costal and sternal muscles.

The **lumbar part** is formed by the two diaphragmatic crura. The right crus is larger than the left. Each crus arises from a long bifurcate tendon, which comprises a long, strong portion arising from the cranial edge of the body of the fourth lumbar vertebra and a shorter, weaker portion arising from the body of the third lumbar vertebra. These tendons unite close to the midline, medial to the psoas minor muscle. Each crus may be differentiated into lateral, intermediate and medial portions.

The **costal part** is formed by fibres radiating from the costal wall to the tendinous centre. It arises peripherally from the proximal 13th rib, distal 12th rib, costochondral junction of the 11th rib, whole length of the 10th and ninth ribs, and the curved portion of the eighth costal cartilage. These fibres run centrally into the lateral borders and columns of the central tendon.

The **sternal part** of the diaphragm is an unpaired medial muscle, continuous with the costal part. It arises from the base of the xiphoid cartilage, the adjacent transversalis fascia and the eight costal cartilages. These fibres run dorsally to the apex of the body of the central tendon (Figure 17.1).

The **aortic hiatus** is bordered ventrally by the diaphragmatic crura and dorsally by the ventral aspects of the lumbar vertebrae. The aorta, azygos and hemiazygos veins and the lumbar cistern of the thoracic duct pass through this hiatus. The **oesophageal hiatus** is bordered by the thick medial edges of the medial part of the crura. The oesophagus, associated vessels and the vagal trunks pass through this hiatus. The **caval hiatus** is located entirely within the central tendon of the diaphragm, although muscle fibres from the costal portion may radiate into the dorsal border of the hiatus. The splanchnic nerves and sympathetic trunk pass dorsal to the dorsal aspect of the lateral part of the crura, in the **lumbocostal arch**.

Nerves and vessels

The main blood supply to the diaphragm is derived from the caudal phrenic arteries. These arise from the paired phrenicoabdominal arteries, which branch from the lateral surface of the abdominal aorta between the cranial mesenteric and renal arteries. These vessels pass along the medial border of the dorsal extension of the central tendon and ramify over the ventrocaudolateral surface of the diaphragm. These vessels follow the course of the muscle fibres peripherally and anastomose with phrenic branches of the 10th, 11th and 12th intercostal arches.

Motor innervation to the diaphragm is provided by the phrenic nerves, which arise from the ventral branches of the fifth, sixth and seventh cervical nerves in the dog and the fourth, fifth and sixth cervical nerves in the cat. A small contribution to the phrenic nerves from the fourth cervical nerve is present in some dogs.

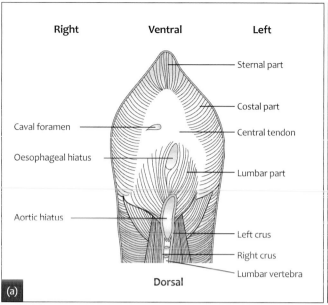

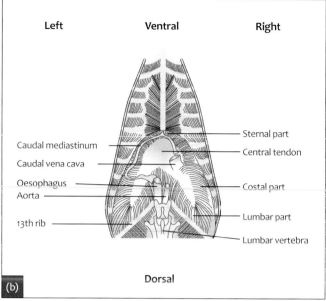

17.1 Anatomy of the diaphragm. (a) Abdominal surface. (b) Thoracic surface.

Embryology

A complex structure such as the diaphragm has a similarly complex embryology. A thorough understanding of the embryological development of the diaphragm allows the congenital abnormalities of the diaphragm to be explained.

The diaphragm is derived from four main structures:

- The septum transversum, ventrally
- The dorsal aspect of the mediastinum (dorsal mesentery of the oesophagus), dorsomedially
- The pleuroperitoneal folds, dorsolaterally
- The posthepatic mesenchymal plate.

In the developing embryo, the initial partition between the thoracic and abdominal cavities is provided by the **septum transversum**. This structure originates in the neck, but migrates to the level of the first lumbar vertebra, where it forms the central tendon. The cervical origin of the septum transversum explains the cervical origin of the phrenic nerves (Figure 17.2).

The **dorsal mesentery of the oesophagus** develops dorsal to the septum transversum and forms the diaphragmatic crura, oesophageal hiatus and aortic hiatus.

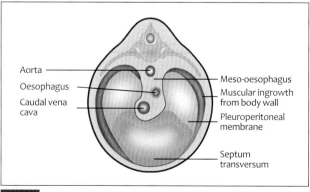

17.2 Embryological development of the diaphragm.

The space between the pleural and peritoneal cavities is partially occluded by the enlargement of the mesonephric organs. As these organs later atrophy, the retroperitoneal flaps they occupied, known as **pleuroperitoneal folds**, continue to enlarge. These folds fuse with the mesentery of the oesophagus and dorsal portion of the septum transversum.

The remaining communication between these two cavities, the pleuroperitoneal canals or foramina of Bochdalek, is then closed by the developing **posthepatic mesenchymal plate**, under the influence of the adjacent developing lung bud.

Once these component parts have fused and the pleural cavity enlarges, myoblasts from the posthepatic mesenchymal plate and abdominal wall invade the peripheral border of the diaphragm to form the costal and sternal parts.

Clinical anatomy

The radiographic appearance of the diaphragm in health (Grandage, 1974) and in disease (Park, 1994) is well documented.

Patient factors such as breed, age, size, body condition, temperament and visceral distension, other clinically induced variables such as sedation or anaesthesia and phase of respiration, and geometric factors associated with the radiographic view, such as positioning, direction of the primary beam, and centring of the primary beam all influence the radiographic appearance of the diaphragm (Grandage, 1974). Although these factors produce an almost limitless number of variations in the appearance, the clinician should be aware of the radiographic appearance of the diaphragm in the standard views and should aim to keep the other variables as constant as possible.

Only a small part of the diaphragm is apparent on any single radiograph. Visualization of the diaphragm is dependent on the adjacent structures being of different radiopacity. Thus, the thoracic surface is easily visualized because of the adjacent air-filled lungs. However, the abdominal surface is less well demarcated because adjacent structures such as the liver and stomach have a soft tissue opacity, although the falciform fat outlines the ventral aspect of the diaphragm on the lateral view.

Radiography may demonstrate the right and left crura, intercrural cleft and the central dome (cupula).

The radiographic appearance alters according to the view:

- Dorsoventral (DV): a single dome-shaped structure
- Ventrodorsal (VD): three separate domed structures
- Right lateral: crura parallel, with the dependent right crus more cranial
- Left lateral: the crura form a Y-shape, with the dependent left crus more cranial.

Function

Contraction of the diaphragmatic muscles causes flattening of the dome of the diaphragm, resulting in caudal displacement of the abdominal viscera and outward displacement of the body wall. Contraction of the costal part also causes expansion of the caudal rib cage. These actions cause enlargement of the thoracic cavity and a reduction in pleural space pressure, resulting in inspiration. Expansion of the chest wall is also provided by contraction of the internal intercostal muscles, which explains why breathing movements may still be made in animals with paralysis of the diaphragm.

Diseases of the diaphragm

Diseases affecting the diaphragm are primarily alterations in its anatomical structure, such as congenital hernias and acquired ruptures, and alterations in its function, such as diaphragmatic paralysis. A hernia is the protrusion of viscera through a normal anatomical opening, which may be pathologically enlarged, and is generally congenital in origin, whereas a rupture is protrusion of viscera through an opening that has been acquired, usually as a result of trauma.

Congenital diseases

Peritoneopericardial diaphragmatic hernia

Anatomy and incidence: Peritoneopericardial diaphragmatic hernia (PPDH) consists of herniation of abdominal organs through a direct communication between the peritoneal cavity and the pericardial sac. It is the most common congenital diaphragmatic and pericardial defect in dogs (Eyster *et al.*, 1977; Evans and Biery, 1980; Bellah *et al.*, 1989a,b) and cats (Frye and Taylor, 1968; Hay *et al.*, 1989). The Weimaraner and Miniature Schnauzer dogs and Persian cat may be predisposed to this anomaly (Evans and Biery, 1980; Hay *et al.*, 1989).

PPDH is often accompanied by other defects (Eyster *et al.*, 1977; Evans and Biery, 1980; Bellah *et al.*, 1989). These include:

- Sternal defects, e.g. reduced number of sternebrae, defects in the sternum, fusion of sternebrae and sternal dysraphism
- Cranial midline abdominal wall hernia
- Umbilical hernia
- Abnormal swirling of the hair in the cranial ventral midline
- Intracardiac defects, e.g. pulmonic stenosis, ventricular septal defects, atrial septal defects, tricuspid dysplasia and tetralogy of Fallot
- Pulmonary vascular disease
- Portosystemic shunts.

These combinations are thought to be sporadic or due to teratogenic events rather than being inherited (Eyster *et al.*, 1977; Bellah *et al.*, 1989).

A variant of the usual PPDH has been described in which defects were present in the cranial abdominal wall, caudal sternum and ventral diaphragm, but abdominal organs which had herniated through the diaphragm were restricted to the caudal mediastinum, and did not enter the pericardial sac (Bellah *et al.*, 1989).

Aetiology: These defects may be caused by the following events:

- Failure of the lateral pleuroperitoneal folds and sternal part of the diaphragm to unite during separation of the thoracic and abdominal cavities
- Faulty development of the dorsolateral septum transversum
- Rupture of a thin tissue membrane in the region of the developing septum transversum
- Prenatal injury to the septum transversum or site of fusion of the septum transversum and pleuroperitoneal folds.

These aetiologies are suggested in view of the consistent location of these defects in the ventral or ventrolateral portions of the diaphragm, that is, the parts contributed by the septum transversum and pleuroperitoneal folds (Evans and Biery, 1980).

In one report, two successive litters from the same two parents had a 1:3 ratio of puppies with PPDH to puppies without PPDH, suggesting an autosomal recessive genetic predisposition (Feldman *et al.*, 1968).

Although trauma has been suggested as a potential cause of acquired peritoneopericardial diaphragmatic hernia, no such cases have been described in small animals. Postnatally, there is no direct contact between the pericardial sac and peritoneal cavity, although they are connected by the caudal mediastinal pleura, and traumatic disruption of these two mesothelial sacs, with subsequent re-establishment of continuity between them, would seem to be a rare, if not impossible, event. However, trauma may worsen a pre-existing hernia.

In the embryo, cardiac septation and sternal fusion take place at the same time as the development of the septum transversum and fusion to the other components of the diaphragm. Hence, any environmental insult during this period might be expected to result in defects in the diaphragm and in the cardiac septa and sternum. Alternatively, abnormal blood flow within the chambers of an abnormally positioned heart may lead directly to septal defects through mechanical teratogenesis.

Pathophysiology: Abdominal organs that herniate into the pericardial sac include the liver, gallbladder, falciform ligament, omentum, spleen, small intestine and, rarely, the stomach.

The pathophysiological changes are similar to those occurring during diaphragmatic rupture, but the organs are constrained by the pericardial sac and are generally located caudal and lateral to the heart. Hence, gross compromise of pulmonary function from direct pressure does not generally occur, but indirect pressure from the enlarged pericardial sac may still cause respiratory compromise. Cardiovascular signs result from pressure on the heart or great vessels. Cardiac tamponade may be caused by compression from the abdominal viscera, bloating of a herniated stomach, or an effusion from an incarcerated liver lobe. Compression of the caudal vena cava may cause transient ascites. Obstruction or strangulation of herniated organs, especially parts of the gastrointestinal tract, will cause additional clinical signs. Myelolipomatosis (multiple firm raised white nodules of adipose tissue) and portal hypertension have also been described when liver lobes have become incarcerated (Frye and Taylor, 1968; Schuh, 1987; Hay et al., 1989).

PPDH has also been suggested as the cause of intra-pericardial cyst formation in dogs and cats, and pericardial cysts may be seen associated with the PPDH, or may be identified following PPDH repair. It is hypothesized that these lesions are cystic haematomas, caused by prenatal herniation of falciform fat or omentum from the peritoneal cavity into the pericardial sac, with subsequent closure of the hernia in some cases. In three of nine cases of intra-pericardial cysts, a small PPDH was also apparent.

Diagnosis: Clinical signs associated with this condition may become apparent at any age and some animals with the disease remain free of signs their whole life. In some animals, physical examination is unremarkable (Evans and Biery, 1980). PPDH was an incidental finding in approximately half the patients in one study (Burns et al., 2013).

Clinical signs are diverse and reflect the range of organ systems that may be affected and the severity of the compromise. Most commonly, cardiorespiratory signs (dyspnoea, tachypnoea, coughing, wheezing and poor exercise tolerance) and gastrointestinal signs (vomiting and diarrhoea) are seen.

Physical examination may reveal abnormalities of the sternum and defects in the cranial abdominal wall (Bellah et al., 1989). Auscultation of the chest may yield muffled heart and lung sounds, and heart murmurs in those animals with coexisting congenital heart disease. Rotation of the heart within the enlarged pericardial sac may be sufficient to cause a murmur in the absence of heart disease (Eyster et al., 1977). Patients may present with overt signs of right-sided heart failure or caudal caval compression, such as ascites (Frye and Taylor, 1968).

Electrocardiographic abnormalities reported include alteration in the mean electrical axis, due to displacement of the heart, and arrhythmias.

Thoracic radiography reveals a grossly enlarged, rounded or ovoid cardiac silhouette, which may be accompanied by an abnormal convex projection at the caudal border (Figure 17.3). The soft tissue opacities of the heart and diaphragm are continuous ventrally (positive silhouette sign). In cats, the identification of the dorsal peritoneopericardial mesothelial remnant between the heart and diaphragm is a common radiographic sign of PPDH (Berry et al., 1990). The existence of sternal abnormalities can be confirmed radiographically.

The presence of other opacities, such as gas (e.g. linear gas-filled bowel), fat (e.g. omentum or falciform ligament), soft tissue (e.g. liver lobes or loops of small intestine) or mixed soft tissue/mineral opacities (e.g. faeces-filled large intestine) confirms the existence of abdominal viscera within the thoracic cavity, and the restriction of these opacities by the pericardium differentiates PPDH from a traumatic diaphragmatic rupture (Evans and Biery, 1980). Changes in the position of the abdominal viscera or an abnormal stomach axis may also suggest herniation.

Ultrasonography is a simple and reliable non-invasive method of confirming the diagnosis. Examination may be performed with the transducer in a subcostal or parasternal position. Herniation of abdominal viscera may be identified and differentiated from pericardial effusion, pericardial

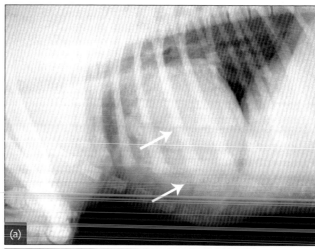

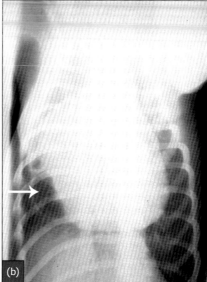

17.3 Peritoneopericardial diaphragmatic hernia. (a) Lateral and (b) ventrodorsal views of the thorax, showing an enlarged cardiac silhouette containing loops of small intestine ventrally and to the right (arrowed). There are also a reduced number of sternebrae and failure of fusion of the caudal sternebra (dysraphism).

masses, cysts and cardiomegaly. The presence of coexisting congenital heart disease may also be identified by these means.

Contrast radiographs are of limited use. A positive contrast barium upper gastrointestinal study may reveal barium-containing loops of small intestine overlying the cardiac shadow, if part of the gastrointestinal tract has herniated (Figure 17.4). Negative and positive contrast peritoneography may demonstrate anatomical continuity between the peritoneal cavity and the pericardium, but a false negative result may occur if the viscera have sealed the defect in the diaphragm (Evans and Biery, 1980).

Treatment: In many animals with PPDH, the hernia is an incidental finding, particularly in mature adult and geriatric cats, and care should be taken when making a decision to manage the condition surgically (Burns et al., 2013). Surgery is more commonly performed in younger cats and in cats with more obvious clinical signs referable to the hernia.

The principles of surgical correction of a PPDH are similar to those for a traumatic diaphragmatic rupture. A ventral midline laparotomy approach gives the best access to the defects in the diaphragm and any associated defects of the cranioventral abdominal wall. Extension of the incision with a caudal median sternotomy may be required if adhesions have developed or if abdominal organs have herniated cranially into the mediastinum from the pericardium (Figure 17.5).

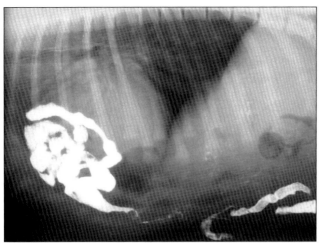

17.4 Peritoneopericardial diaphragmatic hernia: lateral view of the thorax following oral administration of barium suspension to the dog in Figure 17.3. Barium-filled loops of small intestine are present within the pericardium and outline a cranial ventral abdominal hernia.

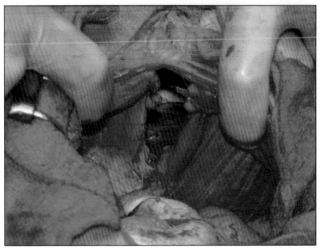

17.5 Peritoneopericardial diaphragmatic hernia: visualization of the heart through the defect in the diaphragm.

The presence of a large volume of pericardial fluid causing cardiovascular compromise may necessitate pericardiocentesis before anaesthesia, but this is not commonly required (Hay *et al.*, 1989). Full cardiac evaluation may not be possible before closing the hernia, and the possibility of concomitant heart disease must be considered (Feldman *et al.*, 1968).

In contrast to a traumatic diaphragmatic rupture, continuity between the pericardial sac and the peritoneal cavity means that the pleural space is not open to the air during the surgery, and therefore intermittent positive pressure ventilation may not be required. However, if the defect has to be enlarged to return the herniated viscera to the abdomen, or if the pericardium has to be incised to use a portion for closure of the defect, then incision of the diaphragm or pericardium will result in iatrogenic pneumothorax and will require ventilatory management.

Adhesions between the herniated viscera and the pericardium or diaphragm are uncommon, but have been described (Hay *et al.*, 1989). Incarcerated liver lobes may be necrotic, fragile or lipomatous, and may need to be resected (Hay *et al.*, 1989).

The hernia is closed with a simple interrupted or continuous suture pattern, running dorsal to ventral. This simultaneously closes the defect in the pericardium and

the diaphragm. If there is tension on the closure, the ventral border of the defect may be approximated to the abdominal fascia over the costal arch with horizontal mattress sutures.

In the majority of animals, there is sufficient tissue to allow closure of the defect without undue tension. In animals with a large defect, the pericardial sac is incised cranial to the junction of the diaphragm and pericardium, and this extra ring of tissue is used to close the defect. Alternatively, the diaphragm may be incised on each side of the defect at its paracostal attachment and bilateral rotation flaps used to close the defect (Bellah *et al.*, 1989). Umbilical hernias and defects in the cranioventral abdominal wall are closed during closure of the laparotomy wound.

Postoperative care and complications: Postoperative recovery is usually uncomplicated. Complications are uncommon, but may include haemorrhage from adhesions between the liver and pericardium, dehiscence of the repair, re-herniation and development of constrictive pericarditis (Wallace *et al.*, 1992; Burns *et al.*, 2013).

Prognosis: The prognosis following closure of an uncomplicated PPDH is good (Evans and Biery, 1980; Hay *et al.*, 1989). The presence of sternal and abdominal wall defects does not adversely affect the prognosis. The prognosis for animals with concurrent congenital heart defects is poorer and the outlook depends on the nature of the heart disease.

Oesophageal hiatal hernia

Anatomy and incidence: Hiatal hernia is the protrusion of abdominal contents through the oesophageal hiatus of the diaphragm into the thoracic cavity. It is uncommon in dogs and rare in cats (Ellison *et al.*, 1987; Waldron *et al.*, 1990). Shar-Peis appear to be predisposed to this condition (Prymak *et al.*, 1989; Williams, 1990; Callan *et al.*, 1993) and it is most commonly seen in young brachycephalic dogs.

Aetiology: The most common classification system favoured in humans (Skinner, 1986) and adopted for small animals is as follows:

* Type I: sliding or axial hiatal hernia
* Type II: rolling or para-oesophageal hiatal hernia
* Type III: combined type I and type II
* Type IV: herniation of other organs into the thorax, e.g. intestine, spleen or pancreas.

All these types have been described in animals, although types III (Williams, 1990) and IV (Brinkley, 1990) are rare. Type I hernias are the most common, representing approximately 90% of the reported cases.

Although they are frequently referred to synonymously, a true para-oesophageal hiatal hernia differs from the type II hernia in that, in the former case, the herniation occurs through a separate defect in the diaphragm, adjacent to the oesophageal hiatus. This defect has not been reported in small animals.

Gastro-oesophageal intussusception (Figure 17.6) is sometimes included in the classification of hiatal hernias. However, although this condition does involve passage of an abdominal organ across the diaphragm into the thoracic cavity, it might be argued that it is not a true hernia. It is not included in human classification systems of hiatal hernia.

An abnormally short oesophagus, which does not allow the stomach to lie in the abdominal cavity, has been

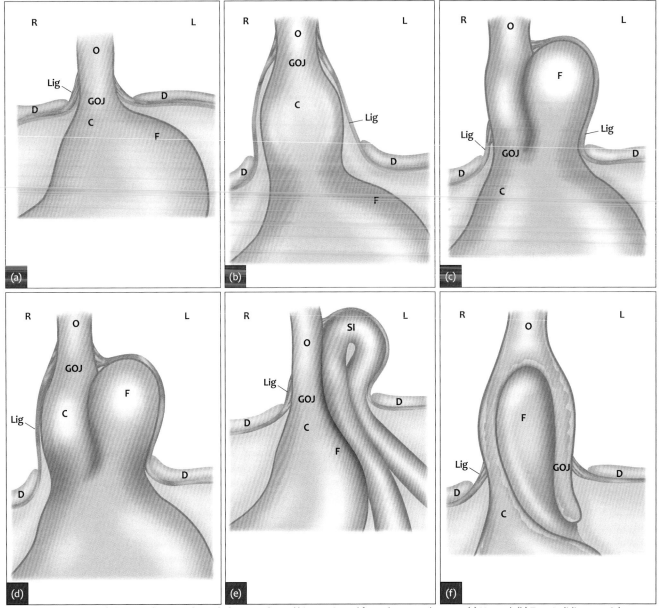

17.6 Protrusion of abdominal organs through the oesophageal hiatus, viewed from the ventral aspect. (a) Normal. (b) Type I: sliding or axial. (c) Type II: rolling or para-oesophageal. (d) Type III: combined types I and II. (e) Type IV: herniation of other organs. (f) Gastro-oesophageal intussusception. C = cardia; D = diaphragm; F = fundus; GOJ = gastro-oesophageal junction; L = left; Lig = phrenico-oesophageal ligament; O = oesophagus; R = right; SI = small intestine.

described as a predisposing factor for hiatal hernia. This is a subtype of type I, but it has been considered as a type IV hernia. Although it has been suggested that this lesion is congenital, it is more likely that the oesophagus shortens secondary to reflux oesophagitis and scarring. This condition has been described in a small number of dogs (Bright *et al.*, 1990) and may result in the permanent fixation of the oesophagus and cardia in the thorax.

Sliding/oesophageal: Sliding hiatal hernia is characterized by axial displacement of the abdominal portion of the oesophagus, the gastro-oesophageal junction and part of the stomach through the oesophageal hiatus (Ellison *et al.*, 1987; Prymak *et al.*, 1989). This type of hernia usually has a sac formed by the stretched phrenico-oesophageal ligament (Merdan Dhein *et al.*, 1980). A larger hernia may also contain the spleen, liver and intestine. Herniated tissues may move in and out of the thoracic cavity with changes in the pleuroperitoneal pressure gradient. These hernias may be further divided into congenital and acquired hernias.

Congenital: Congenital hernias result from a developmental defect in the structures that normally retain these viscera *in situ*, primarily the oesophageal hiatus and phrenico-oesophageal ligament.

Acquired: Acquired hernias may develop in a number of different situations, although a congenital predisposition may be present (Ellison *et al.*, 1987; Burnie *et al.*, 1989; Bright *et al.*, 1990; Waldron *et al.*, 1990; Dieringer and Wolf, 1991; Van Ham and van Bree, 1992; Hardie *et al.*, 1998; Pratschke *et al.*, 1998). They may be seen in animals with severe upper airway obstruction (laryngeal paralysis/ brachycephalic airway disease) that generate a massive pressure gradient in an attempt to get air into their lungs, and passage of the stomach through the oesophageal hiatus can result. Hiatal hernia may also be identified in young brachycephalic dogs with gastric outflow tract obstruction, and it may be difficult to determine which of the lesions identified are clinically relevant. However, it is important to note that an apparently acquired hiatal hernia, identified during evaluation of another disease, may resolve once the underlying disease is addressed (Van Ham and van Bree, 1992).

Causes of acquired hiatal herniation include:

- Trauma
- Inspiratory dyspnoea, e.g. laryngeal paralysis, laryngeal stenosis or brachycephalic airway obstruction syndrome
- Lower respiratory tract disease, e.g. emphysema and bronchogenic carcinoma
- Interference with normal muscular function of the diaphragm, e.g. tetanus or muscular dystrophy
- Loss of abdominal domain following repair of acute and chronic diaphragmatic rupture
- Iatrogenic after cardioplasty for megaoesophagus.

Rolling/para-oesophageal: This type of hernia is characterized by fixation of the gastro-oesophageal junction in its normal position, with protrusion of a part of the stomach, beginning with the fundus, through the hiatus, alongside the normal oesophagus (Miles *et al.* 1988). Gastro-oesophageal reflux is less common with this type of hernia. This type of hernia is usually stationary and does not slide.

Para-oesophageal herniation itself is uncommon and it is normally seen in conjunction with sliding hiatal hernia, as a type III hernia (Williams, 1990). In humans, type II hernias tend to be acquired and to enlarge with time. They are often asymptomatic, but large hernias may allow the herniation of other organs, such as spleen or small intestine, or gastric dilatation, resulting in sudden death.

Pathophysiology: A simplified outline of the pathophysiology is that hiatal hernia causes gastro-oesophageal reflux, which in turn leads to oesophagitis and chronic regurgitation. Chronic regurgitation may lead to aspiration pneumonia. Herniation of other abdominal organs may cause incarceration or gastric tympany. However, the exact nature of the pathophysiological changes in patients with the different types of hiatal hernia is not fully understood. This lack of understanding explains the relatively poor success associated with both medical and surgical therapy.

Gastro-oesophageal reflux: The major consequence of hiatal herniation is gastro-oesophageal reflux, although herniation may occur without reflux (Ellison *et al.*, 1987; Bright *et al.*, 1990; Knowles *et al.*, 1990). However, gastro-oesophageal reflux has been documented as a normal physiological occurrence in dogs, without oesophagitis.

The occurrence and severity of reflux oesophagitis in animals with hiatal hernia depends on two important factors:

- The occurrence of gastro-oesophageal reflux is significantly increased in young animals because of developmental immaturity of the caudal oesophageal sphincter
- The severity of reflux oesophagitis in animals with hiatal hernia depends on the composition of the refluxed material.

Whilst gastro-oesophageal reflux and hiatal hernia can occur independently, with or without clinical signs, when both reflux and a large hernia are present, more severe disease is likely to occur (Hardie *et al.*, 1998). When gastro-oesophageal reflux causes oesophagitis, this has the effect of reducing the tone in the oesophageal muscle and caudal oesophageal sphincter and decreases primary and secondary oesophageal peristalsis, thus making gastro-oesophageal reflux more likely and perpetuating a chronic cycle of reflux–oesophagitis–reflux.

Competence of the gastro-oesophageal junction is maintained primarily by the intrinsic muscle tone of the caudal oesophageal sphincter and various extrinsic factors that act on this region (White, 1993). The extrinsic factors include:

- The pinchcock action of the right diaphragmatic crus surrounding the oesophageal hiatus
- The flap valve effect of the acute angle between the oesophagus and cardia
- The tethering effect of the phrenico-oesophageal ligament
- The mucosal choke formed by mucosal folds of the distal oesophagus
- The length of the abdominal segment of the oesophagus
- The effect of abdominal pressure on the abdominal segment of the oesophagus.

The relative contribution of these factors in normal individuals or individuals with hiatal hernia is not clear (Hardie *et al.*, 1998). However, the intrinsic tone of the oesophagus is likely to be the most important factor and primary incompetence of the caudal oesophageal sphincter has not been demonstrated in dogs or cats. Understanding the relevant importance of these anatomical and functional mechanisms is the key to developing a rational surgical technique.

Other clinical signs: Regurgitation may be caused by the anatomical displacement of the stomach and terminal oesophagus or by the resulting reduction in oesophageal tone or functional length, due to spasm, following oesophagitis. However, megaoesophagus may be a primary lesion rather than a secondary acquired lesion (Prymak *et al.*, 1989).

Dyspnoea may be caused by either aspiration pneumonia or the space-occupying effects of herniated viscera (Waldron *et al.*, 1990). However, hiatal hernia may also be acquired secondary to diseases that cause dyspnoea, because of the increased pleuroperitoneal pressure gradient during respiration.

In most instances, gastro-oesophageal reflux and respiratory disease are mutually reinforcing diseases (Hardie *et al.*, 1998). The association between hiatal hernia and lower respiratory tract disease is well known, but gastro-oesophageal reflux has been considered to be the cause of respiratory disease, primarily bronchitis and aspiration pneumonia (Ellison *et al.*, 1987; Prymak *et al.*, 1989; Bright *et al.*, 1990; Callan *et al.*, 1993). As previously mentioned, however, increased respiratory effort in patients with respiratory disease may predispose to hiatal herniation and gastro-oesophageal reflux. However, the presence of acid reflux in the distal oesophagus may cause bronchospasm, and regurgitation and aspiration may cause laryngospasm, which will worsen respiratory signs (Hardie *et al.*, 1998). Thus, a feedback loop exists whereby respiratory disease can cause gastro-oesophageal disease and gastro-oesophageal disease can worsen respiratory disease.

Oesophageal abnormalities may be observed with hiatal herniation. Within a population of young (3–4-month-old) Shar-Peis, some of which showed vomiting or regurgitation, dogs with a hiatal hernia had slow secondary wave development after swallowing a bolus of food, with poor oesophageal tone and oesophageal redundancy (Stickle *et al.*, 1992). It was hypothesized that the oesophageal disorder was secondary to hiatal hernia because these signs resolved in those animals where surgical correction was performed, but remained in those that were managed medically. However, all of these radiographic signs were also seen in a high proportion (38–69%) of clinically normal Shar-Peis, some of which showed spontaneous resolution of these findings as they grew older (6–12 months old), so the significance is not clear.

Segmental or generalized oesophageal hypomotility and oesophageal redundancy are common in the Shar-Pei breed, but may be incidental radiographic findings, not associated with any clinical signs. In addition, a congenital idiopathic form of megaoesophagus has also been described in the Shar-Pei, with similar clinical signs in young (3-month-old) animals (Knowles *et al.*, 1990). Fluoroscopy should allow differentiation between these conditions.

Diagnosis: The intermittent nature of the herniation makes diagnosis difficult. Clinical signs may be observed any time after weaning in congenital hiatal hernia, and are usually present before 1 year old. Clinical signs associated with acquired hiatal hernia may be seen at any time, depending on the nature of the predisposing factors.

Clinical signs include hypersalivation, regurgitation or vomiting, haematemesis, dysphagia, dyspnoea or orthopnoea and exercise intolerance (Ellison *et al.*, 1987; Prymak *et al.*, 1989; Callan *et al.*, 1993). Regurgitation or vomiting may be exacerbated by excitement or exercise. An attempt should be made to rule out predisposing causes, particularly respiratory tract disease. Some animals show no clinical signs and the hernia is discovered as an incidental clinical or post-mortem finding.

Imaging is the most useful diagnostic test, with survey radiographs, oesophagography and fluoroscopy all playing a useful role. Some reports indicate that a diagnosis can be reached with survey radiographs in all cases (Callan *et al.*, 1993), whereas other reports suggest that contrast radiographic studies are required in a high proportion of cases (White, 1993; Lorinson and Bright, 1998).

The most consistent radiographic sign of herniation is displacement of the stomach. Radiography may reveal a soft tissue opacity in the region of the distal oesophagus, immediately cranial to the left diaphragmatic crus, and a gas-filled oesophagus. This opacity may be identified as stomach if it is gas-filled and reveals rugal folds. The displacement of the stomach produces an abnormal 'stretched' appearance to the remaining portions of the stomach in the abdomen. An alveolar pattern in the dependent portions of the lung lobes, which may progress to lobar consolidation, is consistent with aspiration pneumonia.

A positive contrast oesophagogram, using barium liquid or paste, may show dilatation of the caudal oesophagus and retention of barium in this location, and cranial displacement of the gastro-oesophageal junction, cardia or fundus into the thorax (Figure 17.7). Fluoroscopy, following the administration of barium and food, is the most reliable method for identifying intermittent hiatal herniation and allows assessment of oesophageal motility. Fluoroscopy may reveal gastro-oesophageal reflux, herniation of the stomach, a patulous gastro-oesophageal junction and decreased primary or secondary oesophageal contractions (Prymak *et al.*, 1989). In a para-oesophageal hiatal hernia, the gastro-oesophageal

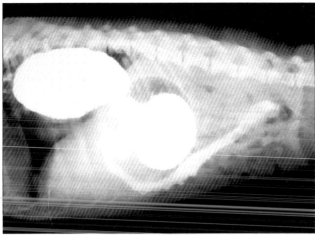

17.7 Hiatal hernia: lateral view of the abdomen and caudal thorax following administration of barium suspension. There is herniation of the stomach through the oesophageal hiatus.

junction remains in its normal position and the stomach protrudes into the thorax (Miles *et al.*, 1988).

Oesophagoscopy may reveal mucosal hyperaemia, inflammation and ulceration of the distal oesophagus (Merdan Dhein *et al.*, 1980). A caudal oesophageal sphincter that lacks tone, or that is displaced to one side, requiring redirection of the tip of the endoscope to enter the stomach, may also be appreciated (Lorinson and Bright, 1998). However, endoscopically apparent oesophagitis is not noted in all cases.

Oesophageal manometry may be used to examine the pressure at the caudal oesophageal sphincter, which is reduced in cases of sliding axial hernias, but not in cases of para-oesophageal hernias (Ellison *et al.*, 1987). However, this is primarily a research tool rather than a clinical diagnostic tool.

Treatment: The difficulty in understanding the complex nature and interplay of the various pathophysiological events is reflected in the relatively poor success of medical and surgical management in many reports. This has been hindered by the rarity of the condition and the tendency to adopt surgical techniques from human medicine, which have subsequently been found to be inappropriate.

General approach to therapy: Gastro-oesophageal reflux associated with hiatal herniation may be treated medically or surgically. In animals with acquired hiatal hernia secondary to other diseases, these diseases should be treated first before considering surgical management of the hiatal hernia. In cases of congenital hiatal hernia, surgery is indicated for animals that show no improvement following medical therapy, or which have frequent relapses following cessation of therapy.

The most appropriate management of the asymptomatic animal with hiatal hernia is not known (Bright *et al.*, 1990). It is not known whether these animals have a non-progressive and potentially self-resolving hernia (e.g. as in some young Shar-Peis), in which case no therapy would be appropriate, or whether clinical signs associated with the hernia may develop, in which case preventive therapy might be appropriate.

The aims of therapy are:

- Amelioration of signs of gastro-oesophageal reflux
- Restoration of normal caudal oesophageal sphincter function

- Prevention of complications arising from chronic oesophagitis, e.g. stricture
- Prevention of complications arising from regurgitation, e.g. aspiration pneumonia
- Prevention of complications arising from herniation of abdominal organs, e.g. gastric tympany.

It is apparent that surgical or medical therapy alone is unlikely to achieve all of these aims, and both medical and surgical management are likely to be appropriate in most individuals. It is suggested that medical therapy is instituted in all animals (Bright *et al.*, 1990; Lorinson and Bright, 1998). A decision regarding surgical management is then taken depending on the success of medical therapy. An initial period of medical therapy is also indicated in animals destined for surgical management, to reduce the signs associated with reflux oesophagitis and to allow treatment for aspiration pneumonia.

Medical therapy: This consists of:

- Establishing a diffusion barrier to peptic mucosal damage, e.g. sucralfate
- Improving the tone of the caudal oesophageal sphincter, e.g. metoclopramide
- Neutralizing or suppressing gastric acid secretion, e.g. antacids, H2-blockers, proton pump inhibitors
- Decreasing gastric emptying time, e.g. metoclopramide, liquid meals, low-fat diet
- Negating the effect of reduced oesophageal tone, e.g. feeding from a height, feeding moist food
- Removal of predisposing causes, e.g. weight loss if obese, treatment of respiratory disease.

In early reports, medical therapy was regarded as unsuccessful (Gaskell *et al.*, 1974; Ellison *et al.*, 1987; Prymak *et al.*, 1989), whereas more recent reports conclude that medical therapy may be successful in a proportion of cases (Bright *et al.*, 1990; Stickle *et al.*, 1992; Lorinson and Bright, 1998). One of the reasons for this is that medical therapy is primarily aimed at reducing the clinical signs associated with reflux oesophagitis. However, this may not be the main cause of the clinical signs in all animals (Prymak *et al.*, 1989; Callan *et al.*, 1993).

Although medical therapy may be successful, it does not completely prevent herniation or gastro-oesophageal reflux, and long-term complications are possible. These include:

- Aspiration pneumonia from chronic regurgitation
- Oesophageal stricture from chronic oesophagitis
- Chronic low-grade or massive acute haemorrhage from oesophageal ulceration
- Massive herniation of organs from persistence or enlargement of a hernia.

Surgical therapy: The indications for surgery are more poorly defined in small animals. In humans, surgery is indicated if:

- Persistent gastro-oesophageal reflux is unresponsive to medical therapy
- Oesophagitis develops
- Aspiration pneumonia occurs
- A large hernia which interferes with cardiorespiratory function is present.

It is likely that similar criteria will apply to small animals. Surgery is recommended for animals that do not respond

to 30 days of medical therapy, or which show frequent relapses following cessation of therapy, or if the owners are unable to comply with the relatively intensive medical regime (Bright *et al.*, 1990; Lorinson and Bright, 1998).

Various surgical techniques have been described in the human and veterinary literature, and fall into the following categories:

- Sphincter-enhancing techniques
- Closure of the hiatus
- Fixation of the stomach and oesophagus.

The surgical principles behind surgical management of any hernia include closure of the hernia ring and fixation of the herniated contents, and therefore techniques that achieve these aims are likely to yield success. In humans, closure of the hiatus and gastropexy (Hill technique) are usually combined with a sphincter-enhancing procedure, and long-term follow up reveals success rates of 80–95%. In small animals, sphincter-enhancing techniques are associated with unacceptable intraoperative and postoperative complications and are no longer recommended.

Surgical technique: The abdominal portion of the oesophagus and the gastro-oesophageal junction are exposed at a cranioventral midline laparotomy. The gastrohepatic ligament, part of the lesser omentum, is incised and the left lobes of the liver are retracted medially. If the stomach is herniated, it is reduced by caudal retraction. The abdominal portion of the oesophagus is further exposed by making a circumferential incision in the phrenico-oesophageal ligament (Figure 17.8), representing the ventral 180 degrees (Prymak *et al.*, 1989) or the full 360 degrees (White, 1993) of the circumference, taking care to avoid the ventral vagal trunk. The caudal 2–3 cm of the oesophagus is retracted into the abdomen and the gastro-oesophageal sphincter is exposed. Placement of an orogastric tube will facilitate identification of the oesophagus.

- **Sphincter-enhancing techniques:** In humans, there is a relatively high prevalence of incompetence of the caudal oesophageal sphincter. Hence, surgical techniques, such as fundoplication, have been designed to augment this region (Merdan Dhein *et al.*, 1980; Miles *et al.*, 1988). However, there is no evidence to suggest that this occurs in the dog, and these techniques do not have a rational basis in this species.

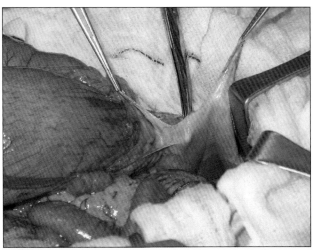

17.8 Hiatal hernia: following reduction of the stomach, the phrenico-oesophageal ligament is incised.

- **Closure of the hiatus:** The oesophageal hiatus cannot be closed completely, because the oesophagus still needs to traverse the diaphragm (Figure 17.9). Sutures placed ventral to the oesophagus will have the effect of moving the oesophagus to a more dorsal position, which has been suggested by White (1993) or dorsal to the oesophagus in the crural muscle, to preserve a more normal position of the hiatus. Previous reports have suggested closing the hiatus to a diameter of 1.5–2 cm, or the width of one or two fingers placed alongside the oesophagus at the hiatus (Ellison *et al.*, 1987; Miles *et al.*, 1988). Care is taken to avoid the dorsal and ventral branches of the vagus nerves and the oesophageal blood vessels.
- **Fixation of the herniated organs:** The abdominal oesophagus is fixed in position by oesophagopexy. Simple interrupted sutures are placed to anchor the oesophagus to the perimeter of the oesophageal hiatus. The fundus of the stomach is fixed in position with a left-sided gastropexy. Gastropexy not only physically prevents the stomach from being displaced cranially, but it also increases the caudal oesophageal barrier pressure, possibly by increasing longitudinal stretch in the distal oesophagus, which causes reflex contraction and reduction in lumen diameter, thus preventing gastro-oesophageal reflux. Stretching of the diaphragmatic crura by gastropexy may also result in an increase in muscle tone at the hiatus.

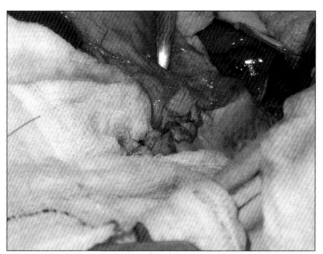

17.9 Hiatal hernia: closure of the oesophageal hiatus. Sutures have been placed in the diaphragmatic crura dorsal to the oesophagus, to maintain its position.

Similar decision-making lies behind the choice of gastropexy technique for hiatal hernia to that employed for gastric dilatation–volvulus, and incisional gastropexy or tube gastrostomy may be selected. However, tube gastrostomy is recommended for the following reasons:

- It is simple and quick to perform
- It allows deflation of the stomach if gastric tympany occurs
- It bypasses the oesophagus, thus reducing regurgitation
- It allows feeding of the anorexic patient.

Choice of procedure: With such an uncommon condition, it is difficult to compare the results of the various studies directly (Prymak *et al.*, 1989; Bright *et al.*, 1990; Callan *et al.*, 1993; White, 1993; Lorinson and Bright, 1998). However,

surgical prudence dictates that the simplest surgery that results in successful resolution of the condition represents the most appropriate choice. The best success rates seem to come from a combination of techniques, rather than any single procedure.

In attempting to evaluate the evidence for a particular method of surgical management, a number of problems are identified:

- Relatively few cases, with fewer large studies, are reported
- The indications for surgery are not always clearly defined
- A consistent surgical technique or combination is not always applied to all animals in a report
- More than one surgical technique is usually applied per operative episode
- The endpoint of hiatal plication is subjective
- Some animals with an acquired hernia have had surgery performed to correct the underlying cause as well as the hernia, with success claimed for surgical management of the hernia (Ellison *et al.*, 1987)
- Some asymptomatic animals have had surgery performed, with success claimed for surgical management of the hernia (Bright *et al.*, 1990)
- Spontaneous remission of clinical and radiographic signs of hiatal herniation are reported in some young dogs (Stickle *et al.*, 1992)
- The definition of 'successful' surgical treatment varies from lack of clinical signs to lack of imaging findings
- There is a relatively short period of follow-up in some reports.

However, the following points can be made:

- Combinations of techniques seem to be more efficacious than single techniques. This is evidenced by the high rate of surgical failure when only one technique is performed (van Sluijs and Happe, 1985; Prymak *et al.*, 1989; Bright *et al.*, 1990) and the failure of the entire procedure if one technique fails
- Plication of the hiatus and pexy of abdominal organs are the mainstays of surgery
- Fundoplication techniques have a low rate of success and high rate of morbidity.

Postoperative care and complications: Medical therapy for gastro-oesophageal reflux should be continued during the immediate postoperative period. Feeding little and often with a low-fat, highly digestible diet may also reduce gastro-oesophageal reflux. Postoperative radiographs and fluoroscopy should confirm the resolution of the oesophageal dilatation, the normal position of the stomach, lack of gastro-oesophageal reflux and improvement in oesophageal motility.

Potential complications include: dehiscence of the repair and recurrence of herniation; gastro-oesophageal reflux; oesophageal obstruction; pneumothorax; and aspiration pneumonia. Aspiration pneumonia and massive herniation with gastric tympany are the most common causes of perioperative mortality (Callan *et al.*, 1993).

Dehiscence is usually the result of poor surgical technique. This is generally due to poor surgical access, resulting in inadequate suture placement. Surgical failure has been attributed to a shortened oesophagus and stricture in one case (Bright *et al.*, 1990). Gastro-oesophageal reflux may continue if the hernia has not been adequately reduced, whereas oesophageal obstruction may result if the diameter of the hiatus is reduced too much, or if a fundoplication procedure is performed. Iatrogenic pneumothorax may follow disruption of the phrenico-oesophageal ligament and adequate measures for controlled ventilation and pleural drainage should be available.

Continued regurgitation or vomiting may be due to unresolved oesophageal motility disorders, continuing gastro-oesophageal reflux, unresolved oesophagitis, mega-oesophagus and gastric hypomotility. Gastric hypomotility may be caused by iatrogenic trauma to the ventral vagus trunk or may be part of generalized gastrointestinal tract hypomotility (Prymak *et al.*, 1989; Callan *et al.*, 1993).

Prognosis: Surgical management of hiatal hernia using sphincter-enhancing techniques has a high rate of failure and frequent complications (Merdan Dhein *et al.*, 1980; Ellison *et al.*, 1987). Operative mortality can be high, up to 64% (Ellison *et al.*, 1987), and success rates are not consistently high; for example, in one study only 25% of animals were relieved of all clinical signs (Ellison *et al.*, 1987). However, if surgical closure of the hiatus and fixation of abdominal organs is performed, and if care is taken to identify and correct predisposing conditions, then the prognosis is good (Burnie *et al.*, 1989; Prymak *et al.*, 1989; Bright *et al.*, 1990; White, 1993; Hardie *et al.*, 1998; Lorinson and Bright, 1998).

Pleuroperitoneal hernia

Anatomy and incidence: This is the least common of the congenital diaphragmatic hernias. A defect is present in the dorsolateral diaphragm, which may range from a lack of the intermediate part of the left lumbar muscle of the crus to absence of both crura and a portion of the central tendon (Feldman *et al.*, 1968; Valentine *et al.*, 1988). These defects do not involve the pericardial sac.

Aetiology: Two aetiologies for these hernias are suggested, which explain their dorsolateral location:

- Incomplete closure of the pleuroperitoneal canals: the pleuroperitoneal folds and posthepatic mesenchymal plate fail to fuse with the septum transversum and dorsal mesentery of the oesophagus, and an opening (foramen of Bochdalek) persists between the thoracic and abdominal cavities (Feldman *et al.*, 1968; Valentine *et al.*, 1988)
- Failure of the pleuroperitoneal folds to incorporate muscular components of the body wall: the pleuroperitoneal canals are closed, but myoblasts from the posthepatic mesenchymal plate and abdominal wall fail to invade this tissue and the lumbar portion of the diaphragm remains membranous rather than muscular, and acts as a hernial sac. This type is referred to as a true pleuroperitoneal hernia (Mann *et al.*, 1991; Voges *et al.*, 1997).

On the basis of finding the defect in litters from repeated matings, an autosomal recessive mode of inheritance has been proposed in the dog (Feldman *et al.*, 1968; Valentine *et al.*, 1988). In humans, the left side of the diaphragm is also more commonly affected and an autosomal mode of inheritance is also suspected. These hernias have also been induced by exposure to various teratogens, such as thalidomide and polybrominated biphenyls, as well as by vitamin A deficiency (Mann *et al.*, 1991).

Failure of the pleuroperitoneal membranes to close may be caused by interference by viscera. For instance, cranial displacement of the liver or caudal displacement of the developing lung bud into the canal may prevent its closure. Alternatively, atrophy of the developing lung bud may fail to guide the posthepatic mesenchymal plate to fusion (Mann *et al.*, 1991). The facts that the left lung bud develops more slowly than the right in many species and that pleuroperitoneal hernias develop predominantly on the left side appear to support the latter hypothesis (Mann *et al.*, 1991).

Pathophysiology: The pathophysiological events in animals with sufficiently large defects are similar to those in animals with traumatic diaphragmatic rupture, with displacement and compression of the thoracic viscera by abdominal organs and, less commonly, incarceration of abdominal viscera in the thorax. Animals may be dead at birth or die soon after with cyanosis and dyspnoea because of an inability to expand the lungs. Organs that commonly herniate include the stomach, liver, spleen, duodenum and pancreas (Feldman *et al.*, 1968). Hernias formed by incomplete muscular invasion of the pleuroperitoneal folds have a hernial sac that limits the extent of herniated organs, compared with hernias formed by incomplete closure of the pleuroperitoneal canals.

Diagnosis: Puppies or kittens may be born dead or may exhibit severe dyspnoea and cyanosis. Less severely affected animals may show mild dyspnoea and abdominal breathing (Feldman *et al.*, 1968; Mann *et al.*, 1991) or no clinical signs (Voges *et al.*, 1997).

Radiography reveals a soft tissue opacity at the cranial extent of the diaphragm (Figure 17.10), which may mimic a mass lesion affecting the diaphragm, lung lobes or pleura. Ultrasonographic examination may reveal an abnormally thin diaphragm with a hernial defect and abdominal organs passing cranial to the diaphragm (Mann *et al.*, 1991).

Differentiating a pleuroperitoneal hernia from a ruptured diaphragm may be difficult if there is no history of trauma. This differentiation is relatively simple for complete tears of the diaphragm. However, this may be difficult in the case of a subtotal diaphragmatic tear, in which there is a traumatically induced rent in the musculotendinous portion of the diaphragm, but the parietal pleura on the thoracic surface of the diaphragm remains intact (Voges *et al.*, 1997). This is sometimes referred to as eventration of the diaphragm. In this situation, the abdominal organs are bounded by a membrane that mimics the hernial sac of the true pleuroperitoneal hernia, although this membrane may be difficult to recognize.

Criteria used to help differentiate a congenital pleuroperitoneal hernia from a ruptured diaphragm are shown in Figure 17.11.

Treatment: Surgical closure of the hernia may be possible, depending on the size of the defect. However, in those animals that survive beyond birth, the hernia is likely to be relatively small and bounded by a hernial sac. Herniorrhaphy is performed in a similar manner to that for a ruptured diaphragm (see below), although the presence of the intact pleuroperitoneal membrane in most cases means that there is no direct continuity between the thoracic and abdominal cavities and intraoperative pneumothorax will not occur unless this membrane is incised or is absent.

Postoperative care and complications: Postoperative recovery is usually uncomplicated. Complications have not been reported.

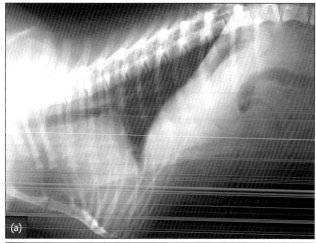

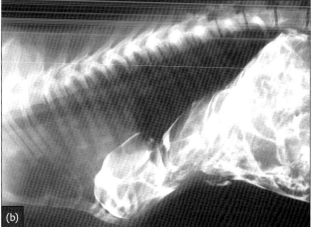

17.10 True pleuroperitoneal hernia. (a) Lateral view of the thorax. The cardiac silhouette is ill-defined ventrally and the trachea is elevated. The caudal sternebrae are fused. (b) Lateral view of the thorax following positive contrast peritoneography. Contrast medium outlines the cranial extent of the parietal peritoneum, which extends into the thorax and contains loops of intestine.
(Courtesy of C Lamb)

Criterion	Congenital hernia	Acquired rupture
Appearance of the opening	Round, smooth border	Irregular border
Association with other abnormalities	Other congenital anomalies possible	Other congenital anomalies unlikely
Extent of herniation and size of defect	Large volume of viscera through a small defect	Volume of viscera tends to approximate size of defect
Histological examination of hernial ring	Lack of inflammation	Inflammatory changes
Hernial sac	Present in true pleuroperitoneal hernia	Absent
Completeness of diaphragm	Portions of diaphragm absent	Diaphragm complete, but torn
Age of animal	Generally young animals	Any age

17.11 Criteria used to help differentiate a congenital pleuroperitoneal hernia from a ruptured diaphragm.
(Kent, 1950)

Prognosis: The prognosis depends on the size and nature of the defect, the degree of visceral displacement and the ability of the lungs to expand. All animals with a pleuroperitoneal hernia that were dead at birth or were euthanased because of severe dyspnoea had a hernia manifested by patent pleuroperitoneal canals (Feldman *et al.*, 1968; Valentine *et al.*, 1988). Those animals that survived beyond a few months with a pleuroperitoneal hernia had a mesothelial membrane limiting herniation of organs into the thoracic cavity and surgical closure was successful (Mann *et al.*, 1991; Auger and Riley, 1997; Voges *et al.*, 1997).

Acquired diseases

Ruptured diaphragm

Anatomy and incidence: Traumatic rupture of the diaphragm is the most common cause of herniation of abdominal organs into the thoracic cavity, representing 77–85% of all cases of herniation (Wilson *et al.*, 1971; Wilson and Hayes, 1986; Boudrieau and Muir, 1987). Young male animals (1–3 years old) are at increased risk for ruptured diaphragm (Stokhof, 1986; Boudrieau and Muir, 1987).

Knowledge of the anatomical structure of the diaphragm helps the clinician understand the common locations of rupture. The weak ventrally located costal muscles are more frequently injured than the stronger central tendon and the large, well protected dorsal lumbar portion (Wilson and Hayes, 1986). Although some studies have shown a predominance of tears on the left or the right side, overall the incidence is probably equal. A single tear is present in most affected animals, but approximately 15% of individuals have either bilateral or multiple tears (Garson *et al.*, 1980; Stokhof, 1986; Wilson and Hayes, 1986). In dogs, the orientation of tears was circumferential in 40%, radial in 40% and a combination of these in the remaining 20%, whereas in cats the majority were circumferential (59%), with fewer radial tears (18%) in one study (Garson *et al.*, 1980).

Aetiology: Ruptured diaphragm is caused by blunt abdominal trauma, primarily from road traffic accidents, although kicks, falls and fights have also been implicated (Walker and Hall, 1965; Wilson and Hayes, 1986; Boudrieau and Muir, 1987). Direct trauma from penetrating injuries (e.g. stab wounds and gunshot wounds) is occasionally seen. Iatrogenic diaphragmatic injury caused by inadvertent incision during cranial extension of a midline laparotomy, or during placement of a thoracostomy tube, and cutaneous asthenia are also rare but possible causes.

Indirect trauma when the glottis is open is the most common cause of diaphragmatic rupture. During normal inspiration, the pleuroperitoneal pressure gradient varies from 7 to 20 cmH₂O, but may increase to over 100 cmH₂O at peak inspiration. Application of force to the abdomen with the glottis open increases this gradient further, which may lead to rupture of the diaphragm. If the glottis is closed, the intrathoracic pressure is higher, the pleuroperitoneal gradient is lower, and rupture of the lung parenchyma, rather than the diaphragm, is the most likely sequel.

Although blunt indirect trauma is well recognized as a cause of ruptured diaphragm, it must be considered that any trauma sufficient to cause rupture of the diaphragm will also result in damage to other thoracic and abdominal organs. In fact, following blunt trauma, such as a road traffic accident, ruptured diaphragm is considerably less common than other injuries, such as rib fractures, pulmonary contusions, pleural disease (e.g. haemothorax, pneumothorax) and myocardial contusions. Approximately 2% of dogs with long bone fractures have a concomitant ruptured diaphragm.

Pathophysiology: Which abdominal organs become displaced into the thoracic cavity is dependent upon their proximity to the diaphragmatic defect and their mobility. Therefore, one or more lobes of the liver are most commonly displaced, being found in the thoracic cavity in approximately 88% of patients with a ruptured diaphragm (Wilson and Hayes, 1986; Boudrieau and Muir, 1987). Other organs that can be displaced into the thoracic cavity following a diaghramatic rupture, in approximate descending order of frequency, include the small intestine, stomach, spleen, omentum, pancreas, colon, caecum and uterus (Garson *et al.*, 1980; Stokhof, 1986; Wilson and Hayes, 1986). When the right side of the diaphragm tears, the liver, small intestine and pancreas herniate, whereas in left-sided tears, herniation of the stomach, spleen and small intestine is more common (Garson *et al.*, 1980).

Gastric tympany may occur following herniation of the stomach; as the stomach expands it compresses the lungs, the heart and venae cavae, reducing alveolar ventilation and cardiac output. These events can be rapidly fatal, and emergency gastric decompression by orogastric intubation or transthoracic needle gastrocentesis should be performed. Obstruction of the small intestine may be partial or complete and may affect the proximal or distal small intestine. Strangulating obstruction may lead to ischaemic necrosis, intestinal perforation and abscessation, peritonitis and pleuritis. Although these complications are not as immediately life-threatening as gastric dilatation, corrective surgical therapy should not be delayed once the animal is stable. Treatment of such patients is very demanding.

Displacement of the liver lobes may result in intrahepatic venous hypertension and cause effusion from the liver surface. Hydrothorax and ascites develop in approximately 30% of animals with herniation of the liver (Wilson *et al.*, 1971; Boudrieau and Muir, 1987).

Pleural effusion is generally from entrapped liver lobes, but may also derive from other organs (e.g. lung lobe torsion). Effusion is typically, therefore, a modified transudate, but haemothorax, chylothorax or bile pleuritis are also occasionally seen.

Proliferation of bacteria normally resident in the liver, such as clostridia, may occur in areas of liver with a poor vascular supply. These organisms may release toxins whilst the lobe is malpositioned or once the lobe has been surgically repositioned. A potential long-term sequelae is abscessation of the liver.

Effects on thoracic viscera are caused by compression or displacement resulting from the presence of abdominal organs, fluid or air in the pleural space. Effects on abdominal viscera include obstruction or strangulation, Incarceration or strangulation may be caused by pressure applied by the edge of the diaphragmatic tear as the organs pass over it, or may be the result of fibrous adhesions.

Filling of the pleural space with air, fluid or abdominal organs will prevent normal coupling between movements of the chest wall and the lungs, resulting in inefficient breathing movements. Furthermore, compression of the lung lobes may lead to atelectasis with resulting hypoventilation, ventilation/perfusion mismatching and hypoxia.

Dyspnoea is the most common clinical sign following acute traumatic rupture of the diaphragm and may be due to:

- Lack of a functioning diaphragm
- Trauma to other accessory components of respiration, e.g. intercostal muscles and ribs
- Filling of the pleural space with air, fluid or abdominal viscera
- Pulmonary contusions
- Pain associated with normal respiratory movements, e.g. in animals with fractured ribs.

Systemic pathophysiological changes: The inciting trauma may also result in circulatory shock, which may be:

- Hypovolaemic, e.g. from bleeding externally or internally into the pleural or peritoneal space
- Cardiogenic, e.g. from myocardial contusions, or release of depressant factors from the hypoxic pancreas if herniated
- Obstructive, e.g. from obstruction of the hepatic veins following herniation of the liver
- Endotoxic, e.g. from liberation of toxins from bacteria proliferating in devitalized herniated organs (e.g. intestine, liver).

Cardiac arrhythmias are present in approximately 12% of patients with a ruptured diaphragm, which may reduce tissue perfusion and exacerbate the shock caused by other pathophysiological changes (Boudrieau and Muir, 1987). Shock may continue as multiple organ system failure. In particular, pulmonary function, which is already compromised, may deteriorate further, with an increase in pulmonary vascular permeability and pulmonary oedema.

Patients with diaphragmatic rupture are often on the edge of fatal cardiopulmonary decompensation and a great deal of care is required in their management. Frequently, these patients benefit from 24–48 hours of stabilization prior to surgical therapy of the diaphragmatic injury. Exceptions to this rule include those with intrathoracic gastric tympany and intestinal entrapment causing obstruction of the bowel.

Diagnosis: The time interval between trauma and diagnosis of diaphragmatic rupture ranges from several hours to several years, with a mean of several weeks in published studies (Garson *et al.*, 1980; Stokhof, 1986; Boudrieau and Muir, 1987). In one report, 20% of cases were diagnosed more than 4 weeks after the injury (Boudrieau and Muir, 1987). The time interval from the traumatic incident to diagnosis may depend on whether or not the trauma was observed, the size and nature of the hernia, the clinical signs shown and the degree of investigation performed.

Any animal with a known history of trauma, or with injuries consistent with a traumatic aetiology, should be considered at risk for diaphragmatic rupture. It is prudent, therefore, to evaluate these animals carefully for the presence of thoracic (and abdominal) disease. These investigations should include thoracic and abdominal imaging, when the patient is stable. This approach will facilitate early diagnosis and treatment of diaphragmatic rupture in particular. Failure to evaluate the patient for the results of thoracic and abdominal trauma often results in a delayed diagnosis and makes surgical therapy more complicated.

It is hypothesized that some individuals may be presented with a diaphragmatic tear and either subtle or no herniation of viscera. Diaphragmatic rupture in these animals may go unnoticed during initial radiographic evaluation. Herniation subsequently develops or worsens over the next few days, particularly if the animal is subjected to sedation, anaesthesia or manipulation for other injuries sustained at the time of trauma. The clinician should therefore remain open to the diagnosis of diaphragmatic rupture, even in a patient that apparently had normal thoracic radiographs shortly after trauma.

History: Historical features include the known occurrence of blunt abdominal trauma or the presence of other injuries that indicate a traumatic incident has occurred. Occasionally, animals with chronic hernias are presented because of progressive exercise intolerance, difficulty breathing or gastrointestinal disease, with no indication of historical trauma other than a ruptured diaphragm.

Clinical signs: There are no pathognomonic signs of diaphragmatic rupture. The clinical signs reflect the extent and severity of the pathophysiological changes outlined above. In acute diaphragmatic rupture, respiratory signs predominate, with dyspnoea, orthopnoea and exercise intolerance present in at least 38% of cases (Stokhof, 1986). Some animals will adopt a sitting or standing position with their elbows abducted and head and neck extended. Animals with pleural space disease usually show a restrictive respiratory breathing pattern, that is, rapid, shallow respiration. In animals with a chronic hernia, gastrointestinal signs may predominate, such as vomiting, diarrhoea, dysphagia and constipation. Other non-specific signs include depression, anorexia, weight loss and difficulty lying down (Stokhof, 1986).

Physical examination: The physical examination may appear to be within normal limits in some individuals.

Palpation of the thorax may elicit pain (e.g. from fractured ribs or bruising) and may reveal a shift of the apex beat of the heart away from the side of the rupture. With experience, thoracic palpation will identify the side of the rupture in 80% of cases (Stokhof, 1986). The abdomen may appear tucked-up and may appear empty on examination or palpation, although this is a subjective and unreliable sign (Garson *et al.*, 1980).

Percussion may reveal hyporesonance if fluid or abdominal organs are present in the ipsilateral pleural space, and hyper-resonance if either free air (e.g. pneumothorax) or circumscribed air (e.g. gastric tympany) is present.

On auscultation of the chest, the heart and lung sounds may be muffled on the side with the rupture. With displacement of the heart, the apex beat may be auscultated in an abnormal location and the heart sounds may be more intense on the side contralateral to the rupture. Auscultation of borborygmi within the chest is an uncommon finding.

Survey radiographs: Thoracic radiography is the most useful screening test for the presence of diaphragmatic rupture, with the lateral view the most useful single view (Sullivan and Lee, 1989). The DV view allows the side of the rupture to be determined and is more sensitive for the detection of small amounts of pleural fluid. The radiographs should also include the cranial abdomen.

Although in ideal circumstances a full radiographic study would comprise a DV and one or two lateral views, care must be taken not to cause the animal undue distress during restraint. The first radiographic view to be taken should be the one that causes least distress. Under no circumstances should a VD view be attempted in the dyspnoeic animal or in a patient where a ruptured diaphragm or other thoracic disease is suspected.

Radiographic signs associated with diaphragmatic rupture (Park, 1994) (Figure 17.12) are:

- Partial or complete loss of the thoracic diaphragmatic surface
- Cranial displacement or angulation of the diaphragmatic line

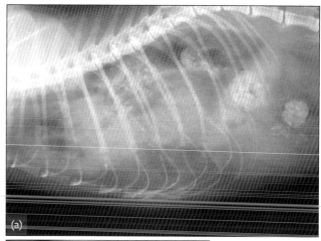

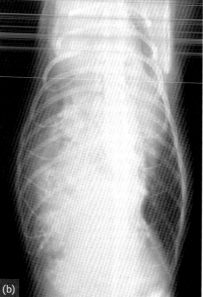

17.12 Ruptured diaphragm. (a) Lateral view of the thorax. The cardiac silhouette and lungs are obscured by an ill-defined heterogeneous soft tissue/fat/gas opacity representing small intestine, colon and liver. The heart is displaced cranially and dorsally. (b) Dorsoventral view of the thorax. The right hemithorax contains an ill-defined heterogeneous soft tissue/fat/gas opacity representing small intestine, colon and liver. The heart is displaced cranially and to the left.

- Abdominal viscera within the thorax, e.g. liver, spleen, stomach, intestine
- Displacement of abdominal structures, e.g. liver, spleen, stomach, intestine
- Displacement of thoracic structures, e.g. heart, mediastinum, lung lobes
- Change in appearance of thoracic structures, e.g. lung lobe collapse
- Loss of demarcation of thoracic structures, e.g. heart shadow
- Pleural fluid.

Abnormal intrathoracic structures may be identified as abdominal in origin if their opacity is different (e.g. fat opacity of the falciform ligament, fat-containing omentum, gas-filled bowel) or if their structure indicates an abdominal organ (e.g. gastric rugal folds, loops of small intestine).

If a diagnosis cannot be obtained from survey radiographs then further procedures may be performed. The simplest procedure should be chosen first. These additional procedures include:

- Repeat survey radiographs following thoracocentesis
- Positional radiographic views made with a horizontal beam
- Contrast radiographs.

Repeat survey radiographs: If there is a significant volume of pleural fluid present, thoracocentesis should be performed (see Chapter 12). Removal of the fluid will alleviate some of the respiratory distress, allow a sample of the fluid to be submitted for analysis to rule out other causes of pleural effusion and improve the detail seen on subsequent radiographs. However, thoracic radiographs taken after thoracocentesis may still not yield a definitive diagnosis (Sullivan and Lee, 1989).

Positional radiography and horizontal beam views: Taking radiographs with the animal in different positions (e.g. a horizontal beam lateral view with the animal in dorsal recumbency), may help to differentiate solid tissue from fluid. Solid tissue will usually remain in place, whereas fluid will move to the dependent part of the thorax. However, it should be stressed that any dyspnoeic patient should not be placed in dorsal recumbency and this is useful only for animals with a small volume of pleural fluid.

Horizontal beam radiography may be required for severely dyspnoeic animals. The patient is allowed to adopt a comfortable sitting or standing position and a radiograph is made with a horizontal beam. Cats may be placed inside a cardboard box on the radiography table to provide minimal restraint. However, this view is not standard, so may be difficult to interpret; positioning is poor, with the forelimbs often obscuring the thoracic cavity, and it requires the use of a horizontal X-ray beam, for which appropriate radiographic safety procedures should be followed.

Contrast radiographs: Various contrast radiographic techniques, such as an upper gastrointestinal barium series, peritoneography (negative and positive contrast), positive contrast pleurography, portography, cholecystography and angiography, have been suggested, although only the first two techniques are recommended. The use of ultrasonography has replaced these techniques and they are only indicated if thoracic radiography is equivocal and ultrasonography is not available.

An upper gastrointestinal barium series, following the administration of 2–4 ml/kg 30% w/v barium sulphate suspension, is relatively simple to perform and non-invasive, but it will only allow a definitive diagnosis to be made if part of the gastrointestinal tract has herniated through the diaphragm (Sullivan and Lee, 1989). Obstruction of the intestinal tract may delay passage of barium and is a further disadvantage. Peritoneography is more invasive and may yield false negative results if the rent in the diaphragm has been sealed by viscera. The use of positive contrast agents (e.g. 1 ml/kg water-soluble iodinated contrast medium) rather than air is more sensitive, although dilution of the medium by pleural fluid may also yield false negative results (Stickle, 1984).

Ultrasonography: Ultrasound examination is a relatively simple, non-invasive, accurate technique for the diagnosis of diaphragmatic rupture (Spattini *et al.*, 2003), which still works well in the presence of pleural fluid. The examination is performed with the probe in a subcostal position, immediately caudal to the xiphisternum, or in a parasternal location, below the costochondral junctions, in an intercostal space selected after evaluation of the thoracic radiograph.

Ultrasonographic examination should always be performed in animals where a diagnosis cannot be made from the radiograph (e.g. if pleural effusion obscures the line of the diaphragm) or where a small tear may be suspected but is not obvious radiographically (e.g. a small tear in the diaphragm with incarceration of a single liver lobe).

Ultrasonography may not always identify the tear in the diaphragm or organs herniating through it, but it will demonstrate the presence of abdominal viscera in the pleural space. The liver, spleen and intestines can all be identified ultrasonographically and their presence in an inappropriate location, such as adjacent to the heart, indicates a diaphragmatic rupture. Asymmetry of the cranial hepatic border may be seen. In some cases, the remnants of the torn diaphragmatic muscle, surrounded by anechoic pleural fluid, may be seen moving in time with respiratory movements. However, mirror image artefact, a common finding that results in the apparent presence of the liver cranial to the diaphragm, should not be misinterpreted as a ruptured diaphragm.

Other diagnostic tests: Arterial blood gas analysis will give further information about the effectiveness of ventilation and gas exchange. Pulse oximetry is a non-invasive tool that will provide information about the saturation of haemoglobin, giving indirect evidence of oxygenation. An electrocardiogram should ideally be performed in all patients to rule out cardiac arrhythmias due to myocardial contusions or hypoxia.

Clinical pathology: In acute cases, there may be little change in routine blood screens. With liver entrapment in the rupture, elevations in serum alanine aminotransferase and alkaline phosphatase may be noted.

Treatment:

Preoperative stabilization: Rupture of the diaphragm is a surgical disease. However, because of the numerous and potentially life-threatening pathophysiological changes, the patient should be stabilized prior to anaesthesia for definitive repair. This will allow an accurate assessment of the severity of the other injuries, and stabilization and treatment of them. If the surgery is carried out too soon, the patient may succumb to other disease processes (e.g. pulmonary oedema). However, if the surgery is delayed the pathophysiological changes may become worse (e.g. worsening atelectasis) and adhesions may start to form between the herniated organs and the contents of the thoracic cavity, thus making reduction of the organs more difficult. Surgical repair within the first 24 hours following trauma has been reported to have the highest mortality rate (33%) (Boudrieau and Muir, 1987), but this finding was not supported by a more recent study where the survival rate was 89.7% (Gibson *et al.*, 2005). It is likely that appropriate patient assessment and stabilization are more important than time *per se*, and some patients with acute life-threatening dyspnoea will benefit from early surgery.

Supplementary oxygen therapy should be provided during the evaluation and initial stabilization of the patient. The need for longer-term therapy can be decided once the patient is stable. This may be provided simply by flow-by, facemask or nasal catheter (see Chapter 2). Intravenous fluid therapy is indicated for patients that are hypovolaemic, in circulatory shock or unlikely to maintain their own voluntary intake. This generally includes all patients following trauma, but care should be taken to avoid volume overload in patients with pre-existing lung contusions so as not to exacerbate pulmonary dysfunction. As previously mentioned, in animals with intrathoracic gastric tympany, the stomach should be deflated with a nasogastric or oro-gastric tube, or by transthoracic gastrocentesis, and an uncapped nasogastric tube should be left in place until surgery is performed. Thoracocentesis should be performed in patients with a significant volume of pleural fluid or a pneumothorax.

The patient should be allowed to assume a comfortable position, which may depend on the side of the rupture and the presence of chest wall pain. However, certain positions will allow more efficient ventilation. The patient should be encouraged to lie in sternal recumbency, so that both lung fields may be used, or in lateral recumbency with the affected side down, so that the less affected lobes are uppermost. The animal should be monitored closely and continuously during this period since rapid decompensation may occur.

Anaesthetic considerations: Oxygen supplementation should be provided in the pre-induction period. Rapid induction with an intravenous agent followed by prompt endotracheal intubation is mandatory. Controlled intermittent positive pressure ventilation, coupled with positive end-expiratory pressure if required, is started soon after induction. If spontaneous breathing is efficient initially, it is important to remember to take control of ventilation as soon as the abdomen is open. Assisted ventilation should not exceed an inspired pressure of 15 mmHg to minimize the likelihood of re-expansion pulmonary oedema. Chronically collapsed lungs should not be forcibly re-expanded during surgery. (For more information on anaesthetic considerations, see Chapter 1.)

Surgical considerations: There are few indications for emergency surgery, but these include:

- Massive organ displacement
- Continuing haemorrhage
- An enlarging gas-filled viscus, particularly the stomach, in the thoracic cavity
- Bowel rupture.

Repair of a ruptured diaphragm has a higher priority than repair of some other injuries sustained during the same traumatic event (e.g. long bone fracture). In a stable animal, definitive fracture repair may be performed following surgical repair of the ruptured diaphragm. However, anaesthetizing the animal a few days later may be a better option.

Although this is a clean or clean-contaminated procedure, perioperative antibiotics are indicated if devitalized tissue (e.g. liver lobes) or significant atelectasis of lung lobes is anticipated.

Surgical approach: A number of surgical approaches have been recommended for gaining access, including ventral midline laparotomy, median sternotomy, intercostal thoracotomy and trans-sternal thoracotomy. However, adequate access can be gained in almost all cases via a cranial ventral midline laparotomy, with extension via a caudal median sternotomy, involving the caudal one to three sternebrae, if required (Figure 17.13).

Surgical technique: An incision is made from the xiphoid to beyond the umbilicus. A large incision makes it considerably easier to expose the diaphragm and abdominal organs. The falciform ligament may be excised to increase exposure, particularly of the ventral diaphragm. Self-retaining retractors are placed to aid exposure, and pleural

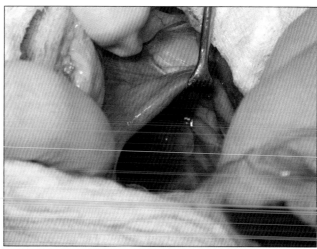

17.13 Ruptured diaphragm: visualization of the left caudal lung lobe through a radial tear in the dorsal aspect of the left side of the diaphragm.

and peritoneal fluid is removed by suction. Long-handled instruments may be useful for suturing the dorsal aspect of the diaphragm, particularly in a deep-chested dog. A thorough examination of the diaphragm and all the abdominal viscera is made.

The abdominal organs can often be reduced by gentle traction. If the herniated organs become engorged or adherent to the edges of the diaphragm, traction may be unsuccessful. In this situation, the rent in the diaphragm may be enlarged to allow careful inspection and reduction of the organs. This is best performed by extending the incision in a radial direction ventrally, taking care to avoid vital structures such as the phrenic vessels, phrenic nerves and caudal vena cava. Adhesions to intrathoracic structures should be divided under direct observation. Adhesions tend to be fibrinous for the first 3 days, becoming more organized with greater quantities of fibrous tissue subsequently. Nevertheless, adhesions of less than 7–14 days old can often be gently peeled apart. More mature adhesions may require division of the affected part, for example, by partial lung lobectomy or complete liver lobectomy. Incarcerated liver lobes and spleen are often friable and should be handled with care. If these appear devitalized, a lobectomy or splenectomy should be performed, ideally before returning these organs to the abdomen. Following reduction, the thoracic cavity is lavaged with warm saline and a thoracostomy tube is placed under direct visualization.

Herniorrhaphy: Once reduced, the abdominal viscera are retracted using saline-soaked laparotomy swabs and malleable ribbon retractors. In animals with an acute diaphragmatic rupture, it is generally easy to determine the correct orientation of the tissues. It is extremely rare to find insufficient tissue for closure of the defect in such animals. In chronic tears, the edges of the defect may have 'rolled over' and mature fibrous tissue may have formed, causing contraction of the tissue. It is not recommended to debride the edges of the tear, because that will increase the size of the defect further and may reduce the holding power of the sutures. However, any scar tissue that prevents movement of the diaphragm should be incised.

Suture technique: The tear is examined and the correct orientation of the edges is determined. In tears of a complex shape, stay sutures may be placed to provide temporary closure in the appropriate manner. Suturing of the hernia is started at the most dorsal aspect, moving ventrally. The ends of the most dorsal sutures are left long and tagged with a haemostat to act as stay sutures for manipulating the rest of the diaphragm in an atraumatic fashion.

Choice of suture material and pattern: Although non-absorbable material has been recommended, the very long-term support this provides is generally not required. In addition, these materials tend to have sharp ends, which may traumatize viscera.

A more rational choice is a synthetic absorbable suture material. Monofilament material, such as polydioxanone, has the advantage that it is relatively long-lasting, but suffers similar disadvantages to the monofilament non-absorbable suture material. Multifilament material is easier to handle and has greater knot security. There is no one single suture material that will be ideal in all cases, and decisions should be made on an individual animal basis.

An appositional suture pattern is recommended, either simple interrupted or continuous. The choice of suture material and pattern is less important than meticulous atraumatic placement of sutures that appose the edges of the diaphragm without tension. The author's preference is to use simple interrupted sutures with a monofilament absorbable material.

Care is taken to avoid constriction of structures running through the diaphragmatic hiati, e.g. the caudal vena cava, during herniorrhaphy. In circumcostal tears, it may be difficult to approximate the diaphragm to the abdominal wall, and in these cases sutures may be passed around the adjacent ribs or the xiphisternum.

Patching: If atrophy and contracture of the diaphragm in a chronic hernia make it impossible to close the defect with appositional sutures, the defect may be patched with autogenous tissue such as omentum, muscle, liver or fascia, or prosthetic materials such as polypropylene mesh, silicone rubber sheeting or lyophilized porcine intestinal submucosa. However, many of these recommendations are based on experimental rather than clinical data.

End of the procedure: Closure of the laparotomy incision is routine. Following reduction of a chronic hernia, replacement of the organs and loss of abdominal domain may cause an increase in intraperitoneal pressure and resulting impairment of venous return. Careful monitoring of cardiovascular haemodynamics is important. Rarely, in a patient with a chronic hernia, the abdominal organs may not fit in the abdomen because of loss of abdominal domain. In this case, an elective splenectomy may reduce the volume of the abdominal viscera.

Postoperative care and complications: Close monitoring of the cardiopulmonary system is important in the postoperative period. Vital signs, mucus membrane colour, capillary refill time, respiratory pattern and pulse volume, quality and rhythm are measured. Supplementary oxygen therapy may be required if there is ventilatory insufficiency. If this persists, aspiration of the chest tube or thoracic radiography should be performed to ensure that this is not due to continuing pneumothorax. Although continuous or intermittent suction may be used, the most simple and practical method is to use intermittent suction with a syringe every 1–4 hours, depending on the volume of fluid or air retrieved. The tube should be removed once no more pleural air is obtained and once the breathing pattern has returned to normal.

Complications in the early postoperative period may be due to pneumothorax, haemothorax, pleural effusion, pulmonary oedema, pulmonary atelectasis, shock and cardiac arrhythmias (Walker and Hall, 1965; Wilson *et al.*, 1971; Garson *et al.*, 1980; Boudrieau and Muir, 1987). Deaths in the later postoperative period may be due to rupture, obstruction or strangulation of the intestinal tract, or other unrelated diseases (Garson *et al.*, 1980; Boudrieau and Muir, 1987).

Ascites may develop after surgery if there is obstruction to the hepatic veins following repositioning of the liver, if herniorrhaphy has resulted in constriction of the caudal vena cava or if there is chronic liver disease (Downs and Bjorling, 1987). Gastric ulceration has been recorded in dogs with chronic ruptures with intrathoracic adhesions to an incarcerated liver (Willard and Aronson, 1981). Dehiscence of the repair and subsequent reherniation of abdominal organs is uncommon and is usually due to faulty surgical technique.

Prognosis: The general prognosis for animals with a ruptured diaphragm is guarded to fair. The overall survival rate has been reported as 52–92% (Wilson *et al.*, 1971; Garson *et al.*, 1980; Stokhof, 1986; Boudrieau and Muir, 1987; Downs and Bjorling, 1987).

A significant proportion, up to 15%, of animals die before presentation for anaesthesia and surgical correction. These deaths are generally due to acute reduction in effective lung volume, hypoventilation, shock, multiple organ system failure and cardiac arrhythmias (Wilson *et al.*, 1971; Garson *et al.*, 1980; Boudrieau and Muir, 1987). Another proportion of animals die because of inappropriate restraint for examination or other diagnostic intervention, such as radiography and peritoneal or pleural drainage (Wilson *et al.*, 1971; Garson *et al.*, 1980; Stokhof, 1986). The other cause of perioperative mortality is induction of anaesthesia. Any delay in intubation and the establishment of controlled ventilation may have adverse effects.

If these animals are removed from the analysis then the overall mean survival rate for animals subject to surgical management of a ruptured diaphragm is 79% for dogs and 76% for cats (Garson *et al.*, 1980; Stokhof, 1986; Boudrieau and Muir, 1987). For animals operated on within 24 hours of the trauma, the survival rate was 67% and for those operated on after 1 year, the survival rate was 37% (Boudrieau and Muir, 1987). In a study of cats with a diaphragmatic rupture, duration of the rupture was not associated with mortality, but older cats, those with low to mildly increased respiratory rates and those with concurrent injuries had a lower survival rate (Schmiedt *et al.*, 2003).

Eventration of the diaphragm

This is an uncommon condition that is manifested by bulging of the diaphragm into the thoracic cavity. It is rare, but it has been described in association with hiatal herniation and gastro-oesophageal reflux (Ayres *et al.*, 1978; Merdan Dhein *et al.*, 1980) and in young cats following anaesthesia for neutering (Gombac *et al.*, 2011). In humans, it may be a congenital abnormality or may be acquired following phrenic nerve injury.

Congenital diaphragmatic eventration is characterized by muscular aplasia of the diaphragm, which may be complete or segmental. Acquired eventrations are caused by injury to the phrenic nerve, with resultant paralysis and displacement of one or both sides of the diaphragm.

The following clinical signs may result:

- Pulmonary function may be compromised by the reduction in intrathoracic volume
- Cardiac insufficiency may result from a mediastinal shift and compression of the vena cava
- Regurgitation may result from the change in gastro-oesophageal angle as the stomach is displaced.

Acquired eventration may respond to symptomatic therapy and may be transient in nature. Congenital eventration has been managed by plication of the atrophic areas of the diaphragm (Merdan Dhein et al., 1980).

Diaphragmatic paralysis

Diaphragmatic paralysis is the most important functional disorder of the diaphragm but is rarely reported (Young et al., 1980; Suter, 1984; Greene et al., 1988; Vignoli et al., 2002). It may be caused by a lesion in the cervical spinal cord, phrenic nerves, neuromuscular junction or diaphragmatic musculature. A number of aetiologies have been suggested. These include: a primary diaphragmatic myopathy; toxoplasmosis; bilateral phrenic neuritis; organophosphate toxicity; external trauma; and iatrogenic trauma during thoracic surgery.

Paralysis may be unilateral or bilateral and temporary or permanent. Diaphragmatic paralysis might be expected to have a major effect on ventilation. However, given that chest wall expansion is also provided by contraction of the internal intercostal muscles, some respiratory movements may be made. Experimental division of both phrenic nerves is claimed not to affect ventilation adversely or to cause respiratory insufficiency (De Troyer and Kelly, 1982). However, diaphragmatic paralysis caused by naturally occurring disease is a cause of respiratory insufficiency (Young et al., 1980; Greene et al., 1988; Vignoli et al., 2002).

The cardinal sign of diaphragmatic paralysis is severe orthopnoea in the absence of abnormal heart or lung sounds. Paradoxical inward movement of the abdominal muscles on inspiration may be seen, particularly in dorsal recumbency. Unilateral paralysis may be asymptomatic. Other clinical signs, representing the underlying disease process, may also be noted.

Thoracic radiography reveals a small thoracic cavity with cranial displacement of the diaphragm. However, the radiographic appearance of the diaphragm is variable depending on patient size, X-ray beam centring, phase of respiration, gravity, age and breed, and a dynamic study may be required to reach a definitive diagnosis. On fluoroscopy, contraction of the diaphragm is absent and paradoxical cranial displacement of the flaccid diaphragm may be seen (Greene et al., 1988). These imaging techniques will differentiate unilateral from bilateral paralysis. Ultrasonography is as sensitive as fluoroscopy, but is less hazardous and more easily performed, and may rule out other lesions of the diaphragm (Vignoli et al., 2002). Percutaneous stimulation of the phrenic nerves may identify denervation of the diaphragm (Greene et al., 1988).

Post-traumatic diaphragmatic paralysis may be a transient phenomenon, requiring only symptomatic and supportive therapy of the respiratory system. Plication of the central tendon of the diaphragm with interlocking interrupted inverting polypropylene sutures has been attempted, which resulted in a taut, non-mobile diaphragm intraoperatively (Greene et al., 1988). This had minimal effect on the radiographic or fluoroscopic appearance 3 weeks postoperatively, but a gradual increase in the size of the thoracic cavity and movement of the diaphragm was recorded over the following year, along with a degree of clinical improvement.

Tumours of the diaphragm

Tumours affecting the diaphragm are rare. There are case reports of the diaphragm being affected by primary tumours (e.g. peripheral nerve sheath tumour), disseminated tumours (e.g. mast cell leukaemia and mesothelioma) and metastases (e.g. bronchogenic adenocarcinoma and haemangiosarcoma). Although rare, mass lesions affecting the diaphragm must be differentiated from mass lesions of the caudal lung lobes and caudal mediastinal structures, rupture of the diaphragm and pleuroperitoneal hernia. Management of these lesions presents a considerable challenge in terms of performing a biopsy, surgical excision and reconstruction of the resulting deficit.

Synchronous diaphragmatic contraction

This condition is rare and only a few cases have been described (Detweiler, 1955; Smith, 1965; Bohn and Patterson, 1970; Mainwaring, 1988), but it may be more frequent than the paucity of case reports suggests.

A number of causes have been suggested and these include: trauma to the thorax; prolonged vomiting; gastric irritation; electrolyte imbalance with alkalosis; uraemia; encephalitis; and post-surgical. Of these, chronic vomiting and thoracic trauma account for the majority of cases.

In this condition, each time the heart beats, one or both phrenic nerves are stimulated and the diaphragm contracts (Suter, 1984). It is hypothesized that if the threshold of excitability of the phrenic nerves is decreased, their pericardial portion may be stimulated by the cardiac action potentials. This reduction in the threshold of excitability may be caused by alkalosis, hypocalcaemia, hypokalaemia and hypochloraemia, which explains the association with chronic vomiting. However, serum electrolyte and blood gas analysis has not been performed in any case thought to be due to these mechanisms.

In addition, thoracic trauma may alter the anatomical relationships between the phrenic nerve and the heart, resulting in stimulation of the phrenic nerves by cardiac action potentials (Mainwaring, 1988). The left phrenic nerve crosses both ventricles as it passes caudally in the thorax, whereas the right phrenic nerve crosses the right atrium but not the ventricles. It is hypothesized that the closer proximity of the left phrenic nerve to the ventricles predisposes to left-sided diaphragmatic contraction. In all cases where this information has been recorded, contraction of the left side only or both sides, with the left side being more forceful, has been noted.

A visible or palpable 'pulse' may be detected over the thoracic wall on one or both sides. Simultaneous auscultation of the heart confirms its association with systole. Subclinical cases may be detected by echocardiography.

This condition is generally self-limiting and no treatment is necessary. Some cases have been treated with intravenous fluids or intravenous phenobarbital, with apparent success (Mainwaring, 1988). In some cases, however, the condition may persist for months (Bohn and Patterson, 1970). The prognosis is determined primarily by the nature and severity of the underlying disease process.

References and further reading

Auger JM and Riley SM (1997) Combined hiatal and pleuroperitoneal hernia in a Shar-pei. *Canadian Veterinary Journal* **38**, 640–642

Ayres CJ, Treharne DF and Eagleson JS (1978) Eventration of the diaphragm in a Great Dane. *Australian Veterinary Practitioner* **8**, 219–221

Bellah JR, Spencer CP and Brown DJ (1989a) Congenital cranioventral abdominal wall, caudal sternal, diaphragmatic, pericardial and intracardiac defects in cocker spaniel littermates. *Journal of the Amrican Veterinary Medical Association* **194**, 1741–1746

Bellah JR, Whitton DL, Ellison GW and Phillips I (1989b) Surgical correction of concomitant cranioventral abdominal wall, caudal sternal, diaphragmatic, and pericardial defects in young dogs. *Journal of the American Veterinary Medical Association* **195**, 1722–1726

Berry CR, Koblik PD and Ticer JW (1990) Dorsal peritoneopericardial mesothelial remnant as an aid to the diagnosis of feline congenital peritoneopericardial diaphragmatic hernia. *Veterinary Radiology* **31**, 239–245

Bohn FK and Patterson DF (1970) Long-standing unilateral contraction of the diaphragm synchronous with the heartbeat. *Journal of the American Veterinary Medical Association* **156**, 1411–1414

Boudrieau SJ and Muir WW (1987) Pathophysiology of traumatic diaphragmatic hernia in dogs. *Compendium on Continuing Education for the Practicing Veterinarian* **9**, 379–385

Bright RM, Sackman JE, Denovo C and Toal C (1990) Hiatal hernia in the dog and cat – a retrospective study of 16 cases. *Journal of Small Animal Practice* **31**, 244–250

Brinkley CH (1990) Hiatus hernia in a cat. *Veterinary Record* **127**, 46–47

Burnie AG, Simpson JW and Corcoran BM (1989) Gastro-oesophageal reflux and hiatus hernia associated with laryngeal paralysis in a dog. *Journal of Small Animal Practice* **30**, 414–416

Burns CG, Bergh MS and McLoughlin MA (2013) Surgical and nonsurgical treatment of peritoneopericardial diaphragmatic hernia in dogs and cats: 58 cases (1999–2008). *Journal of the American Veterinary Medical Association* **242**, 643–650

Callan MB, Washabau RJ, Saunders HM et al. (1993) Congenital esophageal hiatal hernia in the Chinese Shar-Pei dog. *Journal of Veterinary Internal Medicine* **7**, 210–215

De Troyer A and Kelly S (1982). Chest wall mechanics in dogs with acute diaphragm paralysis. *Journal of Applied Physiology* **53**, 373–379

Detweiler DK (1955) Contraction of the diaphragm synchronous with the heartbeat in dogs. *Journal of the American Veterinary Medical Association* **126**, 445–448

Dieringer TM and Wolf AM (1991) Esophageal hiatal hernia and megaesophagus complicating tetanus in two dogs. *Journal of the American Veterinary Medical Association* **199**, 87–89

Downs MC and Bjorling DE (1987) Traumatic diaphragmatic hernias: a review of 1674 cases. *Veterinary Surgery* **16**, 87–87

Ellison GW, Lewis DD, Phillips L and Tarvin GB (1987) Oesophageal hiatal hernia in small animals: literature review and a modified surgical technique. *Journal of the American Animal Hospital Association* **23**, 391–400

Evans SM and Biery DN (1980) Congenital peritoneopericardial diaphragmatic hernia in the dog and cat: a literature review and 17 additional case histories. *Veterinary Radiology* **21**, 108–116

Eyster GJ, Evans AT, Blanchard GL et al. (1977) Congenital pericardial diaphragmatic hernia and multiple cardiac defects in a litter of collies. *Journal of the American Veterinary Medical Association* **170**, 516–520

Feldman DB, Bree MM and Cohen BJ (1968) Congenital diaphragmatic hernia in neonatal dogs. *Journal of the American Veterinary Medical Association* **153**, 942–944

Frye FL and Taylor DON (1968) Pericardial and diaphragmatic defects in a cat. *Journal of the American Veterinary Medical Association* **152**, 1507–1510

Garson HL, Dodman NH and Baker GJ (1980) Diaphragmatic hernia: analysis of 56 cases in dogs and cats. *Journal of Small Animal Practice* **21**, 469–481

Gaskell CJ, Gibbs C and Pearson H (1974) Sliding hiatus hernia with reflux oesophagitis in two dogs. *Journal of Small Animal Practice* **15**, 503–509

Gibson TW, Brisson BA and Sears W (2005) Perioperative survival rates after surgery for diaphragmatic hernia in dogs and cats: 92 cases (1990–2002). *Journal of the American Veterinary Medical Association* **227**, 105–109

Gombac M, Vrecl M and Svara T (2011) Congenital diaphragmatic eventration in two closely related British Shorthair cats. *Journal of Feline Medicine and Surgery* **13**, 276–279

Grandage J (1974) The radiology of the dog's diaphragm. *Journal of Small Animal Practice* **15**, 1–17

Greene CE, Basinger RR and Whitfield JB (1988) Surgical management of bilateral diaphragmatic paralysis in a dog. *Journal of the American Veterinary Medical Association* **193**, 1542–1544

Hardie EM, Ramirez O, Clary EM et al. (1998) Abnormalities of the thoracic bellows: stress fractures of the ribs and hiatal hernia. *Journal of Veterinary Internal Medicine* **12**, 279–287

Hay WH, Woodfield JA and Moon MA (1989) clinical, echocardiographic, and radiographic findings of peritoneopericardial diaphragmatic hernia in two dogs and a cat. *Journal of the American Veterinary Medical Association* **195**, 1245–1248

Kent GC (1950) Feline diaphragmatic hernia. *Journal of the American Veterinary Medical Association* **116**, 348–352

Knowles KE, O'Brien DP and Amann JF (1990) Congenital idiopathic megaoesophagus in a litter of Chinese Shar-peis: Clinical, electrodiagnostic and pathological findings. *Journal of the American Animal Hospital Association* **26**, 313–318

Lorinson D and Bright RM (1998) Long-term outcome of medical and surgical treatment of hiatal hernias in dogs and cats: 27 cases (1978–1996). *Journal of the American Veterinary Medical Association* **213**, 381–384

Mainwaring CJ (1988) Post traumatic contraction of the diaphragm synchronous with the heartbeat in a dog. *Journal of Small Animal Practice* **29**, 299–302

Mann FA, Aronson E and Keller G (1991) Surgical correction of a true congenital pleuroperitoneal diaphragmatic hernia in a cat. *Journal of the American Animal Hospital Association* **27**, 501–507

Merdan Dhein CR, Rawlings CA, Rosin E, Losonsky JM and Chambers JN (1980) Oesophageal hiatal hernia and eventration of the diaphragm with resultant gastro-oesophageal reflux. *Journal of the American Animal Hospital Association* **16**, 517–522

Miles KG, Pope ER and Jergens AE (1988) Paraesophageal hiatal hernia and pyloric obstruction in a dog. *Journal of the American Veterinary Medical Association* **193**, 1437–1439

Park RD (1994) The diaphragm. In: *Textbook of Veterinary Diagnostic Radiology*, ed. DE Thrall, pp. 226–276. WB Saunders, Philadelphia

Pratschke KM, Hughes JML, Skelly C and Bellenger CR (1998) Hiatal herniation as a complication of chronic diaphragmatic herniation. *Journal of Small Animal Practice* **39**, 33–38

Prymak C, Saunders HM and Washabau RJ (1989) Hiatal hernia repair by restoration and stabilization of normal anatomy. An evaluation in four dogs and one cat. *Veterinary Surgery* **18**, 386–391

Schmiedt CW, Tobias KM and Stevenson MAM (2003) Traumatic diaphragmatic hernia in cats: 34 cases (1991–2001). *Journal of the American Veterinary Medical Association* **222**, 1237–1240

Schuh JCL (1987) Hepatic nodular myelolipomatosis (myelolipomas) associated with a peritoneo-pericardial diaphragmatic hernia in cat. *Journal of Comparative Pathology* **97**, 231–235

Skinner DB (1986) Hiatal hernia and gastro-oesophageal reflux. In: *Textbook of Surgery, 13th edn.* ed. DC Sabiston, pp. 704–715. WB Saunders, Philadelphia

Smith LK (1965) Contraction of the diaphragm synchronous with the heartbeat in a dog. *Journal of the American Veterinary Medical Association* **146**, 611–613

Spattini G, Rossi F, Vignoli M and Lamb CR (2003) Use of ultrasound to diagnose diaphragmatic rupture in dogs and cats. *Veterinary Radiology and Ultrasound* **44**, 226–230

Stickle R, Sparschu G, Love N and Walshaw R (1992) Radiographic evaluation of esophageal function in Chinese Shar-Pei pups. *Journal of the American Veterinary Medical Association* **201**, 81–84

Stickle RL (1984) Positive-contrast celiography (peritoneography) for the diagnosis of diaphragmatic hernia in dogs and cats. *Journal of the American Veterinary Medical Association* **185**, 295–298

Stokhof AA (1986) Diagnosis and treatment of acquired diaphragmatic hernia by thoracotomy in 49 dogs and 72 cats. *Veterinary Quarterly* **8**, 177–183

Sullivan M and Lee R (1989) Radiological features of 80 cases of diaphragmatic rupture. *Journal of Small Animal Practice* **30**, 561–566

Suter PF (1984) *Thoracic Radiography: A Text Atlas of Thoracic Diseases of the Dog and Cat.* Suter Wettswil, Switzerland

Valentine BA, Cooper BJ, Dietze AE and Noden DM (1988) Canine congenital diaphragmatic hernia. *Journal of Veterinary Internal Medicine* **2**, 109–112

Van Ham L and van Bree H (1992) Conservative treatment of tetanus associated with hiatus-hernia and gastroesophageal reflux. *Journal of Small Animal Practice* **33**, 289–294

van Sluijs FJ and Happe R (1985) Surgical diseases of the stomach. In: *Textbook of Small Animal Surgery*, ed. DH Slatter, pp. 685–689. WB Saunders, Philadelphia

Vignoli M, Toniato M, Rossi F et al. (2002) Transient post-traumatic hemidiaphragmatic paralysis in two cats. *Journal of Small Animal Practice* **43**, 312–316

Voges AK, Bertrand S, Hill RC, Neuwirth L and Schaer M (1997) True diaphragmatic hernia in a cat. *Veterinary Radiology and Ultrasound* **2**, 116–119

Waldron DR, Moon M, Leib MS, Barber D and Mays KA (1990) Oesophageal hiatal hernia in two cats. *Journal of Small Animal Practice* **31**, 259–263

Walker RG and Hall LW (1965) Rupture of the diaphragm: report of 32 cases in dogs and cats. *Veterinary Record* **77**, 830–837

Wallace J, Mullen HS and Lesser MB (1992) A technique for surgical correction of peritoneal pericardial diaphragmatic hernia in dogs and cats. *Journal of the American Animal Hospital Association* **28**, 503–510

White RN (1993) A modified technique for surgical repair of oesophageal hiatal herniation in the dog. *Journal of Small Animal Practice* **34**, 599–603

Willard MD and Aronson E (1981) Peritoneopericardial diaphragmatic hernia in a cat. *Journal of the American Veterinary Medical Association* **178**, 481–483

Williams JM (1990) Hiatal hernia in a Shar-Pei. *Journal of Small Animal Practice* **31**, 251–254

Wilson GP and Hayes HM (1986) Diaphragmatic hernia in the dog and cat: a 25-year overview. *Seminars in Veterinary Medicine and Surgery: Small Animal* **1**, 318–326

Wilson GP, Newton CD and Burt JK (1971) A review of 116 diaphragmatic hernias in dogs and cats. *Journal of the American Veterinary Medical Association* **159**, 1142–1145

Young PN, Gorgacz EJ and Barsanti JA (1980) Respiratory failure associated with diaphragmatic paralysis in a cat. *Journal of the American Animal Hospital Association* **16**, 933–936

OPERATIVE TECHNIQUE 17.1

Surgery for diaphragmatic rupture

PATIENT PREPARATION AND POSITIONING

The patient is placed in dorsal recumbency with the forelimbs tied cranially. The ventral abdomen is clipped and prepared for a routine ventral midline laparotomy. The ventral thorax should also be clipped and prepared in case a caudal sternotomy has to be performed. Although this is a clean or clean-contaminated procedure, perioperative antibiotics are indicated.

ASSISTANT

It is desirable to have an assistant to help retract the abdominal viscera.

ADDITIONAL INSTRUMENTS

Abdominal retractors, e.g. Balfour or Gossett; a mechanical stapler (in case a liver lobectomy is required); an oscillating saw if a sternotomy is required; long-handled thoracic instruments may be useful for suturing the dorsal aspect of the diaphragm in deep-chested animals.

SURGICAL TECHNIQUE

Approach

A standard ventral midline laparotomy is performed with an incision from the xiphisternum to approximately halfway from the umbilicus to the pubis. This incision may be extended caudally to the pubis if required. A partial or complete median sternotomy may be required if access is difficult or if there are extensive adhesions.

Surgical manipulations

1 Gentle traction is applied to the viscera to reposition the herniated organs into the abdomen as soon as possible, to remove the compression on the lung lobes. If this cannot be performed, it may be due to engorgement of the organs following entrapment, or the formation of adhesions. In this case, the hole in the diaphragm may be enlarged to allow inspection and reduction of the organs. This is best performed by extending the incision in a radial direction ventrally, taking care to avoid vital structures such as the phrenic vessels, phrenic nerves and caudal vena cava.

2 Adhesions to intrathoracic structures should be divided under direct observation if possible. More mature adhesions may require division of the affected part, e.g. by partial lung lobectomy or complete liver lobectomy. Incarcerated liver lobes and spleen are often friable and should be handled with care. If these appear devitalized, lobectomy or splenectomy should be performed, ideally before returning the organs to the abdomen.

3 Once reduced, the abdominal viscera are retracted using saline-soaked laparotomy swabs and malleable ribbon retractors. Following repositioning of the abdominal viscera, a routine exploration of the entire abdomen is performed.

4 The thoracic cavity is lavaged with warm saline and a chest drain is placed into the pleural space under direct visualization before closing the diaphragm.

    With an acute diaphragmatic rupture, it is generally simple to determine the correct orientation of the tissues and rarely is there insufficient tissue to close the defect. In chronic hernias, the edges of the defect may have rolled over and mature fibrous tissue may have formed, causing contraction of the tissue. It is not recommended to debride the edges of the hernia, because that will increase the size of the defect further and may reduce the holding power of the sutures. However, any scar tissue that prevents movement of the diaphragm should be incised.

    The most dorsal suture is placed first and the ends are left long and tagged with a haemostat. Traction on this haemostat allows the rest of the diaphragm to be elevated into the surgical field and facilitates closure, working from dorsal to ventral. Care must be taken to avoid constriction of structures running through the diaphragmatic hiati, e.g. the caudal vena cava, during herniorrhaphy. In circumcostal tears, it may be difficult to approximate the diaphragm to the abdominal wall and, in these cases, sutures may be passed around the adjacent ribs or xiphisternum.

5 Closure of the laparotomy wound is routine. Rarely, in a patient with a chronic hernia, the abdominal organs may not fit into the abdomen because of loss of abdominal domain. In this case, an elective splenectomy may reduce the volume of the abdominal viscera.

→

→ **OPERATIVE TECHNIQUE 17.1 CONTINUED**

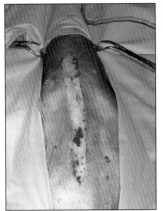
Cranial ventral midline laparotomy.

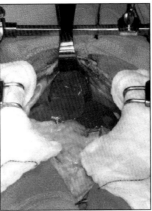
Exposure of the diaphragm.

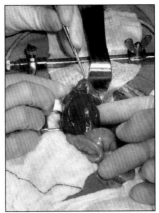
Repositioning liver lobes.

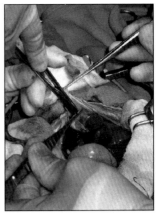
Division of adhesions.

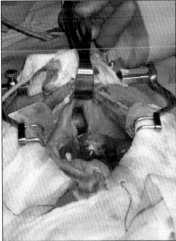
Examination of tear in diaphragm.

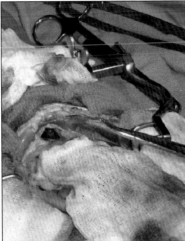
Placement of dorsal suture in diaphragm.

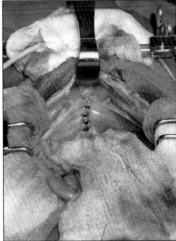
Closure of the defect.

POSTOPERATIVE CARE

Following reduction of a chronic hernia, replacement of the organs and loss of abdominal domain may cause an increase in intraperitoneal pressure and resulting impairment of venous return. Careful monitoring of cardiovascular haemodynamics is important. Supplementary oxygen therapy may be required if there is ventilatory insufficiency. If this persists, aspiration of the chest tube or thoracic radiography should be performed to ensure that this is not due to continuing pneumothorax. The chest drain is aspirated on recovery and every 1–4 hours as required, and is removed once no longer productive, e.g. after 24–48 hours. Analgesia is maintained with systemic opiates and non-steroidal anti-inflammatory drugs.

Index

BSAVA Manual of Canine and Feline Head, Neck and Thoracic Surgery, second edition. Edited by Daniel J. Brockman, David E. Holt and Gert ter Haar. ©BSAVA 2018

Surgical solutions...

BSAVA Manual of Canine and Feline
Abdominal Surgery
Second edition

Editors: John M. Williams, Jacqui D. Niles

This fully revised and updated edition provides a practical surgical reference that is easy to read and follow. Includes step-by-step Operative Techniques.

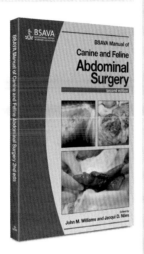

BSAVA Member Price
£49.00
Price to non-members: £79.00

BSAVA Manual of Canine and Feline
Dentistry and Oral Surgery
Fourth edition

Editors: Alexander M. Reiter, Margherita Gracis

This manual provides a practical, up-to-date approach to dentistry and oral surgery in dogs and cats. Includes step-by-step Operative Techniques.

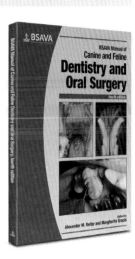

BSAVA Member Price
£49.00
Price to non-members: £79.00

BSAVA Manual of Canine and Feline
Fracture Repair and Management
Second edition

Editors: Toby J. Gemmill, Dylan N. Clements

This manual covers principles of fracture management, repair and management of specific fractures and the treatment and prevention of complications. Includes step-by-step Operative Techniques.

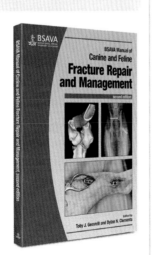

BSAVA Member Price
£59.00
Price to non-members: £89.00

BSAVA Manual of Canine and Feline
Musculoskeletal Disorders
Second edition

Editors: Gareth Arthurs, Gordon Brown, Rob Pettitt

This new edition presents a logically arranged and readily accessible source of practical information for the management of musculoskeletal disorders. Includes step-by-step Operative Techniques.

AVAILABLE SOON

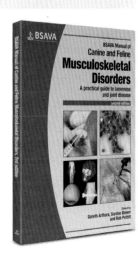

BSAVA Member Price
£59.00
Price to non-members: £89.00

WHERE TO BUY

Order print books at www.bsava.com/shop
or call **01452 726700**
Order online versions at **www.bsavalibrary.com**

BSAVA Publications
COMMUNICATING VETERINARY KNOWLEDGE

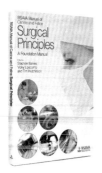 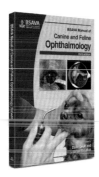 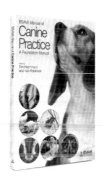 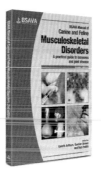 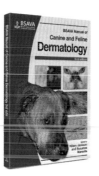 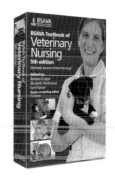
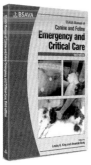 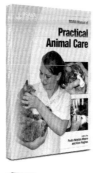 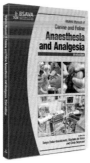 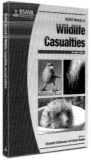 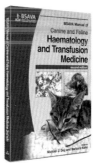 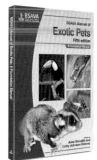
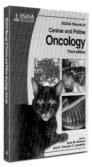 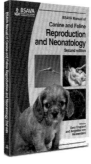 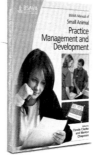 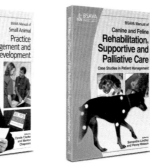 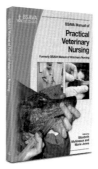 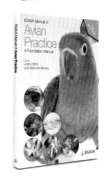
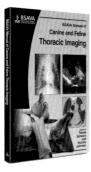 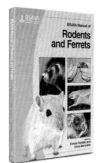 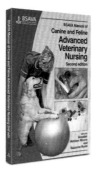 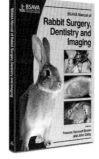 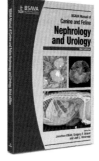 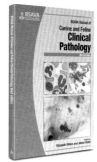
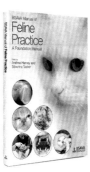 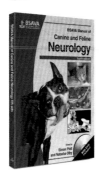 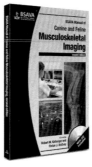 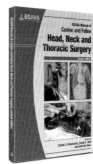 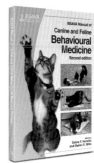 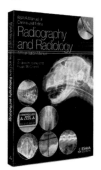